Peritonitis

Edited by

Donald E. Fry, MD

Department of Surgery
University of New Mexico School of Medicine
Albuquerque, New Mexico

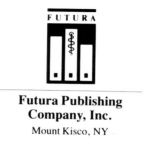

**Futura Publishing
Company, Inc.**
Mount Kisco, NY

Library of Congress Cataloging-in-Publication Data

Peritonitis / edited by Donald E. Fry
    p. cm.
    Includes bibliographical references and index.
    ISBN 0-87993-551-0
    1. Peritonitis, I. Fry, Donald E.
    [DNLM: 1. Peritonitis. WI 575 P4462]
    RC867.P48 1993
    617.5'58—dc20
    DNLM/DLC
    for Library of Congress   92-48289
                                          CIP

Copyright © 1993

Published by
Futura Publishing Company, Inc.
2 Bedford Ridge Road
Mount Kisco, New York 10549

LC #: 92-48289
ISBN #: 0-87993-551-0

Every effort has been made to ensure that the information in this book is as up to date and accurate as possible at the time of publication. However, due to the constant developments in medicine, neither the author, nor the editor, nor the publisher can accept any legal or any other responsibility for any errors or omissions that may occur.

Printed in the United States of America.

Printed on acid-free paper.

Contributors

Marie T. Boyd, MD   Resident in Pathology, University of New Mexico School of Medicine Albuquerque, New Mexico

John A. Carlson, Jr, MD   Professor of Obstetrics and Gynecology, Director, Gynecologic Oncology, Thomas Jefferson Medical College, Philadelphia, Pennsylvania

Thomas G. Day, Jr, MD   Professor of Obstetrics and Gynecology, Director, Gynecologic Oncology, J. Graham Brown Cancer Center University of Louisville School of Medicine Louisville, Kentucky

Donald E. Fry, MD   Professor and Chairman, Department of Surgery, University of New Mexico School of Medicine, Albuquerque, New Mexico

R. Neal Garrison, MD   Professor of Surgery, University of Louisville School of Medicine, Chief, Surgical Service, VA Medical Center, Louisville, Kentucky

Diller B. Groff, MD   Professor of Surgery, University of Louisville School of Medicine, Surgeon-in-Chief, Kosair Children's Hospital, Louisville, Kentucky

Jerry N. King, MD   Clinical Assistant Professor of Radiology, University of New Mexico School of Medicine, Albuquerque, New Mexico

Mark A. Malangoni, MD   Professor and Vice-Chairman, Department of Surgery, Case Western Reserve University School of Medicine, Chief of Surgery, MetroHealth Medical Center, Cleveland, Ohio

Daniel T. Martin, MD   Assistant Professor of Surgery, University of New Mexico School of Medicine, Albuquerque, New Mexico

Byron J. Masterson, MD   Professor and Chairman, Department of Obstetrics and Gynecology, University of Florida College of Medicine, Gainesville, Florida

Hirikati S. Nagaraj, MD   Associate Professor of Surgery, University of Louisville School of Medicine Chief, Pediatric General and Thoracic Surgery, Kosair Children's Hospital, Louisville, Kentucky

David E. Pitcher, MD   Instructor of Surgery, University of New Mexico School of Medicine, Albuquerque, New Mexico

John B. Pietsch, MD   Associate Professor of Surgery, Division of Pediatric Surgery, Vanderbilt University, Nashville, Tennessee

Hiram C. Polk, Jr, MD   Professor and Chairman, Department of Surgery, University of Louisville School of Medicine, Louisville, Kentucky

J. David Richardson, MD   Professor and Vice-Chairman, Department of Surgery, University of Louisville School of Medicine, Louisville, Kentucky

Bruce S. Turlington, MD   Resident in Radiology, University of New Mexico School of Medicine, Albuquerque, New Mexico

Karl A. Zucker, MD   Professor of Surgery, Director, Center for Minimally-Invasive Surgery, University of New Mexico School of Medicine, Albuquerque, New Mexico

Foreword

A major review of peritonitis is timely, and this very timeliness is highly symbolic. There have been measurable advances in the care of patients with peritonitis, including major achievements in diagnosis, specific surgical care, anesthetic techniques, and overall supportive measures, including the wise and judicious use of antibiotics per se. Despite this objective evidence of improvement, there is still a hard core of patients with peritonitis who are recalcitrant to all of these measures. They are typically characterized as presenting late in the course of the disease and may also have other serious illnesses that compromise the patient's physiological resiliency. If a surgeon is to progress further and convert these extremely challenging patients into cures, it will only be by a thorough reassessment of the entire process.

Therefore, the resurgence of interest in peritonitis is particularly gratifying to those of us involved in the front-line care of this prevalent and serious illness. Current inquiries have addressed many different aspects of the process. Sinunons and associates, in an ongoing analysis over most of the last decade, have analyzed many theoretical and experimental aspects of peritonitis and have clearly enhanced our understanding of the basic processes. Major clinical modifications in the care of the patient severely ill with peritonitis have taken place on a worldwide basis, including attempts at systematic radical peritoneal debridement of all fibrin deposits, prolonged intraperitoneal administration of antibiotics in high-volume lavage, and finally in selected cases, the attempt at adequate peritoneal drainage by leaving the cavity virtually open.

These inquiries into the nature of peritonitis itself have two parallel areas of investigation that directly impact upon the patient with peritonitis, but do not deal with the disease process in and of itself. It is quite clear now that the prevalent form of multiple system organ failure that often afflicts the patient with severe and/or continuing peritonitis is much better understood now than a decade ago. It is quite clear that the infective process itself it is responsible for these changes and additional data are now in hand that suggests the remote infective process impairs vital organ function by some manner of particulate debris. Whether this material is fibrin, platelets, polymorphonuclear neutrophils, or combinations thereof, is not yet clearly defined, but it is this microembolic process that is clearly associated with respiratory dysfunction associated with peritonitis. It has even been proposed by some that resuspension and/or elimination of this debris by fibrinectin or related compounds is a feasible therapeutic undertaking. Others continue to focus upon the more definitive treatment of the infection and consider such uses of fibrinectin palliative at best. Here is an area in which much understanding has been accomplished, but much yet remains to be done. Another area that will inevitably impact importantly upon peritonitis is the overall assessment of host defense abnormalities and an attempt to enhance those normal processes in the patient challenged with an infectious process. We have all become convinced there is more to the host-pathogen interaction than is fully appreciated by the "bug-and-drug" mentality. Accordingly, a number of units are assaying the specific abnormalities that may be associated with infectious illness and the responses thereto. Other laboratories are examining the possibility of a nonspecific enhancement of host defenses against infection, an enchanting concept that once again has surfaced after a long period of scientific discredit.

One would not, indeed, be an undue optimist to expect that these multiple levels of inquiry will once again provide an opportunity for the patient with peritonitis and his physician to apply a sounder more sophisticated level of scientific rationale to his care and eventually to improved survival. Finally, it is with no little pride in the maturity of our own surgical unit that one recommends careful study of the following material. The development of a superb broad-based monograph with the sound principles appropriately stressed by a group of faculty, largely from a single department, reflects both a broad and continuing interest in matters related to infection, injury, and physiologic responsiveness of the entire organism.

Hiram C. Polk, Jr, MD

Contents

1

Pathophysiology of Peritonitis

Donald E. Fry, MD

Despite more than four decades of evolution to more potent and broader spectrum antibiotics, improved methods of volume resuscitation, and very sophisticated support technology, the mortality and morbidity from intra-abdominal infection continues to be a major problem. Mortality rates higher than 20% continue to be identified in the severely infected patient.[1-4] The manpower and resource utilization by patients with severe peritonitis indicates that further refinements in the present treatment regimens are necessary.[5]

Peritonitis is a diverse disease and should more appropriately be viewed as a constellation of multiple diseases. A perforated peptic ulcer in a young patient and a perforated colon carcinoma in an octogenarian are both considered to be peritonitis, but the implications of the disease in these two separate settings are entirely different. Indeed, comparisons and interpretations of results in the treatment of peritonitis from different reports in the literature are quite difficult because of the heterogenous mix of patients and the different sources of contamination.

Peritonitis is commonly a complex disease. Refinements in culturing methodology over the last decade have resulted in the appreciation that multiple organisms are participants in the infectious process.[6,7] The host response to peritoneal contamination is equally complex. Finally, numerous adjuvant factors may support bacterial growth, retard the host response, or impede the effectiveness of antimicrobial therapy. Only by having a thorough understanding of the complex pathophysi-

From Fry DE, (ed): *Peritonitis.* Mount Kisco NY, Futura Publishing Co., Inc., © 1993.

ology of peritonitis can conventional treatment be optimally applied and new refinements in treatment be developed.

Definitions

The mesothelial surface of the embryonal coelomic cavity is the peritoneum. By convention the peritoneum is referred to as parietal peritoneum when it covers the posterior surface of the abdominal wall and retroperitoneum, and visceral peritoneum when it reflects onto the intestine and solid visceral organs. The peritoneum is functionally a sac that ordinarily contains only fluid, exfoliated cells, and a few resident phagocytes. Contamination of the sac by microorganisms introduced by trauma, surgical intervention, or spontaneous disruption of the intestine results in an inflammatory response. The resultant infection initially involves the peritoneal lining, and usually progresses to become an active process within the free space of the peritoneal cavity. The severity of the infection may result in direct extension outside of the peritoneal sac with microbial invasion of the peritoneum resulting in extensive soft tissue infection and potentially systemic bacteremia.

Traditionally, peritonitis is referred to as either primary or secondary peritonitis. Primary peritonitis implies that another disease process responsible for bacterial contamination is not present. Microorganisms presumably cause infection following hematogenous or lymphatic "seeding" of the peritoneum from a remote source. In past decades, tuberculous peritonitis was a common cause of primary peritonitis. Currently, the alcoholic patient with ascites probably is the most common victim of primary peritonitis. In these latter patients, pneumococcal peritonitis may be seen from hematogenous dissemination from the respiratory tract, or gram-negative organisms may translocate via the lymphatics into the peritoneal sac. While primary peritonitis receives considerable interest, it represents less than 1% of all cases of peritonitis.

Secondary peritonitis presumes that another disease process within the peritoneal sac is the source of microorganisms. Secondary peritonitis is usually associated with an anatomical defect that requires mechanical control as part of patient management. Diseases of the biliary (eg, acute cholecystitis) and intestinal tracts (eg, perforated ulcers) are the most common sources. Contamination introduced via surgical procedures or from intra-abdominal trauma are similarly viewed as secondary peritonitis. Peritonitis secondary to acute salpingitis does not have an anatomical defect per se, but is generally considered as secondary peritonitis.

Natural History of Peritonitis

Following initial contamination of the peritoneal cavity, the contaminants are rapidly disseminated throughout the peritoneal cavity. Autio[8] has demonstrated that radiopaque substances introduced into the peritoneal cavity are rapidly disseminated. Near complete opacification of the peritoneal cavity occurs within hours, regardless of the specific site of initial placement of the radiopaque material. These movements of peritoneal fluid result in peritonitis being a diffuse process. Certainly the physical examination of patients with a perforated viscus commonly begins with localized physical findings, but rapidly progresses to diffuse signs.

While the movement of peritoneal fluid transforms a localized event to a generalized one, the process of dissemination should properly be viewed as favoring the host in the ensuing efforts to combat potential pathogens. First, the dissemination process reduces the density of microorganisms and facilitates phagocytic cells in the elimination of bacteria. Numerous clinical studies have emphasized the importance of the density of bacterial contamination in determining whether clinical infection occurs in specific anatomical areas.[9-11] In soft tissue and the urinary tract, contaminants greater than 10^5 organisms per gram of tissue or milliliter of urine result in clinical infection, while densities less than 10^5 organisms are within the capability of host mechanisms to manage. While the specific density of microorganisms in the peritoneal cavity that are necessary to result in either death of the host or abscess seems to vary with different species, the dissemination process may be teleologically viewed as acutely reducing bacterial density.

Secondly, dissemination facilitates the removal of bacteria from the peritoneal cavity. Bacteria, or other macromolecules within the peritoneal cavity, can only be removed by two mechanisms: (1) phagocytosis and digestion by macrophages, or (2) removal via the large lymphatic fenestrations on the diaphragmatic surface of the peritoneal cavity. Clearance of macromolecules or bacteria cannot occur through the mesothelial surfaces of the peritoneal cavity. Removal of macromolecule-laden fluid from the peritoneal cavity can only occur through the diaphragm as normal fluid dynamics move the contaminant toward the diaphragm.[12] Indeed, the peritoneal space can be properly viewed as simply a large lymphocele that is in direct communication with the lymphatic system. Of course, excessive transportation of fluid could potentially result in bacteremia, as lymphatic fluid ultimately gains access to the systemic circulation; however, removal of bacteria from the peritoneal cavity is experimentally viewed as favoring the host's management of large concentrations of contaminants.[13,14]

When bacteria lodge in the peritoneal tissues, a nonspecific inflammatory reaction is initiated. Vasoactive substances are released and capillary permeability is increased. Plasma proteins extravasate into the contaminated tissues as interstitial volume increases.[15-16] Complement and fibrinogen are activated, and fibrin deposition is initiated. Neutrophils are drawn to the area by chemoattractants within the primary inflammatory focus. These polymorphonuclear phagocytes are then replaced in 24–48 hours by mononuclear cells. With ingestion of bacteria by various phagocytes, endogenous pyrogen is synthesized within these macrophage cells and released into the inflammatory milieu. Endogenous pyrogen results in fever when it is transported by the systemic circulation to the hypothalamus.[17] Several endogenous pyrogens have been identified with interleukin-1 being the most notable.[18] Interleukin-6[19] and tumor necrosis factor[20] are also identified as having endogenous pyrogen activity.

The redistribution of total extracellular volume into the area of peritoneal inflammation may be enormous. Substantial reduction in plasma volume may occur. Plasma proteins may similarly decrease very rapidly secondary to the altered vascular permeability. Because the peritoneal surface is so extensive, the total redistribution of extracellular water may provoke hypovolemia, oliguria, and even frank clinical shock. Thus, volume resuscitation during the acute phase of inflammation in these patients becomes a cornerstone of management.

Following dissemination and the onset of the acute inflammatory process, the natural history of peritonitis has three potential outcomes (Figure 1). First, the efficiency of host defense mechanisms or the low inoculum of bacterial pathogens may result in complete resolution of the process. The prototype process that usually has complete resolution is the 20–40-year-old patient with a perforated peptic ulcer. Assuming that the source of peritoneal soilage is mechanically repaired, the quantity of contamination is small and the patient is in optimum physiologic condition to handle the infection. Secondly, the quantity of bacterial contaminants may be too great or the integrity of the host sufficiently

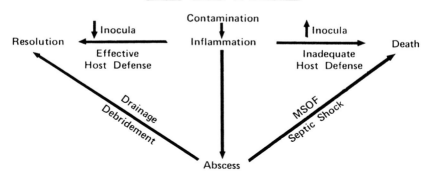

Figure 1: An illustration of the natural history of peritonitis. The specific details of the interactions between the host and pathogen are fully discussed in the text.

inadequate so that fulminant peritonitis results in death. Elderly patients with perforation of a colon carcinoma or patients with perforation of any viscus while on immunosuppression or cancer chemotherapy regimens are especially at risk for death from acute fulminant peritonitis. A third potential outcome is abdominal abscess, which represents a biological stand-off between the host and the pathogen. The young patient that sustains a penetrating injury of the left colon has both a robust host response and a large inoculum of bacterial contamination; thus, intra-abdominal abscess is frequently seen in this clinical circumstance.

Abscesses following the acute phase of peritonitis characteristically occur in the physiologic drainage basins of the abdominal cavity. Those areas that are most dependent generally favor the collection of contaminants that are beyond the capability of the host defense mechanisms to eradicate from the peritoneal sac (Table 1).

Interloop abscesses are relatively uncommon except in cases of multiple abdominal surgeries, where adhesions from previous infection or surgical trauma alter the gravity-dependent movements of peritoneal contaminants.

Local and Systemic Factors

As has been emphasized, the outcome of peritonitis is determined by the consequences of the host-pathogen interaction. However, discus-

Table 1

Physiologic Drainage Basins	
Site	Frequency[4]
Subphrenic space	28%
Subhepatic space	16%
Pelvis	25%
Paracolic gutters	12%
Other areas	19%
(Muliple abscesses)	(15%)

Identifies the physiologic drainage basins of the periotoneal cavity where intra-abdominal abcesses are most likely to be identified.

sion to this point has viewed this host-pathogen interaction in the simple terms of the host's intrinsic immunological competence versus the quantity of bacterial contaminants that have a fixed biological virulence. Numerous local and systemic factors may modify the virulence of the bacterial organism or compromise the host's response to the evolving infection.

An important local factor that enhances bacterial virulence is free hemoglobin.[21,22] The use of hemoglobin has been repeatedly shown to convert nonlethal contamination of the peritoneal cavity into a lethal contaminant. However, the specific mechanism of hemoglobin's adjuvant effect remains unclear. The liberation of ferric iron within the inflammatory environment may simply serve as an important growth factor to accelerate bacterial proliferation. Hemoglobin may saturate transferrin, as a nonspecific opsonic protein, and alter the phagocytic capability of the host's macrophage cells.[23] The release of iron may simply serve as a critical growth factor to stimulate bacterial proliferation. End products of hemoglobin metabolism by bacteria may be toxic to phagocytic cells and may be another mechanism.[24] Still other more complex mechanisms have been hypothesized. Regardless of mechanism, blood in the peritoneal cavity following penetrating injury or surgical intervention may assume special importance in the ultimate outcome of the process.

Foreign bodies within the local inflammatory environment may also enhance bacterial virulence. Studies by Elek and Conen[25] have clearly shown that soft tissue infections require fewer contaminating bacteria to yield an infection when suture material is present. Barium sulfate appears to either potentiate bacterial growth or impair the host response to such contamination. Even the particulate components of fecal material appear to enhance the virulence of a given quantity of bacteria. While the specific mechanisms of the adjuvant effects of foreign material is unclear, the fibers and particles may serve as an environmental haven for bacteria and make them less accessible to phagocytosis.

Nonviable tissue significantly augments bacterial virulence. Necrotic tissue provides an anaerobic environment that favors the facultative pathogen, but impairs the phagocytic cell that requires an oxygen-rich milieu for appropriate function.[26] Additionally, the decomposition of dead tissue may serve as substrate for bacterial proliferation.

Numerous systemic factors that are commonly present in these patients also compromise the host. Patients who are diabetics may have ineffective cellular responses and because of the fundamental microvascular disease may not efficiently deliver host defense elements to the site of contamination.[27] Systemic corticosteroid therapy may alter neutrophil function.[28] Acute or chronic alcoholism may also impair the host response.[29,30] Furthermore, associated factors of systemic hypoxemia or hypovolemia may further serve to augment the pathogenicity of bacteria.[31,32]

Another significant variable in the host's ability to withstand peritonitis is effective systemic reticuloendothelial function. Saba and associates[33,34] have shown the significance of a nonspecific opsonin in the clearance of intravascular aggregates of fibrin and cellular debris. They and others[35] have hypothesized that these aggregates may have pathophysiologic significance in the genesis of multiple organ failure in septic humans. Soft tissue trauma and major surgical interventions appear to exhaust the systemic availability of this nonspecific opsonin and may render the host incapable of managing systemic microaggregates generated by an intercurrent septic process. Thus, these observations would suggest that multiple trauma and major surgery are sources of impairment of the host.

Blood transfusion has recently been identified as having immunosuppressive effects upon the host which may increase the probability of infection. There are both experimental[36,37] and clinical data[38,39] to support that transfusion may increase the severity of infections. While the mechanism of transfusion-associated immunosuppression remains undefined, and the potentiation of peritoneal contamination has not been studied, transfusion appears to be another systemic adjuvant effect that may impact the outcome of patients with peritoneal contamination or infection.

Bacterial Synergism

Koch's postulates have traditionally dictated that each infectious disease process is caused by a single pathogen that can be isolated, inoculated into an experimental model, and re-isolated from the experimental setting. The polymicrobial character of intra-abdominal infection has defied Koch's postulates in that multiple organisms are present and the precarious environmental conditions required for culture (eg, anaerobic organisms) make isolation of all potential pathogens very difficult.

Cultures of intraperitoneal infection may demonstrate up to five microorganisms per patient,[6,7] although most clinical laboratories in a nonresearch setting probably recover only two or three isolates per patient.[40] Examination of the Gram's stain of peritoneal exudates usually demonstrates numerous pleomorphic gram-positive and gram-negative bacteria. One cannot help but speculate that further refinements in culture methodology of bacteria may increase the recognized number of pathogens per peritonitis patient. An especially significant consideration in polymicrobial infection is whether all isolates are necessarily pathogens, or whether some are commensal organisms that are present, but do not contribute to the pathologic process.

Pathogens that have been isolated from peritoneal infection are identified in Table 2.[6,40,41] Organisms of special concern have been (1) the gram-negative enteric rod, (2) the anaerobic species, and (3) the enterococci. First, the prototype gram-negative rod is *Escherichia coli*. This organism is a facultative bacterium that can proliferate in an environment that is either well oxygenated or completely anaerobic. Experimental infections with *Escherichia coli* are quite lethal with this virulence principally attributed to the lipopolysaccharide endotoxin of the outer membrane of these bacteria.

The prototype anaerobic organism of concern in peritoneal infection is *Bacteroides fragilis*. This organism assumes special significance from other anaerobes because it is more frequently cultured from blood in peritonitis patients, it is more tolerant to oxygen than most

Tale 2
Cultures of Patients with Polymicrobial Peritonitis

	Lorber-Swenson[6]	Stone et al.[41]	Mosdell[40]
Aerobes			
E. Coli	57%	45%	42%
Klebsiella	8%	17%	10%
Pseudomonas	3%	18%	12%
Proteus	11%	13%	2%
Enterococcus	12%	40%	6%
Anaerobes			
Bacteroides SP	153%*	65%	27%
Clostridia SP	9%	37%	4%
Peptococcus/ Peptostreptococcus	57%	32%	10%

Identifies the frequency of pathogens isolated in the studies of Lorber and Swenson in 1975, Stone et al. in 1983, and Mosdell et al. in 1991. Percentages were obtained by noting the fequency of isolation of each species and dividing it by total patients. The numbers for each study sum to more than 100% because of multiple isolates per patient. (*) The percentage of 153% indicates there were 1.5 *Bacteroides sp.* identified per patient.

obligate anaerobic species,[42] and it is generally more resistant to antibiotics than other anaerobes. However, experimental bacteremia with *Bacteroides fragilis* does not cause death, hypotension, lactic acidemia, nor other abnormalities identified with *Escherichia coli*.[43] The absence of a potent lipopolysaccharide component of the cell wall may render this organism without pathogenicity in the absence of a synergistic relationship.[44]

The enterococcus is a microorganism that has drawn considerable attention as a potential pathogen in peritonitis.[45,46] This organism has a resilient and relatively impermeable cell wall that permits culturing under very adverse environmental conditions (eg, 6.5% saline). The apparent increased frequency of the enterococcus in inflammatory exudates must relate to an actual increase in the presence of the organism, as opposed to the anaerobic species where increased recognition relates to better culturing techniques. Not unlike the anaerobic species, the enterococcus does not appear to be lethal to experimental animals when monomicrobial bacteremia or intraperitoneal contamination is studied.[47,48]

While the anaerobic species and enterococci do not appear to have virulence consistent with Koch's postulates, that does not mean that they do not have pathogenic potential. The reported mortality rates of higher than 50% in patients with *Bacteroides fragilis*[49] or enterococcal bacteremia[45,46] suggests that pathogenic potential is present nevertheless.

Studies by Onderdonk and associates[48] have demonstrated microbial synergism among the bacterial species found in intraperitoneal infection. These authors used gelatin capsules that contained autoclaved feces and barium sulfate as adjuvant substances to examine the effects of single and combined pathogens in the rat peritoneal cavity. Bacteria were then added to the capsule with the adjuvant substances to permit study of specific organisms and combinations of organisms upon the natural history of the disease. The capsule was then surgically placed in the peritoneal cavity. The capsule then dissolves with resultant peritonitis. When only a single species of bacteria was placed in the capsule, *Escherichia coli* alone proved to have significant virulence. When enterococcus or *Bacteroides fragilis* were the contaminant in the capsule, no virulence was identified. When combined inocula were used in the capsule, acute mortalities were only identified when *Escherichia coli* was present. When *Bacteroides fragilis* was present with *Escherichia coli*, the mortality rate of peritonitis rats was not increased, but all survivors had intra-abdominal abscesses. Enterococcus and *Bacteroides fragilis* together resulted in no acute mortalities but all surviving rats had abdominal abscess, although neither organism caused abscess when used alone. Enterococcus when combined with *Escherichia coli* resulted in a mortality rate identical to *Escherichia coli* alone.

All these experimental data allow formulation of a theoretical basis of microbial synergism (Figure 2). The acute phase mortalities are only identified when a potent bacterial endotoxin, or other virulence factor, is present (eg, *Escherichia coli*). When an oxygen-consuming organism is present (*Escherichia coli* or enterococcus), the pyogenic pathogenicity, thought to be mediated by a polysaccharide component of the cell wall, of *Bacteroides fragilis* can be expressed. Studies by Rink and associates[50] suggest that the lethality of *Escherichia coli* can actually be enhanced by the addition of *Bacteroides fragilis* to the contaminant. Thus, the actual virulence of *Escherichia coli* and other lipopolysaccharide bearing facultative gram-negative rods may be enhanced by the presence of other bacteria within the environment. The exact nature of this bacterial synergism requires further study.

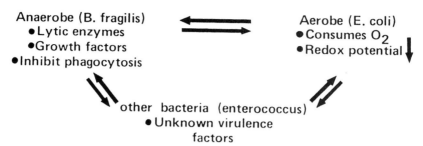

Figure 2: An illustration of a theoretical model of the synergistic relationship among the polymicrobial pathogens that are usually encountered in the patient with peritonitis.

Environment of Intraperitoneal Infection

The complex interaction of bacterial contaminants with the host, and the interactions of bacteria between species results in a local environment that has significant implications upon subsequent therapy in these patients. Once the infection has proceeded to the abscess phase, traditional teaching indicates that antibiotics are not effective and that only surgical drainage is effective, even when comprehensive antimicrobial coverage is used. These observations suggest that either systemic antibiotics do not reach the site of infection or the environment of infection compromises the activity of antibiotics.

Indeed, the environment of established peritoneal infection is dramatically different than conditions used in the laboratory for determination of sensitivities of clinical isolates. The presence of oxygen in the environment is a significant factor in both microbial metabolism and antibiotic activity. The pO_2 of abscess suppuration is 0, since facultative bacteria rapidly use any oxygen that is available.[51] This anaerobic environment significantly affects the activity of the aminoglycoside antibiotics.[52] Because the environment is principally anoxic, acid end products of substrate metabolism reduce the pH. Lower pH values in peritoneal pus have been identified and also may alter antimicrobial activity.[51] Additionally, the altered vascular permeability, fibrin deposition, and disintegrated leukocytes result in a protein-rich environment. This high density of protein may also buffer the effects of antimicrobial agents.

Fibrin is one specific protein that has had special significance in protecting bacteria from both host defense and systemically administered drugs. The condensation of fibrin on the cell wall of bacteria is well known to retard leukocyte phagocytosis. The encasement of bacteria within fibrin makes microorganisms inaccessible to the host cellular elements, in addition to the fact that antibiotics given after the deposition of fibrin penetrate this matrix very poorly.[53]

Finally, the density of bacteria within the infected focus of the peritoneal cavity may also have special significance to subsequent chemotherapy. Quantitative cultures of experimental abdominal abscess indicated that *Escherichia coli* was present in a concentration of 10^8 organisms per milliliter. *Bacteroides fragilis* was present in a concentration of 10^9 microorganisms per milliliter.[50] The significance of bacterial inoculum on antimicrobial sensitivity is illustrated in Figures 3 and 4.[54] Bacterial species consistently demonstrate increased resistance as bacte-

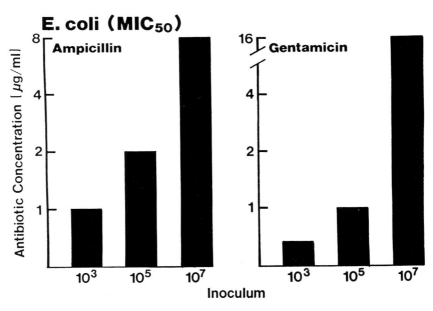

Figure 3: An illustration of how the minimum inhibitory concentration of selected antibiotics is affected by varying the inoculum of *Escherichia coli* used in the tube dilution method of determination of antimicrobial sensitivities.

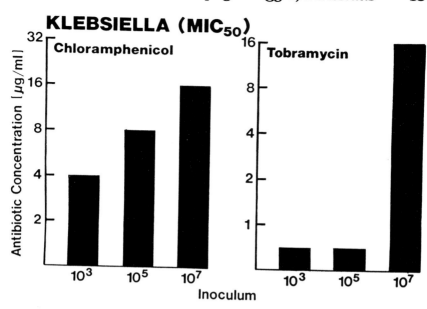

Figure 4: An illustration of how the minimum inhibitory concentration of selected antibiotics is affected by varying the inoculum of *Klebsiella sp.* used in the tube dilution method of determination of antimicrobial sensitivities.

rial density increases. The *Escherichia coli* and *Klebsiella* strains studied were quite sensitive to aminoglycosides at 10^3 or 10^5 organisms per milliliter, but were essentially resistant to the drug at 10^7 organisms per milliliter. While the basis for the inoculum effect remains unclear, β-lactamases are present in much greater concentrations in the environment as the bacterial concentration increases. The elaboration of enzymes that mediate resistance into the environment of the polymicrobial infection means that one resistant strain in high concentrations could generate resistance for all microbes present. Thus, inhibitors of β-lactamases (eg, clavulanic acid, sulbactam) may have a significant role to play in the treatment of these infections.

Inadequate binding of the antimicrobial receptor sites on or within the bacterial cell may account for the inoculum effect. Every antibiotic has a target receptor site on the bacterial cell (eg, ribosomes) and it is likely that a critical number of these target sites must be bound for inhibition of growth or for bactericidal effects to be present. As the number of otherwise sensitive bacteria in the infected environment is increased, the number of potential bacterial receptors is increased. The consequence of the expanded number of potential receptors is that the critical threshold of receptor binding for antibiotic effect will not be achieved.

The true clinical significance and the mechanism of the inoculum effect will require further study. It may be a significant issue which is responsible for the often seen circumstance of the peritonitis patient that has comprehensive coverage of all apparent pathogens, yet still fails to respond to systemic antibiotic therapy.

Summary

The natural history of peritonitis is a complex interaction of the host and the bacterial contaminants. The summed effects of adjuvant substances, adverse environment, and bacterial density suggest that effective mechanical therapy is essential and that systemic antimicrobial chemotherapy has limited effectiveness. A better understanding of these pathophysiologic relationships will hopefully generate better forms of therapy.

References

1. Welch JP, Donaldson GA: Perforative carcinoma of colon and rectum. *Ann Surg* 180:734, 1974.
2. Miller DW, Wichern WA: Perforated sigmoid diverticulitis: appraisal of primary versus delayed resection. *Am J Surg* 121:536, 1971.
3. Stephan M, Loewenthal J: Generalized infective peritonitis. *Surg Gynecol Obstet* 147:231-234, 1978.
4. Fry DE, Garrison RN, Heitsch RC, et al: Determinants of death in patients with intra-abdominal abscess. *Surgery* 89:517-523, 1980.
5. Richardson JD, Polk HC Jr: Newer adjunctive treatments for peritonitis. *Surgery* 90:917-918, 1981.
6. Lorber B, Swenson RM: The bacteriology of intra-abdominal infections. *Surg Clin North Am* 55:1349, 1975.
7. Stone HH, Kolb LD, Geheber CE: Incidence and significance of intraperitoneal anaerobic bacteria. *Ann Surg* 181:705, 1975.
8. Autio V: The spread of intraperitoneal infection. Studies with roentgen contrast medium. *Acta Chir Scand* 123(Suppl 321):5-31, 1964.
9. Krizek TJ, Robson MC, Kho E: Bacterial growth and skin graft survival. *Surg Forum* 18:518, 1967.
10. Kass EH: Bacteriuria and the diagnosis of infection in the urinary tract. *Arch Intern Med* 100:709, 1957.

11. Flemma RJ, Flint LM, Osterhout S, Shingeton WW: Bacteriologic studies of biliary tract infection. *Ann Surg* 166:563, 1967.
12. Tsilibary EC, Wissig SL: Absorption from the peritoneal cavity: SEM study of the mesothelium covering the peritoneal surface of the muscular portion of the diaphragm. *Am J Anat* 149:127, 1977.
13. Hau T, Simmons RL: Heparin in the treatment of experimental peritonitis. *Ann Surg* 187:294-298, 1978.
14. O'Leary JP, Malik FS, Donahoe RP, Johnston AD: The effects of a minidose of heparin on peritonitis in rats. *Surg Gynecol Obstet* 148:571-575, 1979.
15. Manzo G, Palade GE: Studies on inflammation. I. The effect of histamine and serotonins on vascular permeability: an electron microscopic study. *J Biophys Biochem Cytol* II:571, 1961.
16. Spector WG, Willoughby DA: Capillary permeability factors, nucleosides and histamine release. *J Pathol Bacteriol* 73:133, 1957.
17. Dinarello CA, Wolff SM: Pathogenesis of fever in man. *N Engl J Med* 298:607-612, 1978.
18. Dinarello CA: Interleukin-1 and the pathogenesis of the acute phase response. *N Engl J Med* 311:1413-1418, 1984.
19. Nusten MWN, De Groot ER, Ten Duis JH, et al: Serum levels of interleukin-6 and acute phase responses. *Lancet* 2:921, 1987.
20. Dinarello CA, Cannon JG, Wolff SM, et al: Tumor necrosis factor(cachectin) is an endogenous pyrogen and induces the production of interleukin-1. *J Exp Med* 163:1433-1450, 1986.
21. Hau T, Simmons RL: Mechanisms of the adjuvant effect of hemoglobin in experimental peritonitis. III. The influence of hemoglobin on phagocytosis and intracellular killing by human granulocytes. *Surgery* 87:588-592, 1980.
22. Lee JT Jr, Ahrenholz DH, Nelson RD, Simmons RL: Mechanisms of the adjuvant effect of hemoglobin in experimental peritonitis. V. The significance of the coordinated iron component. *Surgery* 86:41-48, 1979.
23. Polk HC Jr, Miles AA: Enhancement of bacterial infection by ferric iron: kinetics, mechanisms, and surgical significance. *Surgery* 70:71-77, 1971.
24. Pruett TL, Rotstein OD, Fiegel VD, et al: Mechanisms of the adjuvant effect of hemoglobin in experimental infections: VIII. A leukotoxin is produced by *Escherichia coli* metabolism of hemoglobin. *Surgery* 96:375-383, 1984.
25. Elek SD, Conen PE: The virulence of Staphylococcus pyogenes for man. A study of the problems of the wound infection. *Br J Exp Pathol* 38:573, 1957.
26. Casciato DA, Goldberg LS, Bluestone R: Polymorphonuclear neutrophil chemotaxis under aerobic and anaerobic conditions. *Infect Immun* 21:381-386, 1978.
27. Robertson HD, Polk HC Jr: The mechanism of infection in patients with diabetes mellitus: a review of leukocyte malfunction. *Surgery* 75:123-128, 1974.
28. Fuenfer MM, Olson GE, Polk HC Jr: Effect of various corticosteroids upon the phagocytic bacteriocidal activity of neutrophils. *Surgery* 78:27-33, 1975.
29. Klepser RG, Neugster WJ: The effect of alcohol upon the chemotactic response of leukocytes. *J Infect Dis* 65:196-199, 1939.
30. Marr JJ, Spilberg I: A mechanism for decreased resistance to infection by

gram-negative organisms during acute alcoholic intoxication. *J Lab Clin Med* 86:253-258, 1975.

31. Hunt TK, Linsey M, Grislis G, et al: The effect of differing ambient oxygen tensions on wound infection. *Ann Surg* 181:35-39, 1975.

32. Esrig BC, Frazee L, Stephenson SF, et al: The predisposition to infection following hemorrhagic shock. *Surg Gynecol Obstet* 144:915-917, 1977.

33. Saba TM, Blumenstock FA, Scovill WA, Bernard H: Cryoprecipitate reversal of opsonic alpha-2 surface binding glycoprotein deficiency in septic surgical and traumatic patients. *Science* 201:622-624, 1978.

34. Saba TM, Jaffe EJ: Plasma fibronectin(opsonic glycoprotein): its synthesis by vascular endothelial cells and role in cardiopulmonary integrity after trauma as related to reticuloendothelial function. *Am J Med* 68:577-594, 1980.

35. Blaisdell FW: Pathophysiology of the respiratory distress syndrome. *Arch Surg* 108:44-49, 1974.

36. Waymack JP, Gallon L, Barcelli U, et al: Effect of blood transfusions on macrophage function in a burned animal model. *Curr Surg* 43:305-307, 1986.

37. Waymack JP, Rapien J, Garnett D, et al: Effect of transfusion on immune function in a traumatized animal model. *Arch Surg* 121:5-54, 1986.

38. Nichols RL, Smith JW, Klein DB, et al: Risk of infection after penetrating abdominal trauma. *N Engl J Med* 311:1065-1069, 1984.

39. Dellinger EP, Oreskovich MR, Wertz MJ, et al: Risk of infection following laparotomy for penetrating abdominal injury. *Arch Surg* 119:20-24, 1984.

40. Mosdell DM, Morris DM, Voltura A, et al: Antibiotic treatment for surgical peritonitis. *Ann Surg* 214:543-549, 1991.

41. Stone HH, Strom PR, Fabian TC, Dunlop WE: Third generation cephalosporins for polymicrobial surgical sepsis. *Arch Surg* 118:193-200, 1983.

42. Tally FP, Stewart PR, Sutter VL, Rosenblatt JE: Oxygen tolerance of fresh clinical anaerobic bacteria. *J Clin Microbiol* 1:161-164, 1975.

43. Fry DE, Kaelin CR, Rink RD: Oxidative metabolism in experimental Bacteroides fragilis bacteremia. *J Surg Res* 28:501-506, 1980.

44. Kasper DL: Chemical and biological characterization of the lipopolysaccharides of Bacteroides fragilis subspecies fragilis. *J Infect Dis* 134:59-66, 1976.

45. Garrison RN, Fry DE, Berberich S, Polk HC Jr: Enterococcal bacteremia: clinical implications and determinants of death. *Ann Surg* 196:43-47, 1982.

46. Dougherty AB, Flohr AB, Simmons RL: "Breakthrough" enterococcal septicemia in surgical patients: 19 cases and a review of the literature. *Arch Surg* 118:232, 1983.

47. Fry DE, Berberich S, Garrison RN: The bacterial synergism of enterococcus and E. coli. *J Trauma* 23:637, 1983.

48. Onderdonk AB, Bartlett JG, Louie TJ, et al: Microbial synergy in experimental intraabdominal abscess. *Infect Immun* 13:22-26, 1976.

49. Fry DE, Garrison RN, Polk HC Jr: Clinical implications in bacteroides bacteremia. *Surg Gynecol Obstet* 149:189-192, 1979.

50. Rink RD, Kaelin CR, Raque G, et al: Effects of pure or combined inocula of E. coli and B. fragilis on the liver and related metabolism. *Lab Invest* 46:282-288, 1982.

51. Fry DE, Garrison RN, Rink RD, et al: An experimental model of intra-abdominal abscess in the rat. *Adv Shock Res* 7:7-11, 1982.

52. Verklin RM, Mandell GL: Alterations of effectiveness of antibiotics by anaerobiosis. *J Lab Clin Med* 89:65-71, 1977.
53. Ahrenholz DH, Simmons RL: Fibrin in peritonitis. I. Beneficial and adverse effects of fibrin in experimental E. coli peritonitis. *Surgery* 88:41-46, 1980.
54. Fry DE, Garrison RN, Trachtenberg L, Polk HC Jr: Bacterial inoculum and the activity of antimicrobial agents. *Surg Gynecol Obstet* 160:105-108, 1985.

2

Hemodynamic and Metabolic Aspects of Peritonitis

Donald E. Fry, MD

The systemic and metabolic response to peritonitis and to the septic state in general represents a complex constellation of physiologic responses. The septic patient has abnormalities of substrate and oxygen metabolism that remain poorly understood. The septic shock patient frequently manifests the paradox of markedly increased cardiac output with hypotension as opposed to shock states identified with hypovolemia or primary cardiogenic failure.[1-5] The sustained septic state results in multiple, or sequential, system organ failure that further supports the concept that an end-organ abnormality at the tissue level is fundamental to the process.[6-10] Not only is the understanding of these fundamental processes necessary for the supportive care of the peritonitis patient, but it is required in order to understand newer forms of therapy as they are introduced.

The Appropriate Stress Response

Following acute trauma, hemorrhage, or major surgical intervention, an appropriate systemic stress response occurs that affects cardiovascular, endocrine, and metabolic homeostasis. Each response can be teleologically viewed as an effort to enhance the peripheral delivery of oxygen and substrate to fuel reparative processes.

Cardiac output increases, but with a minimal yet appropriate reduc-

From Fry DE, (ed): *Peritonitis.* Mount Kisco NY, Futura Publishing Co., Inc., © 1993.

tion in peripheral vascular resistance. Arteriovenous oxygen content remains unchanged, which combined with increased flow from the hyperdynamic circulation, results in increased total oxygen consumption. Increased energy demands of peripheral tissues are thus met. Lactic acidemia is not of significance given normovolemia and adequate hemoglobin saturation, since no oxygen debt is incurred.

The body economy in circumstances of stress shifts to a catabolic mode to provide ample substrate to fuel the demands of host response and tissue repair. Catecholamine concentrations are increased.[11] Glycogenolysis rapidly occurs. Glucagon levels increase as gluconeogenesis in the liver is actively stimulated.[12] Increased concentrations of adrenocortical steroids passively encourage gluconeogenesis.[13] Growth hormone concentrations also rise.[14] Typically, insulin concentrations are increased under such circumstances.[15] The stimulation of gluconeogenesis results in significant skeletal muscle proteolysis for mobilization of amino acids to provide the hydrocarbons necessary for structural synthesis of new glucose in the hepatocyte. Increased glucose synthesis from amino acid precursors results in increased hepatic ureogenesis and an obligatory increase in urinary excretion of nitrogen. Despite increased insulin concentrations, lipolysis results in mobilization of fat stores. While fatty acids cannot directly participate in the gluconeogenic process, the glycerol residue of triglyceride hydrolysis can be used for new glucose synthesis. The fatty acids themselves are oxidized for energy purposes. The Cori cycle represents an indirect method for new glucose to arise from precursor carbon from fatty acids.[16]

The adaptive physiologic and metabolic responses defined above are temporally limited and as such do not represent a sustained disruption to homeostasis. The hypermetabolism and attendant features of stress are limited to 4 to 7 days after major surgical stress and trauma, although some features of increased oxygen consumption and increased substrate metabolism will persist until the reparative process is complete. The self-limiting nature of the stress response assumes that the host is not subjected to an intercurrent insult such as sepsis, hemorrhage, or a major operation.

Response to Peritonitis

The initial physiologic and metabolic response to mild peritonitis is similar to the adaptive response of stress. However, severe peritonitis results in exaggeration of the normal stress response with metabolic decompensation and severe catabolism being the net result.

Cardiovascular Response

A theoretical model of the natural history of the cardiovascular response during the natural history of septic peritonitis is illustrated in Figure 1. Like staging systems similarly used by oncologists, the follow-

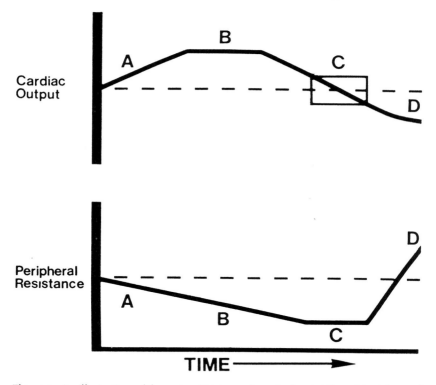

Figure 1: An illustration of the natural history of septic shock. The critical determinants that govern the stages of the illness are the cardiac output and the peripheral vascular resistance. The rectangle at stage C indicates the usual findings of the patient who is called in septic shock. It actually represents only a phase in the overall progression of the problem. However, the patient is considered as in shock at this point in time because of systemic hypotension. Actually, alterations of oxygen consumption are noted much earlier in the process and shock from the perspective of the tissues has occurred before hypotension intervenes.

ing classification scheme is a simplification that basically follows that which has previously been reported by Siegel and associates.[1] During stage A the cardiac output is increased, but with minimal changes in peripheral vascular resistance. Stage A represents the compensated phase of the septic response and is analogous to the appropriate stress response. Patients with mild peritonitis from an acute perforated peptic ulcer would commonly be identified in this group.

However, in stage B, peripheral vascular resistance decreases in an inappropriate fashion and this results in increased cardiac output, probably mediated by the sympathetic nervous system secondary to afterload reduction. The cardiac index in these patients may reach 200–300% of normal. In younger patients with considerable cardiac reserve, this hyperdynamic state can be sustained for days. Older patients and those with organic heart disease may not be able to generate or sustain an increased level of cardiac performance.

Severe peritonitis in a younger patient after a major colon injury will commonly be associated with a period of stage B sepsis. As the natural history of the disease progresses to stage C, cardiac performance declines to levels that under ordinary circumstances would be considered normal. This decline in myocardial performance represents the inability to sustain the high-output stage. The marked reduction of peripheral vascular resistance makes this level of cardiac output inadequate to support systemic arterial blood pressure and hypotension is identified clinically as a result. On the other hand, the patient with severe peritonitis without sufficient cardiac reserve to generate an elevated cardiac output may quickly progress to stage C without proceeding through the previous stages that require a hyperdynamic circulation.

Finally, stage D represents the cardiogenic phase of septic shock, where frank myocardial failure is superimposed upon the primary peripheral abnormality of the septic process. When low cardiac output intervenes, peripheral vascular resistance dramatically increases. In the aggressively treated, normovolemic patient, the development of stage D usually represents a preterminal event.

Oxygen Metabolism

As noted earlier, the appropriate stress response results in increased oxygen consumption. This increased oxygen consumption is characterized by increased blood flow with an unchanged arteriovenous difference in oxygen content. However, as the patient evolves into stage B decompensation with peritonitis, the arteriovenous difference narrows. Total oxygen consumption is reduced at a point in time when systemic cardiac output is increased. Lactic acidemia can be identified in the stage B patient without lactic acidosis. Plasma buffering capacity is reduced. As stage C sepsis develops, the further dissociated relationships between cardiac output and peripheral resistance are accompanied by frank arterial lactic acidosis. Thus, a peripheral defect in oxygen uptake or utilization appears to be a fundamental feature of the septic process.

The pathophysiologic basis for reduced oxygen consumption in the septic patient has been the focus of considerable clinical and experimental investigation. Numerous hypotheses have been proposed to explain the reduction in oxygen consumption. The basic discussions have concerned whether alterations of oxygen metabolism are consequences of a primary cellular injury that render the cell unable to utilize available oxygen, or whether abnormalities of microcirculatory flow result in defective delivery of oxygen to the cell.

The data to support a primary cellular injury have focused on hypothesized injuries to the mitochondrion, since this organelle represents the final stage in the processes of cellular oxidative metabolism. Experimental studies by Mela et al.[17] and Schumer et al.[18] have identified severe uncoupling and inhibition of hepatic mitochondria from rats subjected to lethal endotoxemia. They have suggested that endotoxin may have a direct effect on the cellular oxidative machinery. However, Rink et al.[19] noted that endotoxemia resulted in reduced tissue pO_2 in the liver and Asher et al.[20] identified reduced hepatic nutrient blood flow to the liver in endotoxemia at a point in time when mitochondrial function was unchanged. The pattern of uncoupling and inhibition noted by Mela[17] and Schumer[18] is very similar to patterns noted in hepatic mitochondria following hemorrhagic shock[17,21] and warm ischemia.[22] Thus, the experimental data to support a mitochondrial injury from endotoxemia experiments may be secondary to ischemic changes and may not be fundamental to the primary process.

More compelling evidence for a mitochondrial injury are the studies of Siegel and Cerra.[1,2] Large numbers of septic patients were sequentially studied for numerous physiologic and metabolic parameters. Systemic lactate and pyruvate levels in severely septic patients were both significantly elevated but the lactate:pyruvate ratio was unchanged. If the abnormalities of the septic cell were that of oxygen deficiency, all nicotinamide dinucleotide (NAD^+) in the cell cytoplasm would be in a reduced state (NADH⁺) (Figure 2). All pyruvate from glycolysis would not be able to proceed through aerobic processes in the mitochondria because of the lack of oxygen. Pyruvate would then be rapidly converted to lactate so that NAD⁺ can be regenerated to permit other NAD⁺-dependent reactions of glycolysis to proceed. Indeed, the molar ratio of lactate:pyruvate is thought to reflect the molar ratio of extramitochondrial NADH⁺:NAD⁺. The equimolar increases of both lactate and pyruvate have led to the hypothesis that injury to the mitochondria more appropriately explains the inability of pyruvate to enter the Krebs cycle, with resultant reduced oxygen consumption. Pyruvate dehydrogenase is one enzyme system that may be affected based on these data.[23]

Arguments against the mitochondrial injury hypothesis still persist. Mitochondria that are isolated from liver[24] and kidney[25] during experimental peritonitis demonstrate no injury of oxidative capability. Actually, increased efficiency of hepatic mitochondria have been identified

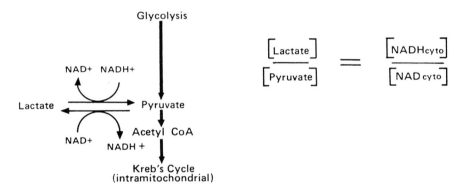

Figure 2: An illustration of the equilibrium between the oxidation-reduction state of nicotinamide adenine dinucleotide (NAD) and the molar relationships of lactate and pyruvate. This figure is only considering NAD that is in the cytoplasm of the cell. When the acetyl coenzyme A groups that are generated by glycolysis are unable to proceed into oxidation in the mitochondria (Kreb's cycle), then the equilibrium between lactate and pyruvate shifts toward lactate production. This equilibrium is governed by the state of oxidized (NAD⁺) or reduced (NADH⁺) nicotinamide adenine dinucleotide. If oxygen availability was the rate-limiting issue for cellular energy production, then increases of lactate would be dramatic with limited changes in pyruvate. Thus, the equimolar increases of lactate:pyruvate have led to the hypothesis of a mitochondrial injury. The author contends that the oxidation-reduction state of NAD is altered in the cytoplasm by ureogenesis and gluconeogenesis within the hepatocyte. Inadequate oxygen delivery to the cell remains a viable explanation for the reduced oxygen metabolism of sepsis.

in peritonitis animals,[24] a response known to be recognized when systemic hypoxemia exists.[26] Pyruvate oxidation appears unaffected when specifically studied.[24]

Secondly, experimental peritonitis results in both reduced effective hepatic[27-29] and renal blood flow.[30] While experimental and clinical studies have demonstrated no reduction in flow in septic extremities,[31,32] flow patterns in the viscera of those organs known to fail as a consequence of the septic process may not correspond to skeletal muscle. Indeed, serum elevations of serum glutamic-oxaloacetic transaminase (SGOT), lactate dehydrogenase (LDH), and alkaline phosphatase are common in the septic patient.[8-10] Increases in serum creatine phosphokinase or myoglobin are not identified.

Finally, while the lactate:pyruvate ratio suggests a potential mitochondrial injury, this assumes that systemic concentrations parallel intracellular levels of these substrates. Examination of the β-hydroxybutyrate:acetoacetate ratio in the data of Siegel[1] as well as the data of Ozawa et al.[33] shows a disproportionate increase in the molar concentration of β-hydroxybutyrate. Increase in this ratio has been correlated with the ratio of $NADH^+:NAD^+$ concentrations within the mitochondrion (Figure 3).[34] This implies a hypoxic intramitochondrial compartment with inadequate electron acceptor to allow dehydrogenase reactions to proceed. Thus, the lactate:pyruvate and β-hydroxybutyrate:acetoacetate data are not consistent with each other.

A plausible explanation to reconcile the apparent paradox of ketone ratios that imply a reduced state, but lactate:pyruvate molar ratios that remain constant, can be found in the experiments by Townsend et al.[28] In these studies with cecal ligation and puncture in the rat, equimolar

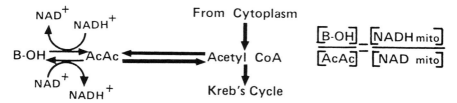

Figure 3: An illustration of the intramitochondrial relationships of the oxidation-reduction state of NAD with β-hydroxybutyrate (B-OH) and acetoacetate (AcAc). Shifts of acetyl coenzyme A to the ketone bodies is partially governed by the oxidized (NAD^+) or reduced ($NADH^+$) state within the mitochondria. The marked molar increases of β-hydroxybutyrate suggest that adequate electron acceptor (oxygen) is not available.

increases in lactate:pyruvate ratios in the blood were identified in a fashion similar to the human septic condition. However, measurements of lactate:pyruvate concentrations in hepatic tissue identified a dramatic increase of lactate concentration over that of pyruvate. The lactate increase was consistent with reduced hepatic nutrient blood flow, even though the animals had a hyperdynamic circulation characterized by a high cardiac output during the study period. Thus, the equimolar systemic concentrations of lactate:pyruvate ratio were dictated by the well perfused, large tissue mass of skeletal muscle, while lactate production was generated from the liver and other ischemic splanchnic tissues. Several other potential mechanisms have been postulated to explain how inadequate oxygen delivery to the cell might occur. Miller and associates[35] have published data that suggest alterations in oxyhemoglobin dissociation may result in increased affinity of hemoglobin for oxygen. This would theoretically result in inadequate cellular oxygenation despite normal or even increased tissue perfusion. However, other studies have indicated that oxyhemoglobin dissociation and concentrations of 2,3- diphosphoglycerate shift in a direction that is favorable to oxygen release.[36,37] Furthermore, systemic or tissue level acidosis acutely changes oxyhemoglobin dissociation to lower pO_2 partial pressures at the 50% level of hemoglobin saturation, and should enhance oxygen delivery.

Another interesting hypothesis with respect to red blood cells and defective oxygen delivery relates to alterations of red cell deformability in the septic state. The red cell that is 6–8 μm in diameter must deform longitudinally to pass through the capillary microcirculation that is only 3–4 μm in diameter. Studies by Hurd et al.[38] have demonstrated reduction in red cell deformability in both human and experimental peritonitis. Membrane rigidification secondary to lipid peroxidation has been a hypothesized mechanism for this change.[39] These data are interesting and require further experiments to ascertain their potential clinical relevance.

Microarteriovenous shunts have been postulated to explain the defective oxygen utilization in septic patients.[40,41] The systemic hemodynamic response of increased cardiac output, reduced peripheral vascular resistance, and reduced oxygen extraction is certainly consistent with shunting. Experimental and clinical studies have not demonstrated shunts in septic extremities.[31,32] The presence of shunts in visceral organs have not been identified. While an attractive hypothesis, there is little scientific evidence to support it.

Finally, reduced oxygen consumption secondary to microaggregates that occlude or embolize the microcirculation and embarrass the nutrient blood flow of tissue have been postulated. Saba and associates[42,43] have demonstrated that a nonspecific, α-2 glycoprotein, opsonin of serum is necessary for clearance of aggregates that form within the circulation. Binding of this opsonin, also known as fibronectin, to microaggregates facilitates their elimination via the reticuloendothelial system, especially the Kupffer cells of the liver. Saba and associates[42,43] have demonstrated that the number of microaggregates seems to increase secondary to shock, trauma, or infection and that the areas of tissue injury result in binding of fibronectin at the injury site. Increased microaggregate formation combined with acute consumptive depletion of circulating fibronectin results in the identification of increased aggregates of platelets, leukocytes, and fibrin in the capillaries of the microcirculation. The impact of these formed aggregates may result in pulmonary failure, multiple system organ failure, and perhaps the altered oxygen consumption of sepsis. Studies by Garrison[27] and Asher[20,44] have noted reduced nutrient blood flow in experimental models of peritonitis and bacteremia. Histopathology in these animals indicates increased aggregates within the sinusoids of the liver. A randomized human trial where human fibronectin replacement was attempted in septic patients has failed to demonstrate any clinical efficacy.[45]

Are aggregates within the microcirculation that are identified histologically[44] the consequences of microembolization or are they de novo aggregates that form at the endothelial surface? Considerable evidence now supports the notion that activated neutrophils marginate to microcirculatory endothelial cells. The fully activated neutrophil, secondary to (1) complement cleavage products,[46] (2) macrophage cytokines (particularly tumor necrosis factor),[47] and (3) potential direct effects of endotoxin,[48] when marginated to the endothelial cell releases reactive oxygen intermediates that creates a microcirculatory inflammatory nidus.[49] Thrombosis of the microcirculation results in focal tissue ischemia. The relationships of leukocyte-endothelial cell interaction require further study.

A generally accepted mechanism to explain the altered oxygen consumption in the septic state remains unclear. The progression of the disease process from stage B to stage C and D results in further compromise of arterial flow and further compromise of both oxygen and substrate delivery. It is the better understanding of the fundamental abnormality of oxygen consumption that will most significantly affect new concepts in the management of these patients.

Substrate Metabolism

All aspects of substrate metabolism become significantly deranged as the patient proceeds from the compensated stage A to the decompensation of stage B. While the subsequent discussion will focus on each individual type of substrate, the biochemical disorders of each fuel are interrelated to each other.

Glucose Metabolism

The septic patient during the hyperdynamic stage B generally has an increased blood glucose. This hyperglycemia has a twofold contribution from (1) relative resistance to insulin in peripheral tissues and (2) marked stimulation of gluconeogenesis in the liver. Circulating levels of insulin are increased, but blood glucose remains at inappropriately high concentrations. Similarly, the septic patient is usually poorly responsive to exogenously administered insulin as well. In addition to insulin resistance, exaggerated stimulation of gluconeogenesis by glucagon results in large amounts of glucose released into the circulation. The circulating levels of glucagon are reported to be 20–60 standard deviations (SD) above normal.[1] This active stimulation of gluconeogenesis has to be fueled by amino acids, especially alanine. The reservoir for the amino acids is skeletal muscle. If unchecked, the totally uncontrolled hepatic gluconeogenesis can exhaust critical masses of the patient's skeletal muscle with biochemical malnutrition becoming a significant risk.

The consequences of the tremendous stimulation of the cell by glucagon create a potential crisis of bioenergy availability for other hepatic metabolic functions. The process of gluconeogenesis requires utilization of reduced nicotinamide dinucleotide ($NADH^+$) for synthesis of new glucose from pyruvate. The process of ureagenesis similarly requires $NADH^+$ to permit elimination of the nitrogenous end products from deamination of amino acids used in the gluconeogenic process. Since one $NADH^+$ molecule ordinarily yields three adenosine triphosphate molecules from oxidative phosphorylation, the utilization of $NADH^+$ might be considered an enormous drain on the energy reserves of the cell. On the other hand, utilization of $NADH^+$ in these synthetic processes permits regeneration of NAD^+ and may be a critical compensatory mechanism to allow glycolysis to continue in the cell that is unable to utilize oxygen appropriately, for whatever reason.

Amino Acid Metabolism

The major changes of amino acid metabolism are (1) increased utilization of branched-chain amino acids by skeletal muscle as a preferred energy substrate, (2) increased ulitilization of glutamine as a preferred fuel by the enterocyte of the small intestine, (3) increased amino acid release from skeletal muscle to fuel gluconeogenesis, and (4) increased circulating levels of aromatic amino acids.

Resting skeletal muscle preferentially uses fatty acids for an energy substrate. With exercise, endogenous glycogen stores and extracellular glucose are used. During the adaptive stress response, branched-chain amino acids (valine, leucine, and isoleucine) are preferentially used with a resultant reduction in the circulating plasma concentrations of these amino acids. However, when stage B sepsis evolves, the circulating concentrations of the branched-chain amino acids increase. The leucine oxidation appears to continue with further progression of the septic process into stage B.[50] Proteolysis becomes dissociated from energy need with massive release of amino acids in proportion to their presence in muscle. At this stage, exogenously administered amino acids and calories do not blunt the muscle catabolism, and exhaustion of the body's substrate reserve continues unless the septic process is controlled.[50]

The glucogenic amino acids, glycine and especially alanine, are released in increased quantities from skeletal muscle during stage A, and this release continues as septic catabolism continues. Not only do the glucogenic amino acids fuel the gluconeogenesis process in the liver but they also serve as a nitrogen shuttle to eliminate NH_3^+ groups that are the consequenses of deamination and oxidation of the branched-chain amino acids in muscle.

Recently, considerable discussion has focused upon the apparent increased oxidation of glutamine by the small intestinal enterocyte.[51] The hypermetabolic state results in increased oxidation of glutamine by the enterocyte that may not be adequately provided by muscle catabolism or from exogenous sources.[52]

Glutamine is a five-carbon amino acid that has two amino groups.

Its oxidation by the enterocyte results in one amino group being eliminated as ammonia into the intestinal lumen. The second amino group is eliminated as alanine into the portal circulation. A net of two carbons is oxidized within the enterocyte for energy purposes. The release of alanine is thought to then be a substrate to further fuel gluconeogenesis in the liver. Atrophy of the intestinal mucosa due to this inadequate delivery of substrate is thought to be a potential issue in the loss of intestinal barrier function.[53]

The uncontrolled proteolysis of the stage B results in release of numerous amino acids, many of which are not readily metabolized during the septic process. Of considerable interest are the aromatic amino acids. Under basal conditions and during the adaptive stress response, aromatic amino acids are metabolized by the liver. However, during septic decompensation the oxidation of tyrosine and phenylalanine is especially impaired and very high incomplete metabolism of these two aromatic amino acids may result in false neurotransmitters that could play an integral role in the marked peripheral vasodilatation of the septic patient.

Fat Metabolism

The adaptive response to stress results in increased lypolysis and mobilization of triglycerides. Triglicerides are readily hydrolized to free fatty acids and glycerol so that circulating levels are not increased. Glycerol may be utilized for gluconeogenesis while free fatty acids undergo β-oxidation for energy purposes. In stage B, hypertriglyceridemia and increased levels of fatty acids develop, but without increases in circulating levels of glycerol. Glycerol levels remain low because of accelerated gluconeogenesis. Serum ketone levels are increased mainly due to increased concentrations of β-hydroxybutyrate, as discussed above.

Summary

The metabolic and physiologic abnormalities of the patient with severe sepsis from peritonitis are especially complex. Much of the data in the laboratory is difficult to assimilate because of the different animal models that are used. Patient data can be obscured by concurrent treatments that may color the interpretation of results. The overall complexity of intermediary metabolism further compounds unraveling the clinical and experimental observations. Nevertheless, significant improvement in the care of the critically-ill peritonitis patient will await further definition of the fundamental mechanisms.

References

1. Siegal JH, Cerra FB, Coleman B, et al: Physiologic and metabolic correlations in human sepsis. *Surgery* 85:163-193, 1979.
2. Cerra FB, Siegal JH, Border JR, et al: The hepatic failure of sepsis: cellular versus substrate. *Surgery* 86:409-422, 1979.
3. Cohn JD, Greenspan M, Goldstein CR, et al: Arteriovenous shunting in high cardiac output shock syndromes. *Surg Gynecol Obstet* 127:282, 1968.
4. Duff JH, Groves AC, McLean AP, et al: Defective oxygen consumption in septic shock. *Surg Gynecol Obstet* 128:1051, 1969.
5. Cerra FB, Siegal JH, Border JR, McMenamy RH: Correlations between metabolic and cardiopulmonary measurements in patients after trauma, general surgery, and sepsis. *J Trauma* 19:621-626, 1979.
6. Border JR, Chenier R, McMenamy RH, et al: Multiple systems organ failure: muscle fuel deficit with visceral protein malnutrition. *Surg Clin North Am* 56:1147-1167, 1976.
7. Eiseman B, Beart R, Norton L: Multiple organ failure. *Surg Gynecol Obstet* 144:323-326, 1977.
8. Fry DE, Pearlstein L, Fulton RL, Polk HC Jr: Multiple system organ failure: the role of uncontrolled infection. *Arch Surg* 115:136-140, 1980.
9. Fry DE, Garrison RN, Polk HC Jr: Clinical implications in bacteroides bacteremia. *Surg Gynecol Obstet* 149:189-192, 1979.
10. Fry DE, Garrison RN, Heitsch RC, et al: Determinants of mortality in patients with intra-abdominal abscess. *Surgery* 89:517-523, 1980.
11. Davies CL, Newman RJ, Molyneux SG, et al: The relationship between plasma catecholamines and severity of injury in man. *J Trauma* 24:99-105, 1984.
12. Wilmore DW, Lindsey CA, Moylan JA, et al: Hyperglucagonaemia after burns. *Lancet* 1:73, 1974.
13. Vaughan GM, Becker RA, Allen JP, et al: Cortisol and corticotrophin in burned patients. *J Trauma* 22:263, 1982.
14. Richardson JD, Rodriguez JL: The metabolic consequences of injury. In: Richardson JD, Polk HC Jr, Flint LM, eds. *Trauma: Clinical Care and Pathophysiology*. Chicago, IL: Year Book Medical Publishers, Inc; 1987:87-101.
15. Black PR, Brooks DC, Bessey PQ, et al: Mechanisms of insulin resistance following injury. *Ann Surg* 196:420-435, 1982.
16. Bhagavan NV: Metabolic homeostasis. In: Bhagavan NV, ed. *Medical Biochemistry*. Boston, MA: Jones and Bartlett Publishing, Inc; 1992:495-527.
17. Mela L, Bacalzo LV Jr, Miller LD: Defective oxidative metabolism of rat liver mitochondria in hemorrhagic and endotoxin shock. *Am J Physiol* 220:571, 1981.

18. Schumer W, Das Gupta TK, Moss GS, et al: Effect of endotoxemia on liver cell mitochondria in man. *Ann Surg* 171:875, 1970.
19. Rink RD, Short BL, Pennington C: Hepatic oxygen supply and plasma lactate and glucose in endotoxic shock. *Circ Shock* 5:105, 1978.
20. Asher EF, Garrison RN, Ratcliffe DJ, Fry DE: Endotoxin, cellular function and nutrient blood flow. *Arch Surg* 118:441-445, 1983.
21. Rhodes RS, DePalma RG, Robinson AV: Relationship of critical uptake volume to energy production and endotoxemia in late hemorrhagic shock. *Am J Surg* 130:560-564, 1975.
22. Daniel AM, Beaudoin J: Evaluation of mitochondrial function in the ischemic rat liver. *J Surg Res* 17:19-25, 1974.
23. Vary TC, Siegel JH, Nakatani T, et al: Effect of sepsis on activity of pyruvate dehydrogenase complex in skeletal muscle and liver. *Am J Physiol* 250:E634-E640, 1986.
24. Fry DE, Silver BB, Rink RD, et al; Hepatic cellular hypoxia in murine peritonitis. *Surgery* 85:652-661, 1979.
25. Garrison RN, Ratcliffe DJ, Fry DE: The effects of peritonitis on murine renal mitochondria. *Adv Shock Res* 7:71-76, 1982.
26. Mela L, Olofsson K, Miller LD, et al: Effect of lysosomes and hypoxia in shock. *Surg Forum* 22:19-21, 1971.
27. Garrison RN, Ratcliffe DJ, Fry DE: Hepatocellular function and nutrient blood flow in experimental peritonitis. *Surgery* 92:713-719, 1982.
28. Townsend MC, Hampton WW, Haybron DM, et al: Effective organ blood flow and bioenergy status in murine peritonitis. *Surgery* 100:205-213, 1986.
29. Schirmer WJ, Townsend MC, Schirmer JM, et al: Galactose elimination kinetics in sepsis: correlation of liver blood flow with function. *Arch Surg* 122:349-354, 1987.
30. Haybron DM, Townsend MC, Hampton WW, et al: Alterations in renal perfusion and renal energy charge in murine peritonitis. *Arch Surg* 122:328-331, 1987.
31. Wright CJ, Duff JH, McLean APH, MacLean LD: Regional capillary blood flow and oxygen uptake in severe sepsis. *Surg Gynecol Obstet* 132:637-644, 1971.
32. Clowes GHA Jr, O'Donnell TF Jr, Ryan NT, et al: Energy metabolism in sepsis: treatment based on different patterns in shock and high output stage. *Ann Surg* 179:684, 1974.
33. Ozawa K, Aoyama H, Yasuda K, et al: Metabolic abnormalities associated with postoperative organ failure. *Arch Surg* 118:1245-1251, 1983.
34. Klingenberg M, von Hafen H: Wege des Wasserstoffs in mitochondrien. I Die Wasserstoffubertragung von succinat zu acetacetat. *Biochem Z* 337:120, 1963.
35. Miller LD, Oski FA, Diaco JF, et al: The affinity of hemoglobin for oxygen: its control and in vivo significance. *Surgery* 68:187, 1970.
36. Valeri CR, Kopriva CJ: Oxyhemoglobin dissociation curve in hemorrhage and septic shock. *Adv Exp Med Biol* 23:177, 1971.
37. Watkins GM, Rabelo A, Plzak LF, Sheldon GF: The left shifted oxyhemoglobin curve in sepsis: a preventable defect. *Ann Surg* 180:213, 1974.
38. Hurd T, Dasmahapatra K, Rush B, et al: Red blood cell deformability in human and experimental sepsis. *Arch Surg* 123:217-220, 1988.

39. Powell RJ, Machiedo GW, Rush BF Jr, Dikdan G: Oxygen free radicals: effect on red cell deformability in sepsis. *Crit Care Med* 19:732-735, 1991.
40. Border JR, Gallo E, Schenk WG: Systemic arteriovenous shunts in patients under severe stress: a common cause of high output cardiac failure. *Surgery* 60:225-229, 1966.
41. Siegal JH, Greenspan M, Del Guercio LR: Abnormal vascular tone, defective oxygen transport and myocardial failure in human septic shock. *Ann Surg* 165:504, 1967.
42. Scovill WA, Saba TM, Kaplan JE, et al: Disturbances in circulating opsonic activity in man after operative and blunt trauma. *J Surg Res* 22:709, 1977.
43. Scovill WA, Saba TM, Kaplan JE, et al: Deficits in reticuloendothelial humoral mechanisms after trauma. *J Trauma* 16:898, 1976.
44. Asher EF, Rowe RL, Garrison RN, Fry DE: The effects of experimental bacteremia on hepatic nutrient blood flow. *Circ Shock* 9:173, 1982.
45. Mansburger AR, Doran JE, Treat R, et al: The influence of fibronectin administration on the incidence of sepsis and septic morbidity in severely injured patients. *Ann Surg* 210:297-306, 1989.
46. Schirmer WJ, Schirmer JM, Naff GB, Fry DE: Complement activation produces hemodynamic changes characteristic of sepsis. *Arch Surg* 123:316-321, 1988.
47. Schirmer WJ, Schirmer JM, Fry DE: Recombinant human tumor necrosis factor produces hemodynamic changes characteristic of sepsis and endotoxemia. *Arch Surg* 124:445-448, 1989.
48. Wright SD, Ramos RA, Tobias PS, et al: CD-14 serves as the cellular receptor for complexes of lipopolysaccharide with lipopolysaccharide binding protein. *Science* 249:1431-1433, 1991.
49. Schirmer WJ, Fry DE: Microcirculatory arrest. In: Fry DE, ed. *Multiple System Organ Failure*. Chicago, IL: Mosby Year Book Publishers; 1992:73-85.
50. Cerra FB, Siegal JH, Coleman B, et al: Septic autocannibalism: a failure of exogenous nutritional support. *Ann Surg* 192:570-580, 1980.
51. Windmueller HG: Glutamine utilization by the small intestine. *Adv Enzymol* 53:201, 1982.
52. Souba WW, Wilmore DW: Postoperative alteration of arteriovenous exchange of amino acids across the gastrointestinal tract. *Surgery* 94:342, 1983.
53. Wilmore DW, Smith RJ, O'Dwyer ST, et al: The gut: a central organ after surgical stress. *Surgery* 104:917-923, 1988.

3

Diagnosis of Peritonitis

R. Neal Garrison, MD

The peritoneal cavity is the largest extravascular space in the body, containing less than 100 mL of sterile lubricating fluid. The inflammatory response of this large peritoneal surface to bacteria or chemicals is termed peritonitis. Such inflammation usually results from gastrointestinal, biliary, or genitourinary tract contamination, but follows every abdominal operation to some extent. When contamination occurs, the clinical presentation is variable, tempered by the amount and location of spillage along with the local and systemic ability of the patient to respond to the soilage. Generalized peritonitis is the usual initial result of a large acute free perforation, and the resulting "acute abdomen" presents few diagnostic dilemmas even for the novice physician. Conversely, a small occult lesion in a debilitated postoperative patient, especially at extremes of age, taxes the diagnostic acumen of even the most astute experienced clinician. Only when the possibility of intra-abdominal infection is seriously considered will attempts at a thorough diagnosis be made. The effective management of this lethal condition mandates an early accurate diagnosis.

A careful history is the initial step toward this early and accurate working diagnosis. Peritonitis produces pain as its main symptom due to the inflammatory reaction of the visceral and parietal peritoneal surfaces to the noxious agents. The character, time, and mode of onset and distribution of the pain alert the physician not only to the possibility of peritonitis, but also give him hints as to its etiology. Nausea, vomiting, and anorexia are very nonspecific findings, but when these symptoms are absent, the diagnosis of peritonitis should be questioned. Overall, the history alone is helpful in establishing the diagnosis of intra-abdomi-

From Fry DE, (ed): *Peritonitis.* Mount Kisco NY, Futura Publishing Co., Inc., © 1993.

nal infection when the onset is acute. However, because of the difficulty in obtaining a detailed history at the extremes of age, the physician usually has to depend primarily on the physical examination to alert him to the presence of peritonitis.

The general appearance of the patient can at times give a clue to the examiner as to the serious nature of the problem. A pale, sweating, anxious individual portrays the initial shock from a catastrophic abdominal event. Although anxious, the patient has a dislike for body movement, and the knees are usually flexed in order to relieve abdominal wall pressure. Stimulation of the psoas muscles from local inflammation flexes the corresponding thigh. Pulse, blood pressure, temperature, and respiratory rate should always be noted as indicators of the severity of the situation, but if they are abnormal, they do not point specifically to the abdominal culprit.

The examination itself must always be performed as painlessly as possible. Patience, gentleness, warm hands, and a warm stethoscope go a long way in allaying the patient's anxiety. If the patient is hurt, evidence may become obscure in that he may resist further examination. Auscultation should be done first to detect the presence and degree of peristalsis, as bowel sounds are usually absent when diffuse peritonitis exists. After this, palpation is carried out with the extended fingertips gently placed on the abdomen as far as possible from the spot of pain indicated by the patient. Initial light palpation is needed to assess the degree of muscular resistance and to compare this involuntary guarding to the contralateral side. Palpation over the oblique muscles places the fingers nearer to the peritoneum itself, and less voluntary guarding is encountered as these muscles are not as strong as the anterior rectus abdominus muscles.

Light percussion of the abdomen is the best method to check for peritoneal irritation. This should be a gentle maneuver in contrast to the sudden mass release technique so often indulged in through deep palpation with rebound. Other valuable information, such as fluid accumulation or abnormal liver dullness seen at times when free air is present within the abdominal cavity, can be elicited with this technique. If signs of peritoneal irritation are not demonstrated by percussion, the examiner can then try to evoke the rebound phenomena in a more standard fashion.

No abdominal examination would be complete without an index finger inserted into the rectum, as this point is nearest to the peritoneum where masses and tenderness can best be detected. Tension placed on a rectal fold moves peritoneal surfaces against one another, and in a patient with true pelvic peritonitis, a definite response will be elicited. Similarly, a bimanual pelvic exam in female patients is essential to detect pelvic masses or tenderness.

Several other physical findings should be mentioned only in passing. The iliopsoas and obturator tests, where pain is elicited when these muscles are placed on stretch, are occasionally helpful although very nonspecific and, in the absence of other findings, are not diagnostic for peritonitis. Similarly, hyperesthesia of the abdominal wall skin to pinprick cannot be elicited in many patients and, thus, by itself is of little value. Murphy's sign, that of pain with inspiration to deep palpation in the right upper quadrant, is quite helpful in patients with suspected acute cholecystitis.

Laboratory tests can generally be minimized in patients with an "acute abdomen" as the diagnosis rests primarily with the physical findings. Studies should first include a hemogram and white blood cell count with a differential. The hematocrit forms a baseline for comparison of later values. In severe long-standing acute peritonitis, this value may actually be elevated, reflective of the massive transfer of extracellular fluid into the inflamed area from the intravascular space. The white cell count is highly variable but may indicate the need for some concern if elevated with acute inflammatory cells. Certainly, some hematologic malignancies present with a component of abdominal pain and sepsis, and here the total and differential white blood cell counts are of primary diagnostic importance.

A urinalysis should also be done to obtain gross evidence of a possible urinary tract cause for the peritoneal findings. The specific gravity of the sample gives some assessment of the degree of dehydration, while the presence of blood, bile or reducing agents gives some insight as to the underlying etiology of the abdominal pain. In the young black patient, a test for sickle cell anemia should be included, while a serum amylase, although very nonspecific, is of value in the patient where the pancreas or biliary tract is the suspected source of the peritonitis. Serum electrolyte determination and other blood tests, such as serum calcium or arterial blood gases, are seldom of diagnostic importance. These blood tests may be quite helpful, however, in the perioperative fluid and pulmonary management of patients.

A judicious paracentesis with a large-bore needle is helpful at times, especially if purulent fluid is obtained. All fluid should be submitted for immediate Gram's stain, cell count differential, and culture. When organisms or an elevated cell count are found, a laparotomy is usually indicated regardless of other physical or laboratory findings. Inability to aspirate purulent fluid does not eliminate the possibility that peritonitis is present, but a positive tap is very helpful in the decision for celiotomy.

Recently, peritoneal lavage has been shown to be quite helpful in the surgeon's evaluation for intra-abdominal infection. This technique involves irrigation of the peritoneal cavity with 1,000 mL of a saline solution via a catheter placed through a small lower midline incision. This approach to diagnosis is very helpful in the patient with an altered sensorium, such as the comatose or paralyzed individual. The presence of bile or 500 white blood cells per milliliter of effluent would indicate the need for operative treatment. An aliquot of fluid should always be sent for bacterial and yeast culture. Absolute contraindications to this procedure include a distended urinary bladder, a gravid uterus, recent abdominal surgery, or the existence of enough evidence that the surgeon intends to explore the patient regardless of the lavage findings. Multiple previous abdominal incisions are relative deterrents to the use of this diagnostic modality. It is, however, easily performed at the bedside under local anesthesia and appears to be highly sensitive in many difficult diagnostic situations.

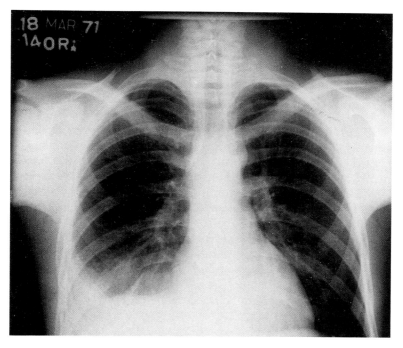

Figure 1: This chest roentgenogram demonstrates a large right pleural effusion in a patient with a subsequently proven right subphrenic abscess.

Radiographic examinations are of definite diagnostic value in the patient with evidence of peritonitis. While the diagnosis in the "acute abdomen" setting rests primarily with the history and physical findings, corroborative information can be derived from several simple x-ray procedures. A chest film should be done initially on all patients with suspected peritonitis to eliminate or better define supradiaphragmatic causes for the abdominal signs. Similarly, the basilar segments of the lungs are frequently secondarily inflamed from a subdiaphragmatic inflammatory process. Upright posteroanterior and lateral views are needed to record these segments of lung and are the best method for assessing the presence of free air within the peritoneal cavity. On occasion, it may be necessary to introduce a contrast agent into the gastrointestinal tract to better define the subphrenic space. A high hemidiaphragm accompanied by a pleural effusion and infiltrate or atelectasis in the adjoining lung segments is the most common sign of a subphrenic abscess (Figure 1). Demonstration of limited or paradoxical movement of the affected diaphragm with fluoroscopy confirms the diagnosis.

Flat, upright, and left lateral decubitus views of the abdomen can be of definite value in the diagnosis of intra-abdominal infection. The finding of one or more extraluminal gas bubbles, which do not move when the patient's position is changed, is pathognomonic for an abscess, although this is demonstrated in only a small percentage of cases (Figures 2, 3, and 4). At times, contrast studies or sinograms of fistulous tracts may be needed to confirm the extravisceral location of such gas collections (Figures 5 and 6). More frequently seen is the mass effect of an abscess (Figures 7, 8, and 9). When large enough, displacement of the neighboring bowel from its normal position occurs along with localized intestinal ileus. A partial bowel obstruction may result if the mass is of sufficient size. A more subtle finding is the obliteration of the fat strip along the lateral margin of the psoas muscle shadow by inflammation (Figure 9).

Overall, plain abdominal x-rays are helpful in only a small percentage of patients. The classic findings of extraluminal air or bowel displacement indicative of intra-abdominal sepsis are seen infrequently and usually only when quite large and obvious on several exams. Seldom is operative therapy planned solely on the plain radiographic findings. Similarly, barium contrast examinations either by the oral or rectal route are helpful only in outlining intestinal displacement or paralytic ileus. Such indirect findings of abdominal infection are usually insufficient to warrant definitive surgical intervention without further corroborative evidence.

The diagnosis of intra-abdominal infection must be made clinically, and the limitations of conventional radiographic studies are well known. This presents a diagnostic dilemma for the surgeon called to treat such patients since most abscesses follow either from an initial episode of diffuse peritonitis or as the result of operative therapy. The surgeon is loath to proceed with further operative procedures based on vague abdominal symptoms masked by postoperative pain and analgesics unless confirmative evidence is found. A variety of new diagnostic techniques has altered the investigative approach in these patients and is now used routinely to bolster a clinical suspicion. The new noninvasive cross-sectional imaging modalities of ultrasonography and computed tomography are quite accurate for abscess detection. Other scanning techniques are less sensitive but helpful in certain patients. Considerable judgment must be exercised when using these new techniques as conflicting results often lead to a delay in definitive therapy. There is a tendency to repeat the same examination when studies or clinical opinion conflict.

Gray-scale ultrasonography is the preferred technique for an initial examination. In skilled hands, it is accurate, rapid, and completely noninvasive, and it does not expose the patient to irradiation (Figure 10). Cross-sectional ultrasonographic studies allow detailed anatomical location of fluid collections, but the sound beam cannot penetrate air or bone and requires an intact abdominal wall overlying the fluid collection. Obesity, postoperative ileus, and the presence of metal ligatures scatter the sound beam and give unsatisfactory results. Areas beneath the costal margin and behind air-filled organs remain relatively inaccessible. Open wounds, colostomies, and dressings also limit sonographic survey; however, in experienced hands, the accuracy of this procedure is noteworthy. Taylor[1] reports an overall accuracy of 96.8% in 220 patients in whom intraperitoneal abscess was suspected. Although this success is remarkable, other centers have not found this procedure as clinically useful in patient management of abscess detection.

Computed tomography is another new noninvasive technique that appears to be even more accurate than ultrasound. Very high resolution, the ability to see beneath bone or gas-filled structures, a standard procedure eliminating operator skill interpretation, and the absence of the requirement for an intact abdominal wall are the major advantages of this diagnostic modality. Radiation exposure is the only major disadvantage of note. A purulent collection appears as a low-density extraluminal area (Figure 11). Intralesional gas is an important finding seen in 30% to 50% of intra-abdominal abscesses found by this technique. Opacification of the intestinal tract is usually necessary to assure the extra-alimentary location of the density in question. At times, a well-defined hypervascular abscess wall can be defined following the intravenous administration of contrast solutions.

The accuracy for abscess detection by computed tomography is excellent with 90% to 95% true abnormal rates being reported. In a large series, Koehler and Moss[2] identified 78 to 79 abscesses correctly while missing only 1 abscess in 32 normal examinations where an abdominal collection was suspected. It appears that, unlike sonography, false normal computed tomographic scans are extremely uncommon. An occasional small abscess or phlegmon can be missed. False-positive exams are more frequent as nonpurulent collections and bowel loops can at times produce confusion in the interpretation of the study. However, a normal exam in a patient with suspected intra-abdominal infections appears to yield fairly reliable data.

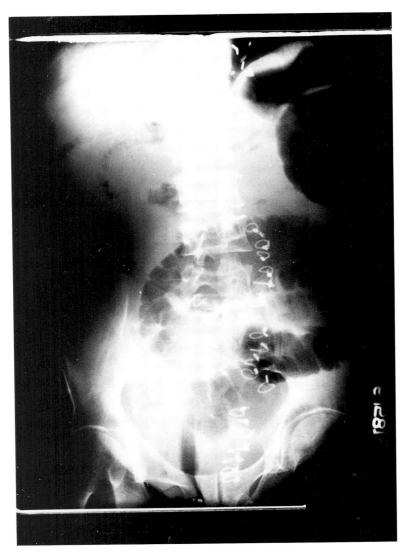

Figure 2: These roentgenograms are from a 60-year-old male who had a distended abdomen and clinical small bowel obstruction after a right hemicolectomy for a perforated cecal carcinoma. (A) shows extraluminal gas in the right upper quadrant in this supine film. (B) demonstrates muitiple air-fluid levels within the small intestine in an upright film.

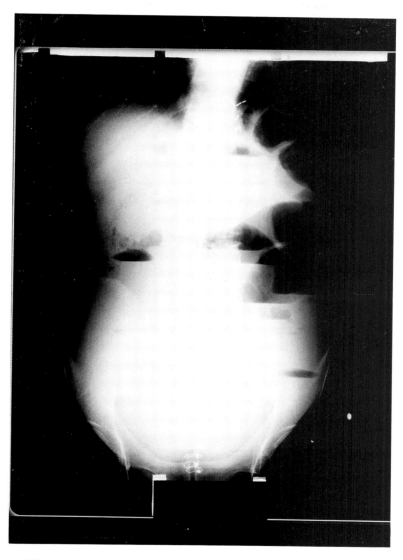

Figure 2B.

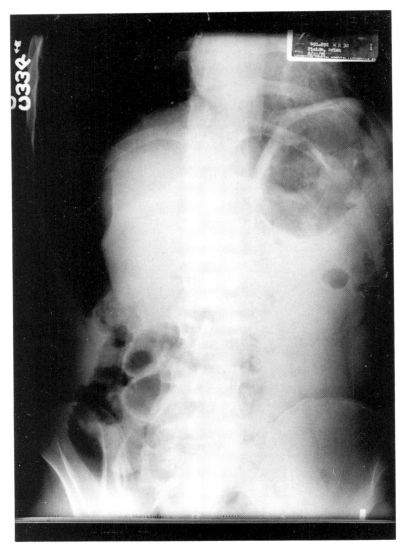

Figure 3: Free air along the right colon and liver with loss of the psoas shadow on the right is noted on this plain abdominal roentgenogram from a 30-year-old male with clinical signs and symptoms of acute appendicitis.

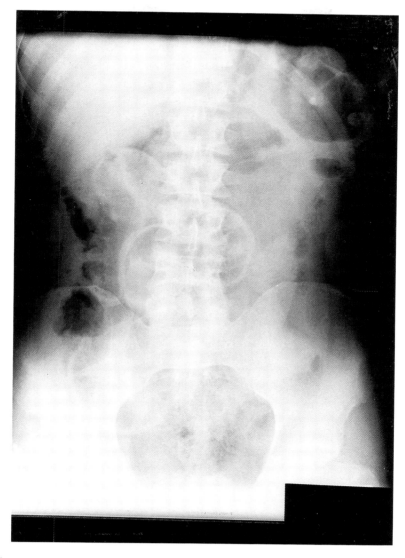

Figure 4: Extraluminal air and thickening of the small bowel shadows are noted in this patient with a gangrenous, perforated gallbladder.

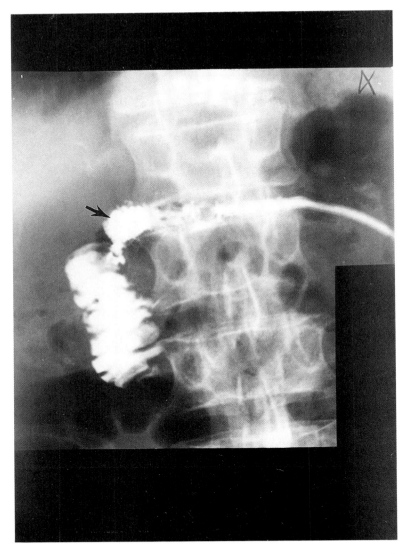

Figure 5: These roentgenograms illustrate a sinogram of a drain tract site 10 days after a subtotal gastrectomy and distal pancreatectomy for a perforated gastric ulcer. (A) identifies an abscess cavity (arrow) leading to the disrupted end of the duodenal stump. (B) is a later film in the sequence that identifies contrast within the pancreatic duct.

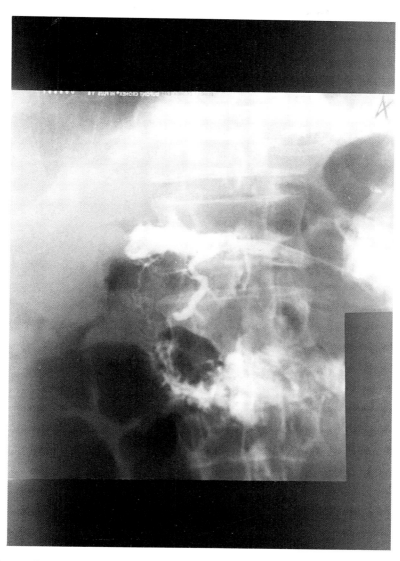

Figure 5B.

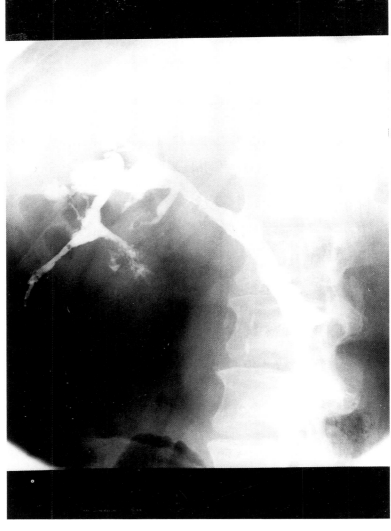

Figure 6: A sinogram of a drain tract shows a large abscess cavity and communication with the bile duct system 3 months after a right colectomy for a perforated appendix with necrosis of the cecum.

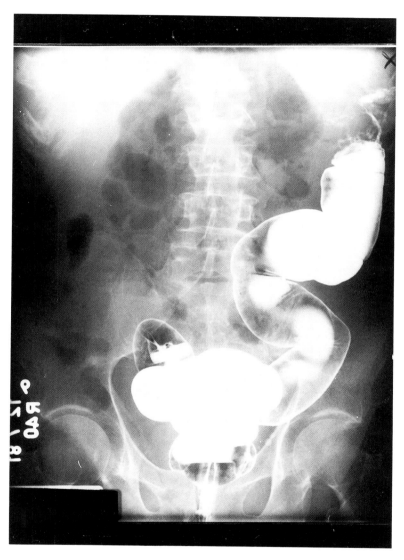

Figure 7: These films are from a 62-year-old male, 14 days after a left hemicolectomy for carcinoma, who is now septic with multiple organ failure. (A) demonstrates a barium enema film with downward displacement of the colon. (B) is an anterior chest roentgenogram with a left pleural effusion. (C) is a lateral chest roentgenogram with the same pleural effusion illustrated.

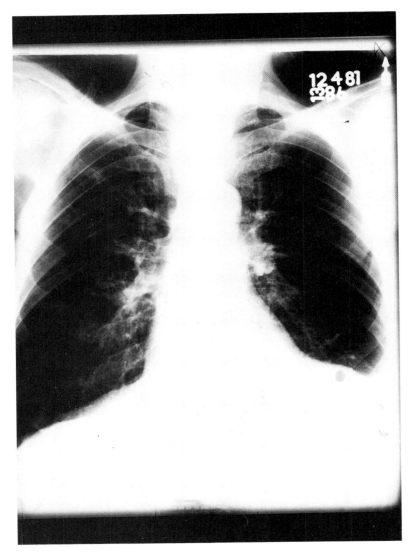

Figure 7B.

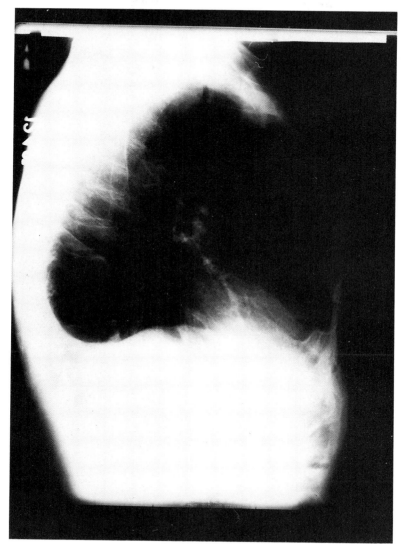

Figure 7C.

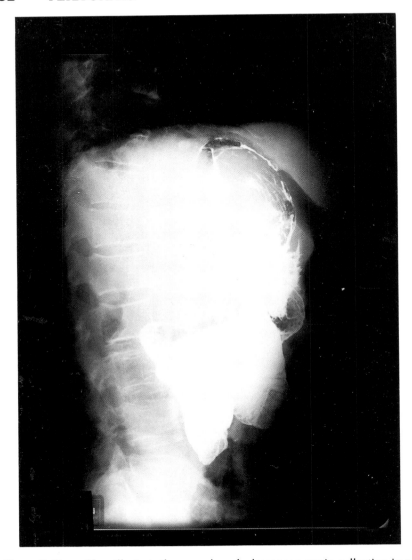

Figure 8: These films illustrate the sequelae of a lesser sac septic collection in an alcoholic patient with severe pancreatitis. (A) is a lateral abdominal film that demonstrates anterior displacement of the stomach. (B) demomstrates the superior and lateral displacement of the stomach on an anterior roentgenogram of the abdomen after a barium swallow. (C) illustrates the inferior compression of the tramsverse colon on a barium enema. (D) is a computed tomography scan of the abdomen that clearly illustrates the lesser sac collection.

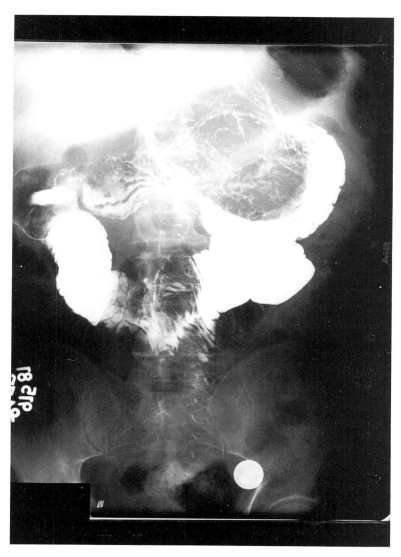

Figure 8B.

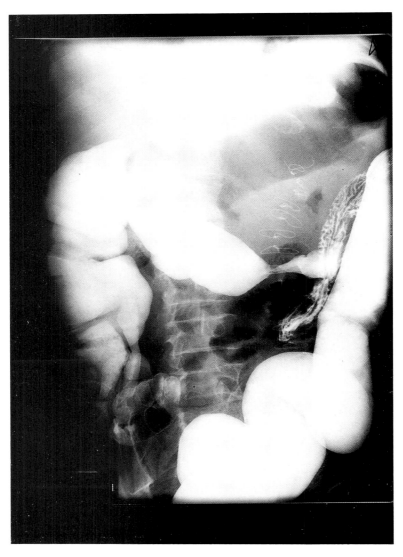

Figure 8C.

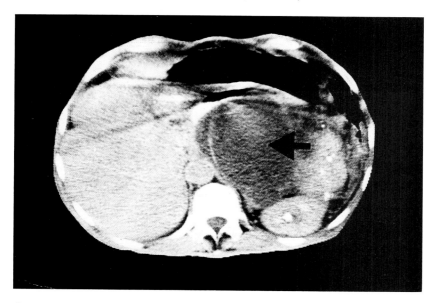

Figure 8D.

Radionuclide scintigraphy techniques are used more as localization procedures rather than for diagnosis. The time honored simultaneous liver and lung scanning to outline the subphrenic spaces is well known; however, it is of only limited use. At times, specific organ scans can detail large intra-organ collections, but add little to the overall localization of intra-abdominal abscess.

Gallium-67 scanning has been used in the diagnosis and localization of inflammatory foci. Increased radionuclide uptake by discrete areas of inflammation can be shown in 80% to 90% of patients studied. However, uptake occurs over a 48-hour period and the material is excreted into the gastrointestinal tract, so adequate bowel preparation is a prerequisite. Both of these problems can be major hurdles in a septic individual. Specificity for this modality is not good because tumors, areas of inflammation, and fresh wounds all show various degrees of uptake, which limits the usefulness of this procedure in postoperative patients.

In order to improve the specificity of scanning for inflammatory

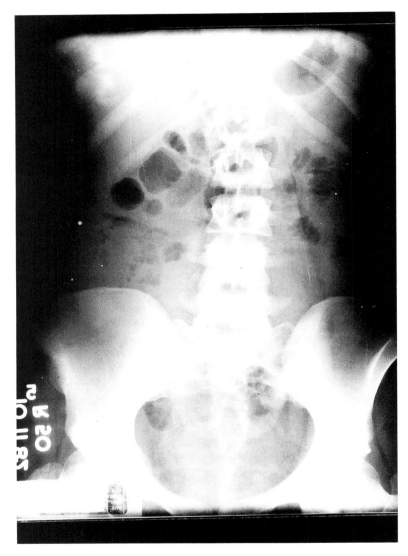

Figure 9: These films are the preoperative abdominal roentgenograms of a young woman who was being treated for pelvic inflammatory disease for 2 weeks with antibiotics. (A) illustrates loss of the right psoas shadow. (B) is an oblique projection from a barium enema that shows anterior displacement of the colon. (C) is an anterior view of the barium enema that shows extreme compression of the right colon.

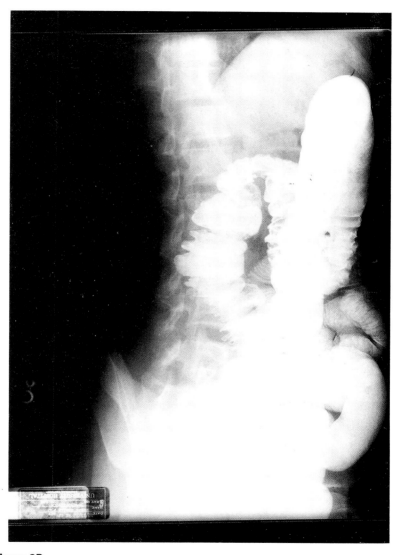

Figure 9B.

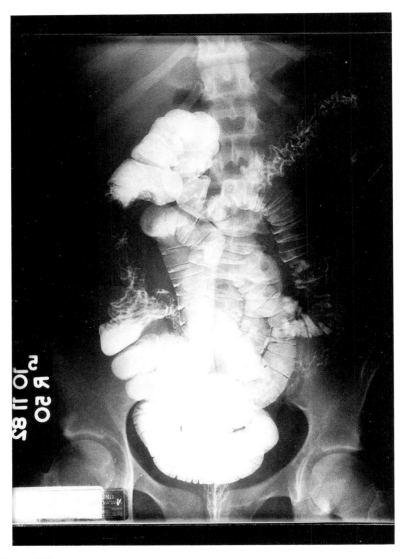

Figure 9C.

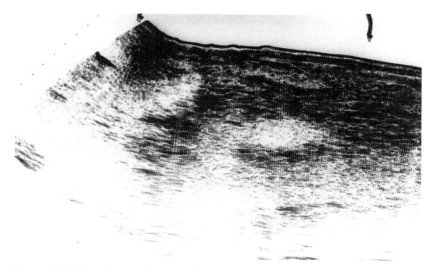

Figure 10: This ultrasound study shows a right lower quadrant fluid collection anterior to the rectus muscle in the abdominal wall.

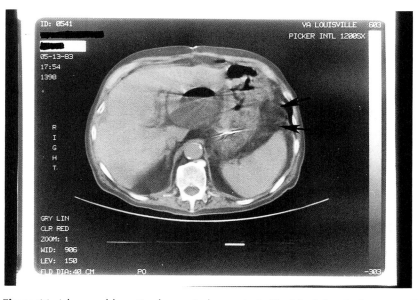

Figure 11: A large subhepatic abscess is demonstrated in this abdominal computed tomography scan from a patient with atrial arrhythmias and renal dysfunction 12 days after a gastrectomy for an obstructing duodenal ulcer.

sites, autologous leukocytes labeled with indium-111 have been introduced as the isotope source. Labeled white blood cells are not accumulated in large numbers by tumors or excreted by the kidneys or into the gut, and recent surgical wounds do not appear to take up these cells preferentially. Twenty-four hours of delay is necessary for cells to localize, and there is a moderate amount of radiation exposure for the patient. It should be emphasized that scanning techniques should only be used for localization of an inflammatory focus. An abnormal radionuclide scan should then direct either ultrasonographic or computed tomographic examination for better definition of the area in question.

When other methods fail, an exploratory laparotomy may at times be indicated as both a diagnostic and therapeutic maneuver. Unfortunately, there is very little in the literature to guide the surgeon in his decision to proceed along this avenue. Certainly, the subtle appearance of multiple system organ failure with respiratory, renal, and liver dysfunction has been shown to correlate with ongoing sepsis. In the absence of extra-abdominal sources of infection, such as infected transvenous catheters, or ongoing urinary or respiratory tract infections, a judicious laparotomy might be indicated. Certainly, if such occult sepsis is not diagnosed and controlled, these organ dysfunctions are predictive of a poor outcome. Similar statements can be made for polymicrobial bacteremia when *Bacteroides* bacteremia is virtually diagnostic for a septic focus in need of surgical therapy. Overall, these subtle findings require the utmost in experience and clinical judgment to be effective as diagnostic tools of value for the patient.

The effective management of intra-abdominal sepsis clearly rests squarely on the shoulders of a timely, accurate diagnosis. Only when the physician becomes aware that peritonitis might be the cause of the complaints or the illness of a patient can a diagnosis be made. This awareness may come quickly in the case of the classic "acute abdomen" presentation, while occult sepsis, multiple organ failure, or the vague impression that a postoperative patient is not progressing at an appropriate rate of recovery may be quite subtle and require an astute diagnostic acumen. Special diagnostic tests may be required and the interpretation that follows must be tempered by institutional variability in the performance of these studies. Ultimately, the diagnosis of intra-abdominal infection is an empirical process, which relies solely on the physician's physical, analytical and interpretive skills.

References

1. Taylor KJ, Wasson JF, de Graaff C, et al: Accuracy of gray-scale ultrasound diagnosis of abdominal and pelvic abscesses in 220 patients. *Lancet* 1:83-84, 1978.
2. Koehler PR, Moss AA: Diagnosis of intra-abdominal and pelvic abscesses by computerized tomography. *JAMA* 244:49-52, 1980.

4

Supportive Care of the Peritonitis Patient

Donald E. Fry, MD

The overall results in the treatment of peritonitis have improved during the last century. Because the improved results in the care of the patient with intraperitoneal infection have been paralleled by more potent and readily available antimicrobial chemotherapeutic agents, one might conclude that a cause-and-effect relationship exists. However, some have suggested that the improved treatment and results of peritonitis have not been affected by antibiotics at all; rather, the rapidly evolving technologies of supportive care for these patients have been more significant variables than antibiotics have been.

The changing pattern of death in the patient with severe infection similarly reflects the pharmacological and technological evolution in care (Figure 1). Improved monitoring, refined volume resuscitation, and effective cardiovascular support have resulted in fewer peritonitis patients dying from hypovolemia or septic shock. Rather, multiple or sequential organ system failure currently represents the common pathway of death in infected surgical patients. The support of specific organ function in these patients is necessary to provide a temporary reprieve in the natural history of the disease and thus permit the treatment modalities of drainage, debridement, and specific antimicrobial therapy an opportunity to reverse the septic process.

Pulmonary Support

The maintenance of systemic oxygenation assumes primary importance for the patients with peritonitis. The fundamental physiologic

From Fry DE, (ed): *Peritonitis.* Mount Kisco NY, Futura Publishing Co., Inc., © 1993.

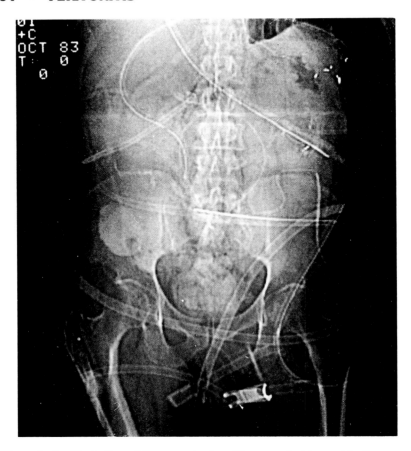

Figure 1: An illustration of the complexity of the care that is used in the severe peritonitis patient. This abdominal roentgenogram shows the enormous numbers of tubes, catheters, and drains that are used in these severely ill patients.

abnormality of the septic process is inefficient extraction or inadequate utilization of oxygen in the periphery. Observations of narrowed arteriovenous oxygen differences and lactic acidemia further emphasize the presence of an oxygen debt.[1,2] Even transient hypoxemia will significantly add to this peripheral deficit.

Inadequate systemic oxygenation may be the consequence of multiple variables. Prolonged anesthesia for repair of the primary source of contamination may depress respiratory activity. Painful, large abdominal incisions may result in significant splinting of ventilation with reduction in tidal volume. Large volumes of resuscitation fluid are commonly required during the acute phase of peritonitis and when combined with alterations of capillary permeability result in significant interstitial edema. These increases in lung water result in reduction of both oxygenation and pulmonary compliance. Aspiration is yet another potential pulmonary insult. The risks of a secondary pneumonitis are always present in the peritonitis patient and will pose major risks of sustained pulmonary failure.

Insurance of a patent airway may even be necessary prior to corrective celiotomy and is usually required for at least a brief period of time following operation. Obvious tachypnea or frank cyanosis are clear clinical indicators that control of the airway is necessary. The auscultatory examination of the chest may demonstrate diffuse rales that indicate early evidence of altered capillary permeability and impending pulmonary compromise. Arterial blood gases are very helpful with low pO_2 indicating problems of oxygenation, and increased pCO_2 indicating inadequate minute volume. Because pulmonary failure can appear to be quite fulminant, endotracheal intubation and ventilator assistance are recommended at the first sign of dysfunction.

Another aspect of pulmonary support in the peritonitis patient is the maintenance of gastrointestinal decompression. Gastrointestinal ileus is a uniform component of peritonitis regardless of cause. Yet delays in the placement of nasogastric tubes prior to definitive laparotomy or overly zealous efforts to remove the tube in the postoperative patient may subject these patients to undue risks of vomiting and aspiration. In the elderly patient or the patient with altered sensorium for any reason, the removal of the nasogastric tube renders these patients quite vulnerable to aspiration. A major aspiration insult in combination with acute bacterial peritonitis is a lethal combination. While nasogastric tube decompression is not complete protection, it will reduce the frequency and severity of aspiration.

Following institution of ventilatory assistance, effective monitoring must be used to ensure the adequacy of pulmonary support. Arterial blood gases continue to be the most readily available and reliable means for the assessment of support measures. Sequential blood gas observations serve as an objective means of monitoring improvement or deterioration of arterial-alveolar gas exchange (pO_2) and tidal volume (pCO_2). While comprehensive interpretation of arterial blood gases is beyond the scope of this chapter, the serial monitoring of arterial pO_2,

pCO_2, and pH has become a very important aspect in the comprehensive management of both ventilatory and metabolic support.

Assumptions about normal pO_2 may pose a special problem in the ventilatory management of the peritonitis patient. Students of medicine are accustomed to considering a normal pO_2 as above 90 mm Hg and hypoxia as pO_2 below 70 mm Hg. However, the aging process significantly affects the normal pO_2 for patients (Figure 2). Historical information about tobacco habits and prior lung status should be obtained whenever possible, since acceptable levels of pO_2 may not need to be so

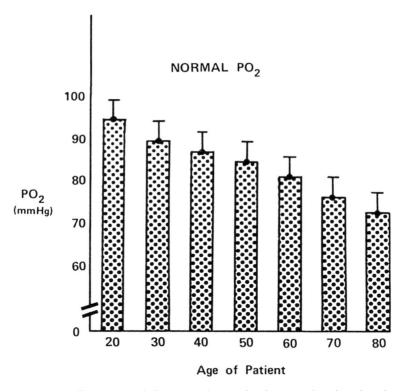

Figure 2: An illustration of the normal pO_2 for humans by decade of age. Preoperative arterial blood gases may prove very useful so that if postoperative pulmonary support is necessary, the norms for that patient will be known. Knowledge of the normal decline of the resting pO_2 will prevent attempts to achieve unrealistic oxygenation while weaning the patient from the ventilator. This graph was designed from the regression equation $pO_2 = 100.1 - 0.323 \times$ (patient age).

high in those patients who normally have ventilation-perfusion abnormalities from emphysema or other intrinsic lung disease. Failure to appreciate norms for a given patient population may result in unrealistic goals for oxygenation and pose very special problems when removal of ventilatory assistance becomes desirable.

Volume Ventilator Management

Following the implementation of mechanically assisted ventilation, the objectives of management are to maintain and carefully monitor systemic oxygenation, and to withdraw the assisted ventilation at the earliest possible time. Sustained ventilatory support places the peritonitis patient at extraordinary risk for the acquisition of a nosocomial, respirator-associated pneumonitis. Mortality rates for such infections exceed 50%.[3] Erosion of the tracheal mucosa from endotracheal tubes or tracheostomy appliances may acutely result in fatal exsanguination or long-term morbidity from tracheal stenosis. Chronic changes from barotrauma are less well defined but are certainly a source of concern.

Normal pulmonary compliance is invariably altered in the severe peritonitis patient as interstitial lung water accumulates. Large tidal volumes become necessary to sustain alveolar ventilation. While normal tidal volume for an adult is 7–8 mL/kg of body weight, tidal volumes of 10–15 mL/kg are commonly required for the ventilator-dependent peritonitis patient. When carbon dioxide retention becomes evident, alveolar minute volume is best achieved by increases in tidal volume rather than respiratory rate.

Initial management for the hypoxemic patient is to increase the oxygen fraction of inspired air (FiO_2). Patients are started at an FiO_2 = 0.4 (40% oxygen) and oxygenation is then monitored with arterial blood gases after appropriate time for equilibration (10–15 minutes). A higher FiO_2 may be warranted if cyanosis, tachypnea, or progressive hypoxemia continues. Special problems are encountered if the FiO_2 is equal to or greater than 0.7. As the FiO_2 increases, there is less nitrogen and more oxygen in the alveolar space. This relative preponderance of completely diffusible gas will increase the risk of alveolar collapse. Furthermore, persistently increased FiO_2 may result in long-term complication of interstitial pulmonary fibrosis. Positive end-expiratory pressure (PEEP) should be used when the FiO_2 exceeds 0.5.

Positive end-expiratory pressure consists of maintaining positive pressure within the patient's airway at the end of expiration, rather than permitting atmospheric equilibration as normally occurs.[4-6] By using PEEP, alveoli that collapse with expiration are kept inflated secondary to the end-expiratory pressure. Maintenance of alveolar inflation improves ventilation-perfusion relationships, reduces the shunt fraction of pulmonary blood flow, and facilitates arterial oxygenation. Positive end-expiratory pressure of 5–10 cm H_2O is commonly used. More enthusiastic proponents have recommended PEEP in excess 20 cm H_2O be used.[7,8]

The use of PEEP has intrinsic risks. The increase in intrathoracic pressure may embarrass venous return to the heart. This is particularly significant in the hypovolemic patient. Monitoring of pulmonary capillary wedge pressure (discussed subsequently) is very useful for patients on PEEP, especially if hypotension or oliguria develops. The combination of high pressures with PEEP, and diseased or injured lung, places the patient at risk for precipitous tension pneumothorax. Awareness of this possible complication is essential for patients on PEEP. While prophylactic chest tubes have been recommended for patients on PEEP,[9] the risks of chest tube complications (by injuring the lung, and resultant bronchopleural fistula or empyema) do not justify this approach.

Periodically, selected patients are not effectively ventilated because of agitation and resistance to acceptance of ventilatory support. This is most often seen when patients are on PEEP. Patient resistance to acceptance of ventilator support results in inadequate ventilation and risks of exaggerated high airway pressure provoking a pneumothorax. The use of neuromuscular blockade with an agent such as pancuroneum (Pavulon® [Organon, Inc., West Orange, NJ, USA]) may be necessary.

The cutting edge of technology in pulmonary support is extracorporeal membrane oxygenation (ECMO).[10,11] This experimental method circulates the patient's blood via femoral vascular access into a membrane oxygenator. This relieves the severely injured lung of its ventilatory function and permits an opportunity for the lung to have complete rest. In patients with severe acute respiratory failure, but potentially reversible primary injury, ECMO has the prospect for providing maximum pulmonary support. Unfortunately the poorest results with ECMO have been seen in the septic patient, such that its use in peritonitis remains unlikely. At the present time, ECMO appears to only be of clinical value in the pediatric patient.

Discontinuation of Ventilator Support

As clinical evidence of improved oxygenation and pulmonary compliance develops, efforts to withdraw ventilator support should be initiated. The patients should by "weaned" in a graduated fashion. The weaning process is necessary since the peritonitis patient may continue to splint ventilatory activity because of the painful abdominal incision. If sepsis and catabolism have been sustained for a period of time, diaphragmatic and intercostal musculature may also be compromised, and will require time to resume normal activity.

Traditional methods of withdrawing ventilator support have used a gradual reduction of FiO_2 and tidal volume. The patient is then given a "trial by fire" and placed on a t-piece. Such weaning regimens have had catastrophic consequences as the patient rapidly tires from the acute responsibility of all ventilatory activity.

Intermittent mandatory ventilation (IMV) represents a superior method for the orderly withdrawal of ventilatory support.[12-14] Intermittent mandatory ventilation permits a gradual reduction in the cycle rate of the ventilator and allows spontaneous breathing between cycles. Thus, a patient with mechanically-assisted respirations of 16 per minute can initially have IMV set at a rate of 8–12 per minute. The rate of IMV can then be further reduced as the patient demonstrates tolerance to resume more spontaneous ventilation.

Classification of Pulmonary Dysfunction

The severity of pulmonary abnormalities in patients with severe intraperitoneal infection or multiple trauma covers a broad continuum. The extremes include transient hypoxia in the perioperative period to persistent, relentless pulmonary failure and death of the patient. Failure to appreciate these differences has led to considerable confusion in the interpretation of shock lung, septic lung, or adult respiratory distress syndrome. The following classification scheme represents an attempt to categorize pulmonary dysfunction by degree of severity (Table 1).

Mild Acute Hypoxia

These patients are representative of the mildest form of pulmonary dysfunction following injury, surgery, and peritonitis. An uneventful

Table 1
Categorizes Pulmonary Abnormalities That are Identified in Peritonitis Patients. The Severity of the Disease and the Magnitude of the Treatment are Quite Variable

Category	Physiologic Insult	Support Modality
Mild Acute Hypoxia	Perforated Ulcer	Mask Oxygen
Severe Acute Hypoxia	Severe Pancreatitis	Short-term (< 96 hrs) Ventilator Support
Progressive Acute Hypoxia	Massive Aspiration	Long-term Ventilator Support (± PEEP)
Adult Respiratory Distress Syndrome	Uncontrolled Peritonitis	Long-term Ventilator Support with PEEP; Increased FiO_2

recovery is the rule rather than the exception. This condition is characterized by mild hypoxia (pO_2 = 50–70 mm Hg on room air) and modest tachypnea is present. The uncomplicated patient with peritonitis secondary to a perforated peptic ulcer is identified in this group. This peritonitis is basically chemical in nature. The patient has a definitive operation, but may have received several liters of resuscitation volume. Pulmonary compliance is essentially unaffected. Mild interstitial pulmonary edema is a likely pathophysiologic cause. Mask oxygen is sufficient treatment when coupled with rational systemic volume administration. Progression of hypoxia is rarely seen. In the absence of intercurrent pulmonary infection, the prognosis is quite favorable.

Severe Acute Hypoxemia

This is the patient with severe peritonitis who requires a major resuscitation effort to combat hypovolemia. Severe pancreatitis is a prototype clinical presentation. The resuscitation may entail many liters of crystalloid given rapidly to manage oliguria or frank hypotension. Once hemodynamic stabilization is achieved, these patients usually have severe hypoxia and have major compliance changes. The capillary permeability and resistance changes within the lung vasculature result in major interstitial edema. In the pancreatitis patient, humoral substances have been postulated to further aggravate changes in pulmonary vascular permeability. This interstitial edema appears to be the cause of hypoxemia and reduced compliance. High FiO_2 and even PEEP may be necessary for initial support. However, the capillary permeability and resistance changes in the lung vasculature will normalize if hemodynamic stabilization is achieved and effective therapy for the fundamental process is instituted. In severe pancreatitis, peritoneal lavage is reported to blunt the pulmonary dysfunction of severe pancreatitis.[15] Withdrawal from pulmonary support can usually be achieved within 72 hours, particularly in younger patients. The prognosis for this transient pulmonary dysfunction is favorable assuming that a second physiologic insult (eg, recrudescence of pancreatitis or pancreatic abscess) does not occur during the resolution phase. Intercurrent insults from the fundamental intra-abdominal pathology or from pulmonary sepsis will compound the severity and duration of pulmonary dysfunction and will result in the evolution of the true adult respiratory distress syndrome.

Progressive Acute Hypoxemia

Patients within this group are similar to those patients with severe acute hypoxemia in that the initial insult results in severe pulmonary compromise and may require increased FiO_2 and PEEP to provide adequate oxygenation. However, these patients are different from the previously described group of patients because the pulmonary dysfunction progresses even though the principal provocation has concluded. Severe physiochemical insults of the lung most commonly initiate these hypoxemic crises. Among trauma patients, those with severe pulmonary contusions or major inhalation injuries are most common. Massive aspiration represents the clinical setting for the peritonitis patient with progressive severe hypoxia. The chemical pneumonitis results in major interstitial edema, intra-alveolar proteinosis, and major airway injury. Mechanically-assisted ventilation, high FiO_2 and increased levels of PEEP are required sometimes for weeks in these patients. Tracheostomy is generally necessary. The high probability of intercurrent pulmonary sepsis in a chemically injured lung makes the prognosis for these patients quite poor. Neither systemic corticosteroids nor systemic prophylactic antibiotics appear to influence either the acute progression of hypoxia nor the intercurrent frequency of pulmonary infection. Indeed, prophylactic antibiotics may only insure that the ultimate pathogen will be resistant to those drugs chosen for prevention.

Adult Respiratory Distress Syndrome

The adult respiratory distress syndrome is pulmonary failure secondary to the septic response. While a relationship between infection and respiratory failure has been identified in several studies,[16-18] it is clear that not all clinical cases have a defined primary infection. It is now apparent that any biologic stimulus that activates the inflammatory mechanisms of the lung can be responsible for the evolution of pulmonary failure.

Adult respiratory distress syndrome consists of progressive relentless hypoxia, increased vascular resistance, altered capillary permeability, reduced functional residual capacity of the lung, and progressive deterioration of pulmonary compliance. Histopathologically interstitial edema, alveolar consolidation, and frank destruction of pulmonary parenchyma are readily noted.

The peritonitis patient is in double jeopardy of developing infection-associated pulmonary failure. First, pulmonary failure may evolve because of the intra-abdominal infection. Respiratory distress from remote sites of infection are initially characterized by the evolution of marked ventilation-perfusion abnormalities.[2] These abnormalities are thought to arise from microembolic or microaggregation events,[19,20] but also may be consequences of endothelial injury or other undefined systemically mediated humoral events. Pulmonary vascular resistance increases, interstitial edema emerges, and pulmonary compliance deteriorates.

Following the events above, the lung is now vulnerable to secondary infection. Richardson and associates[3,21] have noted clinical and experimental evidence that the peritonitis patient is especially vulnerable to developing secondary pulmonary infection. Hunt and associates[22] have noted more deaths in peritonitis patients from intercurrent pulmonary infection than from the primary intra-abdominal process.

Mortality rates from adult respiratory distress syndrome are in excess of 50%.[23,24] Survival requires aggressive pulmonary support with high FiO_2 and PEEP levels for oxygenation. Unless better control of the primary infection is achieved, all supportive efforts are doomed to failure.

Cardiovascular Support

The patient with peritonitis is at risk of cardiovascular instability from multiple causes. Hypovolemia, severe vasodilatation from the septic response, and frank myocardial failure are all potential risks in these patients. Diagnosis of the basic reasons for hemodynamic instability may not be easily achieved. Monitoring of the peritonitis patient becomes very important in instituting proper support.

The hourly monitoring of urine output remains the most significant measure of overall cardiovascular adequacy. However, specific circumstances may render urine output invalid. Elderly patients will frequently have an abnormal creatinine clearance and urine output may not correlate well with renal perfusion. Hyperosmolarity from the abnormalities of glucose metabolism in the septic state or from poorly managed, total parenteral nutrition may provoke an osmolar diuresis. Septic patients may have an inappropriate polyuria that may reflect intrarenal redistribution of blood flow, with normal or increased urine output being the result even when severe hypovolemia coexists. Finally, acute tubular necrosis with either an oliguric or polyuric response may be present.

For monitoring intravascular volume, the central venous pressure (CVP) monitor has been generally popular. Unfortunately, filling pressures of the heart are not accurately reflected by this method, with pulmonary vascular resistance being a particularly significant variable. The CVP proves to be the least reliable in those situations where accurate information is most needed.[25,26]

The Swan-Ganz catheter has replaced CVP monitoring in severe peritonitis patients.[27-29] This balloon-tipped, flow-directed catheter can easily be passed into the pulmonary artery at the patient's bedside in the intensive care unit usually via a subclavian introducer. Fluoroscopic assistance is seldom needed. Once the catheter is positioned within the pulmonary artery, it can be advanced into the wedged position. Documentation of the wedged position is determined by having the catheter connected to a pressure monitor, the balloon inflated, and recognition of the characteristic wedged-pressure tracing as the catheter is slowly advanced. Once positioned, the catheter is anchored at skin level to prevent movement. The balloon is always deflated when the pulmonary capillary wedge pressure is not being measured to prevent pulmonary infarction.

The pulmonary capillary wedge pressure is an estimate of left atrial filling pressure. Pascal's law states that pressure is evenly distributed throughout a fluid-filled container. By occlusion of a branch of the pulmonary artery with the air-filled balloon of the Swan-Ganz catheter, the fluid-filled container of evenly distributed pressure becomes the left atrial pressure measured via the pulmonary capillary conduit. This estimation of left atrial pressure is quite accurate in assisting clinical judgment with respect to volume resuscitation. Furthermore, the Swan-Ganz catheters are now equipped with thermistor probes that permit rapid and accurate determinations of cardiac output by the thermodilution technique. The ability to monitor cardiac output becomes particularly meaningful in the care of the septic patient where systemic pressure and peripheral vascular resistance relationships become grossly distorted.

Hemodynamically unstable patients from all causes that require inotropic support or pharmacologic manipulation of vascular resistance (either vasoconstrictors or vasodilators) should have placement of an arterial line for monitoring of the systemic blood pressure. Arterial lines with continuous pressure monitoring permit recognition of rapidly changing patterns of pressure, provide more accurate pressure determinations than traditional cuff techniques (particularly in obese patients), and may also serve for access to the arterial circulation for repeated sampling of blood gases.

Using the necessary clinical monitors, specific decisions in the care of the patient with peritonitis can be made. The cardiovascular support of these patients is classified as (1) preload support, (2) direct inotropic support, and (3) afterload support.

Preload support in the peritonitis patient poses special problems. Intravascular volume is regulated by total extracellular fluid volume, red cell mass, and Starling's law of the capillary. During peritonitis, Starling's law is acutely repealed as the semipermeability of the capilliary is altered. Plasma volume is lost into the interstitial space and the area within the peritoneal cavity becomes a physiologic sponge in response to inflammation. The pronounced vasodilation of sepsis markedly increases vascular capacitance and further exaggerates volume needs. Tachycardia, oliguria, and even hypotension may result. Pulmonary capillary wedge pressure diminishes (< 5 mm Hg) and cardiac output declines during the hypovolemic phase.

Preload support consists of expansion of extracellular fluid volume and red cell mass if needed. Extracellular volume is best restored by an isotonic sodium solution. Plasmonate, albumin, dextran, and hetastarch have the risks of extravasation into the interstitum and can aggravate pulmonary dysfunction. These colloidal solutions should be used with caution and probably not at all in the acute resuscitation of peritonitis. For many patients, maintenance of urine output is satisfactory for monitoring the effectiveness of preload support. When a Swan-Ganz catheter is necessary, the pulmonary capillary wedge pressure should be targeted for a goal of 15 mm Hg.

A major issue in the maintenance of intravascular volume and peripheral oxygen delivery is the appropriate hematocrit for a peritonitis patient. The issue has now been further compounded by the evolving clinical[30,31] and experimental[32,33] data that identify increased infectious morbidity and immunosuppression with transfusion. For most patients, a hematocrit of 28%–30% is suitable and appears to have optimum rheological properties.[34] In younger patients, still lower hematocrits can be tolerated without difficulty. Because the peritonitis patient with a septic response already has a peripheral defect in oxygen utilization and because the physiologic compensatory mechanism for hemodilution is to elevate an already elevated cardiac output, maintenance of hematocrit at 28%–30% range is generally desirable.

In the patient with peritonitis, volume considerations must constantly be remembered both during the acute and subacute phases of the disease as the principal or contributing cause to oliguria or hypotension. In severe cases, the clinical course can be very difficult with episodic deterioration if the intraperitoneal process is not under control. All subsequent therapy for peritonitis will prove ineffective if intravascular volume is not replete.

A decision for inotropic support is necessary when left ventricular performance is unable to support an adequate cardiac output in the face of an adequate preload. In these complex patients, that decision usually requires evidence from Swan-Ganz measurements of a low cardiac output and an elevated pulmonary capillary wedge pressure.

There are several potential inotropic agents that can be used in the septic patient (Table 2). Dopamine has been a very popular agent, but poses some special problems in this group of patients.[35,36] Dopamine is really three drugs in one, in that it has a different physiologic effect depending upon the rate of infusion. Dopamine at infusion rates of 2-4 μg/kg per minute has primarily a dopaminergic effect upon the microcirculation of the kidney. These dopaminergic rates of infusion have been advocated to enhance renal blood flow in the critically ill and may be of value in the prevention of renal failure. Dopamine infusion rates of 5–12 μg/kg per minute are inotropic concentrations and will increase cardiac output. At the inotropic infusion rate, the dopaminergic effects are lost. At infusion rates greater than 15 μg/kg per minute, dopamine

Table 2
Identifies the Potential Inotropic Agents That May be Used in the Peritonitis Patient With Inadequate Cardiac Output or Frank Septic Shock

Drug	Dosage	Effects in the Peritonitis Patient
Dobutamine	5–20 μg/kg per minute	β-Adrenergic agent; only shows chronotropic effects or vasoconstriction at high doses; is the preferred choice.
Dopamine	4–12 μg/kg per minute	β-Adrenergic agent at this dose; not a β-adrenergic agent at higher doses.
Dopamine	> 12 μg/kg per minute	α-Adrenergic agent; vasoconstrictive effects are not appropriate for the septic patient.
Epinephrine	1–4 μg/min	β-Adrenergic agent at low doses but has significant vasoconstriction at higher doses; commonly used as the last drug of desperation in severe septic shock.
Norepinephrine	2–8 μg/min	Primarily an α-adrenergic agent, but has high dose beta effects; not desirable for septic patients.
Isoproterenol	1–4 μg/min	β-adrenergic agent; marked chronotropic effects; vasodilator; arrhythmia potential.

becomes a purely α-adrenergic agent without β-adrenergic nor dopaminergic effects. Thus, the window for positive inotropic benefits for dopamine is quite limited.

Dobutamine is essentially a pure β-adrenergic agent,[37] which is the author's preference in the treatment of the septic shock patient. Infusion rates can be increased to 20–30 μg/kg per minute to achieve a desired clinical response. Dobutamine is associated with a mild vasodilatory effect at high concentrations, but does not have an α-adrenergic effect that would not be desirable in the septic peritonitis patient.

Other agents have been used for the management of the inadequate cardiac output septic state. Norepinephrine may be employed and is frequently effective in increasing cardiac output. However, the significant α-adrenergic effects of norepinephrine will potentiate the peripheral vasoconstriction of low output sepsis and may embarrass visceral perfusion (eg, renal blood flow). Isoproterenol is a potent β-adrenergic agent that may favorably affect cardiac output. The severe chronotropic effects of this agent may provoke tachyarrhythmias, and dramatically accelerate myocardial oxygen consumption.[38,39] The overall poor results of therapy for patients with low cardiac output septic shock underscores the general ineffectiveness of current management.

Modification of afterload, or peripheral vascular resistance, can assume two roles in the septic patient. Since profound vasodilation is a consistent feature of the septic state, and may be associated with an otherwise normal cardiac output, the elevation of peripheral resistance might seem to be an appropriate endeavor. As has been emphasized, vasoconstriction is not a desirable endpoint. The stage C septic patient actually needs the cardiac output elevated to supranormal levels to meet the peripheral demand of the vasodilated state.

In the stage D septic patient, elevation of cardiac output and restoration of effective tissue perfusion may not be achievable by inotropic support alone because of the profound peripheral vasoconstiction that is present in these patients.[40] Trimethaphan camsylate (Arfonad®, [Roche Laboratories, Nutley, NJ, USA]) or phentolamine (Regitene®, Ciba Pharmaceutical Company, Summit, NJ, USA]) have been used to reduce peripheral resistance in these patients. Nitroprusside and nitroglycerin have been more popular for afterload reduction therapy in recent years. Afterload reduction with these vasodilatory agents has a highly variable response between patients and must be used with caution. An arterial line for online arterial pressure monitoring is essential for patients who are receiving afterload reduction.

Cardiac Arrhythmias

Supraventricular tachyarrhythmias have been periodically seen by the author in patients with acute septic crises. Therapeutic use of a calcium channel blocker is usually required in conjuction with intensive therapy of the primary septic process. Acute hypoxia, pulmonary embolus, and acute myocardial infarction may also provoke paroxysmal atrial tachycardia or acute atrial fibrillation.

Renal Support

The evolution of renal failure in the patient with peritonitis has major life-threatening implications. The disruption of efficient excretion of the nitrogenous end products of metabolism is obvious. Sodium and water retention may provoke pulmonary or cardiovascular decompensation. Cardiac arrhythmias may accompany hyperkalemia. Metabolic acidosis may further compromise the clinical situation.

The peritonitis patient is at risk for multiple variables that may provoke renal failure. Hypovolemia is usually present during the acute phase of diffuse peritoneal inflammation. General anesthesia and a major surgical insult are additional risk factors. Antibiotics commonly used in the treatment of polymicrobial intra-abdominal infection frequently have nephrotoxicity as an associated risk. The consequences of systemic sepsis even without these other variables may represent the most common cause of renal failure in the contemporary surgical patient.

The complexity of renal failure in the patient with peritonitis is compounded by the fact that urine volume is not a completely reliable indicator of renal perfusion. While oliguric renal failure is often seen, normal urine volumes or even frank polyuria may be identified while blood urea nitrogen and serum creatinine concentrations progressively increase. The polyuric variant of sepsis may occur secondary to either corticomedullary redistribution of renal blood flow or may be the consequences of an unidentified osmolar substance in the blood of these patients. The hyperglycemia from sepsis or parenteral nutrition may also result in normal or increased urine output in the face of evolving renal failure.[41,42]

Pre-Renal Support

The reduction in hourly urine output to less than 30 cc/h usually indicates reduced renal blood flow from hypovolemia. Reduction in plasma volume in peritonitis activates the aldosterone mechanism to conserve sodium ion in the distal tubule. Antidiuretic hormone is released and water is similarly conserved with a resultant reduction in urine volume. Persistant reduction in renal blood flow will result in acute tubular necrosis.

The diagnosis of pre-renal azotemia is usually easy. Oliguria with a blood urea nitrogen:creatinine ratio of greater than 20:1 is usually seen. When significant delay is observed in the initial treatment of peritonitis, creatinine levels can be quite high (> 5 mg%), but acute tubular necrosis may still be obviated. The minimal urine output in these circumstances usually has a high specific gravity and a low (> 5 mEq/L) urinary sodium concentration. Urinary sodium concentrations greater than 30–40 mEq/L in a hypovolemic patient indicates tubular damage.

When confronted with pre-renal azotemia, cardiac assessment is very important in the selection of management. Younger patients may be given a volume challenge of isotonic crystalloid solution. Older patients and those with known cardiac problems must have resuscitation guided by the pulmonary capillary wedge pressure and cardiac output. Potent loop diuretics should rarely be used in those patients and only after intravascular volume has been restored by objective criteria. The premature use of furosemide obscures the significance of urine output in the resuscitation phase of peritonitis, compounds hypovolemia, and may only cloud the entire clinical issue.

Intrinsic Renal Failure

Frank renal failure in the peritonitis patient most commonly represents acute tubular necrosis secondary to the septic process. Despite normal intravascular volume, adequate arterial pressure, and even elevated cardiac output, redistribution of renal blood flow away from the cortex results in this ischemic injury of the kidney. With acute renal failure, supportive efforts are designed to manage the life-threatening complication until the renal tubular epithelium is regenerated.

Dialysis is the cornerstone of management in these patients. Peritoneal dialysis with a surgically placed intraperitoneal catheter may be feasible, but generally hemodialysis is the preferred route in the peritonitis patient. Hemodialysis is indicated with rapid increases in blood urea nitrogen and creatinine, hyperkalemia, and metabolic acidosis. When some degree of urine volume persists during the acute failure, hyperkalemia and acid-base balance may not become problems. In a few such patients, creatinine levels may rise very slowly and hemodialysis may not be needed. Anuric renal failure always requires hemodialysis for survival. Even with hemodialysis, results of the management of septic renal failure are extremely poor (> 75% mortality).

Acute hyperkalemia can evolve in these patients and requires specific management when hemodialysis is not immediately available. Systemic administration of sodium bicarbonate will shift the blood pH in an alkaline direction and shift potassium intracellularly. Glucose and insulin administration may similarly move potassium ions into the intracellular compartment and provide time for more definitive measures to be implemented. Polystyrene sulfonate (Kayexelate® [Sanofi Winthrop Pharmaceuticals, New York, NY, USA]) may be given, usually by retention enemas in the peritonitis patient, as an exchange resin to exchange sodium ions for potassium ions across the gastrointestinal mucosa. Systemically administered calcium chloride will increase the ionized calcium concentration and antagonize potassium effects on the myocardium.

Finally, hemodialysis is symptomatic treatment of renal failure in the peritonitis patient. Unless the fundamental septic process is brought under control, survival will not occur. Evolving renal failure in the peritonitis patient requires that the surgeon reevaluate the adequacy of mechanical drainage and debridement. Of course, the role of nephrotoxic antimicrobial agents must similarly be reviewed in these circumstances.

Postrenal Azotemia

Urinary tract obstruction should always be remembered as a potential cause of oliguria in the surgical patient. Prostatic hypertrophy or occlusion of the Foley catheter has been known to provoke either the administration of an intravenous fluid challenge or the use of diuretics needlessly. A judgment of oliguria in these patients requires knowledge that the urinary tract conduit is patent.

Hepatic Support

Liver dysfunction in the patient with peritonitis may be caused by multiple clinical variables. Hypovolemia, reduced cardiac output, and systemic hypoxemia are associated with hepatic injury secondary to inadequate liver oxygenation. Associated diseases of alcoholism or drug abuse may reduce hepatic tolerance of peritonitis, anesthesia, and operation. Prolonged parenteral nutrition and selected antimicrobial agents may result in apparent hepatic dysfunction. Frequent or mismatched transfusions may increase the bilirubin load presented to the liver as well. However, the fundamental septic process will most commonly be responsible for hepatic abnormalities in these patients (Figure 3).

The severity of hepatic dysfunction in peritonitis is quite variable. Some patients have only mild chemical hyperbilirubinemia while other

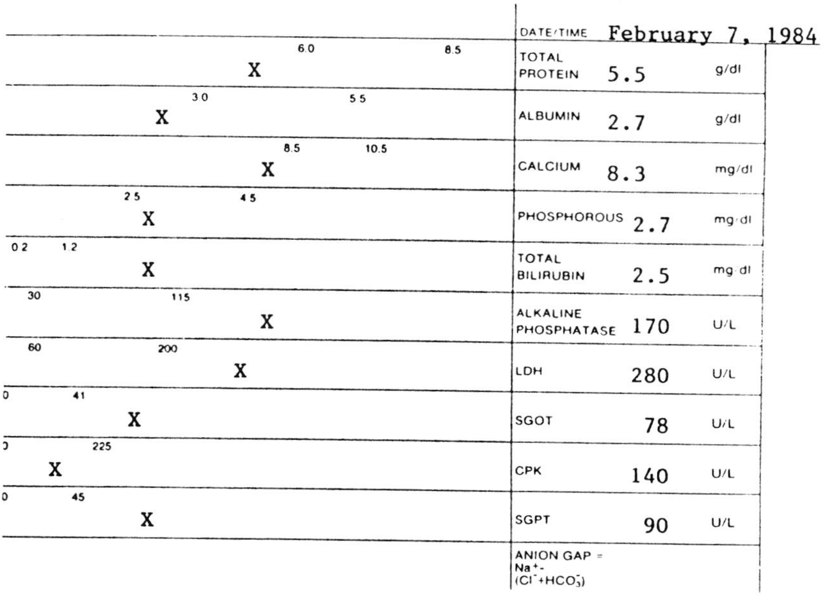

			DATE/TIME	February 7, 1984	
6.0	8.5	X	TOTAL PROTEIN	5.5	g/dl
3.0	5.5	X	ALBUMIN	2.7	g/dl
8.5	10.5	X	CALCIUM	8.3	mg/dl
2.5	4.5	X	PHOSPHOROUS	2.7	mg/dl
0.2	1.2	X	TOTAL BILIRUBIN	2.5	mg/dl
30	115	X	ALKALINE PHOSPHATASE	170	U/L
60	200	X	LDH	280	U/L
0	41	X	SGOT	78	U/L
0	225	X	CPK	140	U/L
0	45	X	SGPT	90	U/L
			ANION GAP = $Na^+ - (Cl^- + HCO_3^-)$		

Figure 3: An illustration of the serum chemistries that are commonly identified in the patient with peritonitis. The modest elevations of bilirubin and hepatic enzymes are commonly early indicators that an abdominal abscess is an emerging problem for the patient.

patients may have florid jaundice and frank hepatic coma. The frequency and magnitude of hepatic dysfunction in peritonitis are difficult to evaluate because of confusion surrounding a proper definition. Parameters such as the prothrombin time and serum albumin may be affected by factors other than intrinsic hepatic function. Thus, in previous investigations the author has chosen to use both increases in the liver enzymes and chemical hyperbilirubinemia as being indicative of hepatic dysfunction.[24,43] Increases in serum liver emzyme concentrations indicate cellular injury while chemical hyperbilirubinemia reflects functional impairment of the liver to deal with circulating bile pigment loads.

The management of hepatic dysfunction requires a comprehensive knowledge of those factors that may be of significance. Patients having severe hypotensive or hypoxic episodes may have transient periods of hyperbilirubinemia that characteristically peak and then regress by the seventh to tenth day. Hepatic dysfunction that coincides with such events usually resolves with comprehensive systemic care. Potentially hepatotoxic drugs such as the tetracycline antibiotics and the phenothiazine sedatives should be discontinued. Patients on long-term parenteral hyperalimentation may develop the so-called hyperalimentation hepatitis.[44] Modification of the protein:calorie ratio must be evaluated in these patients. The most common cause of clinical hepatic dysfunction in the peritonitis patient is poorly controlled infection.[45] The need for better control of infection is generally required in these patients. Unfortunately hepatic abnormalities progress in many of these patients despite application of all appropriate modes of therapy.

Supportive care for the failing liver has not achieved the sophistication seen with the ventilator for pulmonary failure or dialysis for renal failure. Extracorporeal hepatic support remains an unrealized dream.[46,47] Specific measures for metabolic support of the liver have included infusions of glucose and albumin to relieve the liver of both gluconeogenesis and albumin synthesis. The merits of these particular measures in the septic patient are questionable at best. The use of branched-chain amino acid infusions as a means of alleviating the systemic manifestations of severe hepatic dysfunction has been recommended. Hyperalimentation using modified compositions of amino acids has been advocated for patients with severe hepatic failure.[48,49] The value of many of these methods of hepatic support in the septic patient remains uncertain.[50]

Stress Gastrointestinal Bleeding

Significant hemorrhage from acute erosive gastritis continues to be a major complication in the peritonitis patient.[51] The pathophysiology of stress ulceration remains unclear, despite numerous experimental and clinical studies.[52-55] The mechanism includes the following postulated factors: (1) reduced blood flow of the gastric mucosa; (2) back-diffusion of intraluminal acid; and (3) alterations of the mucus barrier of the stomach. While hypersecretion of hydrogen ion does not appear to be necessary, it does appear that the presence of acid within the lumen is a requirement for acute erosive gastritis.

Even though the fundamental pathophysiology of stress gastrointestinal bleeding remains unknown, most efforts at prevention have centered around measures designed to reduce the concentrations of acid within the gastric lumen. Antacids administered by nasogastric tube have been shown to be effective in keeping the intragastric pH above 4.0 and reducing the incidence of stress hemorrhage.[56,57] Cimetidine has also been similarly useful in the prevention of stress bleeding, although some data have shown cimetidine to be significantly less effective at controlling gastric pH than are antacids in those patients with sepsis.[58,59] Furthermore, despite effective prevention of stress gastrointestinal bleeding, prospective randomized trials have not shown prophylaxis to improve the survival rate in the patients studied.[56]

While prevention of stress-associated gastric mucosal bleeding has generally been recognized as an important objective for the critically-ill patient, recent concerns about nosocomial pneumonia secondary to the use of antacids and H-2 blockers has raised serious concerns. Driks et al.[60] published information that demonstrated an increased nosocomial pneumonia rate when upper aerodigestive tract alkalinization was attempted with antacids and with antacids plus H-2 blockade of hydrogen ion secretion by the gastric parietal cell. They demonstrated a lower rate of pneumonia with the use of sucralfate, an agent designed to protect the barrier of the mucosa, but does not affect acid production nor gastric pH. However, a close examination of their data indicates that the lowest rate of nosocomial infection occurred in those patients receiving H-2 blockade alone. Thus, while sucralfate appears to be an effective agent in the prevention of stress-associated mucosal bleeding, it probably does not have the special benefits in the prevention of nosocomial pneumonia.

When upper gastrointestinal (GI) bleeding is first identified, diagnostic confirmation of stress ulceration is required. Flexible upper GI endoscopy is ideal for this purpose. The flexible endoscopy can be conveniently done in the intensive care unit and can usually pinpoint the many potential causes of upper GI bleeding.

The management of bleeding from acute erosive gastritis in peritonitis requires better control of fundamental causes. Hypovolemia must be corrected. Systemic oxygenation must be adequate. Uncontrolled infection must have a reevaluation of both the mechanical and pharmacological means of treatment. Management of the specific bleeding complication requires vigorous gastric lavage and systemic volume replacement. Temporary control can be sustained by efforts to maintain the gastric pH above 4.0 with antacids.

When clinical bleeding does not respond to conservative methods of management, minimally invasive methods with flexible upper GI endoscopy have been used to control bleeding with less than satisfactory results. Local electrocoagulation, heater probes, and even lasers have been used through the fiberoptic endoscope to control bleeding. These methods to control upper GI bleeding have generally been successful in acute peptic ulcer bleeding or in bleeding from acute gastric ulcers. Stress mucosal hemorrhage of the gastric mucosa is generally a diffuse process with multiple bleeding sites. The bleeding is commonly a persistent "ooze" rather than overt arterial bleeding. Endoscopic methods have not been especially promising in this area.

For the rare patient requiring surgery for exsanguinating hemorrhage, no surgical choice is particularly ideal. Vagotomy and pyloroplasty, usually combined with local attempts to suture, ligate, or electrocoagulate specific bleeding sites, have been commonly used because of a generally perceived lower surgical risk for this procedure. Total or near-total gastrectomy will stop the bleeding, but carries with it a much higher surgical risk and potentially more severe long-term consequences if the patient survives. Vagotomy with antrectomy or subtotal gastrectomy moderates the above two positions by yielding fewer acute mortalities but presents increased risks of rebleeding.

No surgical procedure has been satisfactory in these patients; surgery for control of bleeding should only be undertaken when all conservative measures have been exhausted. However, reoperation because of an undrained focus of intra-abdominal infection must not be deferred because of the patient's overall circumstance, because the most important objective in the management of stress gastrointestinal bleeding is better control of the fundamental septic process.

Nutritional Support

The widespread utilization of nutritional support in the peritonitis patient has been one of the most significant additions to the management of the critically-ill patient in the last decade. The septic patient has a disordered metabolic crisis that results in exhaustion of the body reservoir of proteins. While exogenous calories may not have major effects in alteration of the catabolic process, continued research in the appropriate composition and route of delivery of nutritional support is an area that may have a major impact in the future. Certainly the recovery of the peritonitis patient is particularly hastened by nutritional support after the principal septic process is controlled.

The caloric utilization by the peritonitis patient is significantly increased over basal requirements. Basal coloric requirements in the absence of exercise are approximately 20–25 Kcal/kg body weight per day. Requirements increase 25–30% by major trauma or surgical procedures, and the severe peritonitis patient may have caloric requirements that increase by 50% over the basal state. During the physiologic stress and septic state it is generally desirable to provide 2 gm protein per kilogram per day for these patients.[61]

The relationship between nonprotein and protein calories changes in the peritonitis patient. In the basal state, 300–350 nonprotein kilocalories per gram of nitrogen intake (6.25 grams protein = 1 gram nitrogen) usually provide adequate protein sparing. In major nonseptic surgical stress, such as would be encountered following major surgical procedures, the nonprotein calorie-to-nitrogen relationship changes to 125–150 kilocalories per gram of nitrogen. In the severe stress of peritonitis and the septic response, calorie-to-protein ratios of 80–100 are reasonable objectives. The relative increase in the need for protein in these patients is secondary to the increased role that protein plays as an energy substrate (Table 3).

Caloric administration of excessive nonprotein calories will result in hepatic dysfunction and fatty metamorphosis.[44] Inadequate nonprotein administration will result in oxidation of the exogenously given

Table 3
Identifies the Role of Amino Acids as Substrates in the Septic Response Patient. Note That the Role of Aromatic Amino Acids in the Production of False Neurotransmitters is a Very Deleterious Effect for the Host

Amino Acid	Target Cell	Substrate Function
Alanine, Glycine	Hepatocyte	Provides carbon structure for hepatic gluconeogenesis
Branched-Chains (valine, leucine isoleucine)	Muscle cell	Oxidative substrate; alanine production
Glutamine	Enterocyte	Oxidative substrate; alanine production
Arginine	Lymphocyte; Endothelial cell	Thymotrophic effect; Nitric oxide production
Aromatic group (eg, phenylalanine)	Hepatocyte	False neurotransmitter

protein, with increased urea synthesis and elevation of blood urea nitrogen.

The branched-chain amino acids appear to have advantages over other amino acids in the severely stressed surgical patient. Current evidence indicates that the branch-chains (valine, leucine, and isoleucine) may serve as preferential substrates by skeletal muscle, and as such may inhibit the catabolic process.[62] Additional research is required to see whether the severe peritonitis patient will genuinely benefit from the branched-chain amino acids or whether the septic "auto-cannibalism" of this process will not be inhibited.[50]

With recent information that has again focused attention upon the gastrointestinal tract as being a potential source for the septic response, enteral nutrition is now receiving increased attention.[63-66] While a traditional axiom in the care of surgical patients has been "if the gut works, then use it," the reality has been that surgeons have become quite comfortable with using parenteral nutrition. Concerns about the translocation of bacteria or endotoxin, and the attendant interest in preserving the gut barrier function, have led to some considerable debate about enteral nutrition being preferable because of its beneficial effects upon the mucosal barrier function.

The benefits of enteral nutrition presumably are for two reasons. The gut mucosa obtains much of its energy substrates directly from the lumen of the intestine and not from the circulation. Parenteral nutrition obviously denies the enterocyte this potential source of nutrients. By the administration of nutrients via the intestinal tract, enterocyte nutrition appears to be better supported than by comparable isocaloric, isonitrogenous parenteral administration.[67] Secondly, intraluminal nutrients foster proliferation of normal colonization of bacteria within the gut lumen. Normal colonization, particularly the anaerobic species, is felt to be an important component of the gut barrier function.[68] Thus, maintenance of the gut barrier by enteral nutrition prevents bacteria and bacterial cell products from becoming disseminated stimuli for the septic response, and also prevents the dissemination of resistant bacteria from the GI tract as potential nosocomial pathogens at distant sites.

The discussion about gut barrier function and microbial translocation has been further compounded by the potential role of glutamine as a preferred fuel for oxidation by the gut enterocyte.[69] Glutamine is a 5-carbon amino acid with two amino groups. The absence of glutamine in the diet under circumstances of stress is thought to promote gut atrophy and loss of the gastrointestinal barrier. Since glutamine is essentially absent from parenteral nutritional support systems, one school of thought would contend that gut atrophy is a consequence of nutritional composition and not necessarily the route of nutritional delivery. Further research will obviously need to be undertaken to resolve the issue of the optimum route of nutrition support and the desirability of glutamine enrichment.

Other Organ Systems

The discussions in this chapter have principally focused upon the major organ systems and how they are affected by the septic process during peritonitis. Other important organ systems are obviously involved. The endocrine system undergoes enormous changes during peritonitis, with these many metabolic aberrations being the center of a separate chapter. Pancreatic failure has been identified as part of the sequential organ failure syndrome of shock and may similarly be involved in peritonitis.[70] Coagulation dysfunction is certainly identified with thrombocytopenia, hypoprothrombinemia, and disseminated intravascular coagulation noted in many of these patients. Perhaps the most critical failure of organ systems in peritonitis is neurological failure, with altered sensorium in these patients being the clearest evidence of central nervous system involvement.[71] The role of each of these systems in the natural history of peritonitis remains unclear. The absence of data on many of these areas makes specific recommendations in supportive care not possible.

While all discussions to this point have addressed each organ system as an isolated entity, most organ failure complexes occur as the multiple organ failure syndrome.[23,24] Multiple organ failure will be discussed separately in a subsequent chapter. In terms of supportive care, most critically-ill peritonitis patients will have multiple systems that will require simultaneous management. Indeed, the extensive nature of the support systems for the management of these patients is complex indeed.

In conclusion, the supportive care of the patient with peritonitis requires attention to each of the major organ systems that are targeted by the septic process. The support technology that is available for this purpose is quite extensive; the time and expense for such efforts can prove to be a major stress on health care resources. Supportive care must always be viewed as an adjunct to the primary treatment of the infectious process.

References

1. Clowes GHA Jr, O'Donnell TF, Ryan NT, Blackburn GL: Energy metabolism in sepsis: treatment based on different patterns in shock and high output stage. *Ann Surg* 179:684-696, 1974.
2. Siegel JH, Cerra FB, Coleman B, et al: Physiologic and metabolic correlations in human sepsis. *Surgery* 86:163-193, 1979.
3. Richardson JD, DeCamp MM, Garrison RN, Fry DE: Pulmonary infection complicating intra-abdominal sepsis: clinical and experimental observations. *Ann Surg* 195:732-738, 1982.
4. Craig DB, McCarthy DS: Airway closure and lung volumes during breathing with maintained airway positive pressures. *Anesthesiology* 36:540-543, 1972.
5. Feeley TW, Saumarez R, Klick JM, et al: Positive end- expiratory pressure in weaning patients from controlled ventilation. *Lancet* 2:725-728, 1975.
6. Powers SR: The use of positive end-expiratory pressure (PEEP) for respiratory support. *Surg Clin North Am* 54:1125-1136, 1974.
7. Civetta JM, Flor RJ, Smith CD: Aggressive treatment of acute respiratory insufficiency. *South Med J* 69:749-751, 1976.
8. Kirby RR, Downs JB, Civetta JM, et al: High-level positive end-expiratory pressure (PEEP) in acute respiratory insufficiency. *Chest* 67:156-163, 1975.
9. Hayes DF, Lucas CE: Bilateral tube thoracostomy to preclude fatal tension pneumothorax in patients with acute respiratory insufficiency. *Am Surg* 42:330-331, 1976.
10. Hanson EL, Drinker PA, Don HF, et al: Venoarterial bypass with a membrane oxygenator: successful respiratory support in a woman following pulmonary hemorrhage secondary to renal failure. *Surgery* 75:557-565, 1974.
11. Hanson EL: Membrane oxygenator support for pulmonary insufficiency. *Surg Clin North Am* 54:1171-1178, 1974.
12. Downs JB, Klein EF, Desautels DA, et al: Intermittant mandatory ventilation: a new approach to weaning patients from mechanical ventilation. *Chest* 64:331-335, 1973.
13. Gabel JC, Julett WB, Glass DD, Poirier J: Intermittant mandatory ventilation. *South Med J* 70:274-276, 1977.
14. Millbern SM, Downs JB, Jumper LC, Modell JH: Evaluation of criteria for discontinuing mechanical ventilatory support. *Arch Surg* 113:1441-1443, 1978.
15. Ransom JHC, Spencer FC: The role of peritoneal lavage in severe acute pancreatitis. *Ann Surg* 187:565-575, 1978.
16. Clowes GHA, Hirsch E, Williams L, et al: Septic lung and shock lung in man. *Ann Surg* 181:681-692, 1975.
17. Fulton RL, Jones CE: The cause of post-traumatic pulmonary insufficiency in man. *Surg Gynecol Obstet* 140:179-186, 1975.
18. Walker L, Eiseman B: The changing pattern of post-traumatic respiratory distress syndrome. *Ann Surg* 181:693-697, 1975.
19. Blaisdell WF: Pathophysiology of the respiratory distress syndrome. *Arch Surg* 108:44-49, 1974.

20. Robb HJ, Margulis RR, Jabs CM: Role of pulmonary microembolism in the hemodynamics of endotoxin shock. *Surg Gynecol Obstet* 135:777-783, 1972.
21. Richardson JD, Fry DE, Van Arsdall L, Flint LM Jr: Delayed pulmonary clearance of gram negative bacteria: the role of intraperitoneal sepsis. *J Surg Res* 26:499-503, 1979.
22. Hunt JL: Generalized peritonitis: to irrigate or not to irrigate the abdominal cavity. *Arch Surg* 117:209-212, 1982.
23. Eiseman B, Beart R, Norton L: Multiple organ failure. *Surg Gynecol Obstet* 144:323-326, 1977.
24. Fry DE, Pearlstein L, Fulton RL, Polk HC Jr: Multiple system organ failure: the role of uncontrolled infection. *Arch Surg* 115:136-140, 1980.
25. Forrester JS, Diamond G, McHugh T, Swan HJC: Filling pressures in the right and left sides of the heart in acute myocardial infarction: a reappraisal of central venous pressure monitoring. *N Engl J Med* 285:190-193, 1971.
26. Swan HJC: Central venous pressure monitoring is an outmoded procedure of limited practical value. In: Ingelfinger F. ed. *Controversey in Internal Medicine*. Philadelphia, PA: WB Saunders; 1974:185-193.
27. Civetta JM, Gabel J: Flow-directed pulmonary artery catheterization in surgical patients: indications and modifications of technique. *Ann Surg* 176:753-756, 1972.
28. Swan HJC, Ganz W: Use of balloon flotation catheters in critically ill patients. *Surg Clin North Am* 55:501-520, 1975.
29. Swan HJC, Ganz W, Forrester JS, et al: Catheterization of the heart in man with the use of a flow-directed balloon-tipped catheter. *N Engl J Med* 283:447-451, 1970.
30. Nichols RL, Smith JW, Klein DB, et al: Risk of infection after penetrating abdominal trauma. *N Engl J Med* 311:1065, 1984.
31. Dellinger EP, Oreskovich MR, Wertz MJ, et al: Risk of infection following laparotomy for penetrating abdominal injury. *Arch Surg* 119:20, 1984.
32. Waymack JP, Gallon L, Barcelli U, et al: Effect of blood transfusion on macrophage function in a burned animal model. *Curr Surg* 43:305-307, 1986.
33. Waymack JP, Rapien J, Garnett D, et al: Effect of transfusion on immune function in a traumatized animal model. *Arch Surg* 121:50, 1986.
34. Messmer K: Hemodilution. *Surg Clin North Am* 55:659-677, 1975.
35. MacCannell KL, McNay JL, Meyer MB, et al: Dopamine in the treatment of hypotension and shock. *N Engl J Med* 275:1389-1392, 1966.
36. Goldberg LI: Dopamine-clinical uses of an endogenous catecholamine. *N Engl J Med* 291:707-710, 1974.
37. Jewitt D, Birkhead J, Mitchell A, et al: Clinical cardiovascular pharmacology of dobutamine: a selective inotropic catecholamine. *Lancet* 2:363, 1974.
38. Tally RC, Goldberg LI, Johnson CE, McRay JL: A hemodynamic comparison of dopamine and isoproterenol in patients in shock. *Circulation* 39:361-378, 1969.
39. Tarazi RC: Sympathomimetic agents in the treatment of shock. *Ann Intern Med* 81:364-370, 1974.
40. Cerra FB, Hassett JM, Siegel JH: Vasodilator therapy in clinical sepsis with low cardiac output syndrome. *J Surg Res* 25:180-183, 1978.

41. Lucas CE, Rector FE, Werner M, Rosenberg IK: Altered renal homeostasis with acute sepsis. *Arch Surg* 106:444-449, 1973.
42. Rector F, Gayal S, Rosenberg IK, Lucas CE: Sepsis: a mechanism for vasodilation in the kidney. *Ann Surg* 178:222-226, 1973.
43. Fry DE, Garrison RN, Heitsch RC, et al: Determinants of death in patients with intra-abdominal abscess. *Surgery* 88:517-523, 1980.
44. Sheldon GS, Petersen SR, Sanders R: Hepatic dysfunction during hyperalimentation. *Arch Surg* 113:504-508, 1978.
45. Norton L, Moore G, Eiseman B: Liver failure in the postoperative patient: the role of sepsis and immunologic failure. *Surgery* 78:6-13, 1975.
46. Eiseman B, Norton L, Kralias NC: Hepatocyte perfusion within a centrifuge. *Surg Gynecol Obstet* 142:21-28, 1976.
47. Eiseman B, Van Wyk J, Griffen WO: Methods for extracorporeal hepatic assist. *Surg Gynecol Obstet* 123:522-527, 1966.
48. Fischer JE, Rosen HM, Ebeid AM, et al: The effect of normalization of plasma amino acids on hepatic encephalopathy in man. *Surgery* 80:77-83, 1976.
49. Freund H, Hoover HC Jr, Atamian S, Fischer JE: Infusion of the branched chain amino acids in postoperative patients. *Ann Surg* 190:18-23, 1979.
50. Cerra FB, Siegal JH, Coleman B, et al: Septic autocannibalism: a failure of exogenous nutritional support. *Ann Surg* 192:570-580, 1980.
51. Skillman JJ, Bushnell IS, Goldman H, et al: Respiratory failure, hypotension, sepsis and jaundice. A clincial syndrome associated with lethal hemorrhage from acute stress ulceration of the stomach. *Am J Surg* 117:523-531, 1969.
52. Ivey KJ: Acute hemorrhagic gastritis: modern concepts based on pathogenesis. *Gut* 12:750-757, 1971.
53. Moody FG, Aldrete JS: Hydrogen permeability of canine gastric secretory epithelium during formation of acute superficial erosions. *Surgery* 70:154-160, 1974.
54. Robbins R, Idjadi F, Stahl WH, et al: Studies of gastric secretion in stressed patients. *Ann Surg* 175:555-562, 1972.
55. Skillman JJ, Gould SA, Chung RS, et al: The gastric mucosal barrier: clinical and experimental studies in critically ill and normal man, and in the rabbit. *Ann Surg* 172:564-584, 1970.
56. Hastings PR, Skillman JJ, Bushness LS, et al: Antacid prophylaxis of bleeding in the critically ill. *N Engl J Med* 298:1041-1045, 1978.
57. McAlhany JC Jr, Czaja AJ, Pruitt BA Jr: Antacid control of complications from acute gastroduodenal disease after burns. *J Trauma* 16:645-649, 1976.
58. Martin LF, Max MM, Polk HC Jr: Failure of gastric pH control by antacids or cimetidine in the critically ill: a valid sign of sepsis. *Surgery* 88:59-68, 1980.
59. Martin LF, Stalock DK, Simonowitz DA, et al: Failure of cimetidine prophylaxis in the critically ill. *Arch Surg* 114:492-496, 1979.
60. Driks MR, Craven DE, Celli BR, et al: Nosocomial pneumonia in intubated patients given sucralfate as compared with antacids or histamine type 2 blockers: role of gastric colonization. *N Engl J Med* 317:1376-1381, 1987.
61. Cerra FB, Blackburn GK, Hirsch J, et al: The effect of stress level, amino acid formula, and nitrogen dose on nitrogen retention in traumatic and septic stress. *Ann Surg* 206:282-287, 1987.

62. Cerra FB, Upson D, Angelico R, et al: Branched chains support postoperative protein synthesis. *Surgery* 92:192-199, 1982.
63. Deitch EA, Winterton J, Li M, et al: The gut as a portal of entry for bacteremia: role of protein malnutrition. *Ann Surg* 205:681-692, 1987.
64. Deitch EA, Berg R, Specian R: Endotoxin promotes the translocation of bacteria from the gut. *Arch Surg* 122:185-190, 1987.
65. Rush BF Jr, Sori AJ, Murphy TF, et al: Endotoxemia and bacteremia during hemorrhagic shock. *Ann Surg* 207:549-554, 1988.
66. Rush BF Jr, Redan JA, Flanagan JJ, et al: Does bacteremia in hemorrhagic shock have clinical significance? *Ann Surg* 210:342-347, 1989.
67. Mochizuki H, Trocki O, Dominioni L, et al: Mechanism of prevention of post burn hypermetabolism and catabolism by early enteral feeding. *Ann Surg* 200:297-310, 1984.
68. van der Waaij D: colonization resistance of the digestive tract: clinical consequences and implications. *J Antimicrob Chemother* 10:263-270, 1982.
69. Wilmore DW, Smith RJ, O'Dwyer ST, et al: The gut: a central organ after surgical stress. *Surgery* 104:917-923, 1988.
70. Tilney NL, Bailey GL, Morgan AP: Sequential system failure after rupture of abdominal aortic aneurysms: an unsolved problem in postoperative care. *Ann Surg* 178:117-122, 1973.
71. Baue AE: Multiple, progressive, or sequential system failure after rupture of abdominal aortic aneurysms: an unsolved problem in postoperative care. *Arch Surg* 110:779-781, 1975.

5

Antimicrobial Chemotherapy for Peritonitis

Mark A. Malangoni, MD

Antimicrobial agents are given in conjunction with surgery or other interventional treatment for the complete therapy for peritonitis. The exception to this is the unusual occurrence of primary peritonitis when antibiotics alone will suffice for treatment. The goals of surgical treatment of secondary bacterial peritonitis are to control the source of contamination, reduce the size of the microbial inoculum, remove adjuvant materials that accentuate the disease process, and decrease the effect of bacterial by-products. If the source of contamination is controlled, radiologically guided drainage can also be used for treatment of an intra-abdominal abscess in selected circumstances.[1] While antimicrobial agents are relegated to an adjunctive role in the management of secondary bacterial peritonitis, the proper use of these drugs is crucial for successful treatment.

This chapter will concentrate on the role that antibiotics have in the treatment of secondary bacterial peritonitis. Therefore, surgical techniques will be mentioned only as they relate to antibiotic management. It is important to understand that antibiotic use will not replace appropriate surgical techniques nor will it replace appropriate judgment and overall management of the patient. In order to fully understand the rationale that supports the prudent use of antimicrobial chemotherapy, a brief review of the pathophysiology of peritonitis and the experiments and clinical studies that provide the foundation for treatment of this disease will follow.

From Fry DE, (ed): *Peritonitis.* Mount Kisco NY, Futura Publishing Co., Inc., © 1993.

Pathophysiology and the Local Response to Peritonitis

In the normal state, the peritoneal cavity is a contracted space in which the serosal surfaces of the intestines, solid viscera, and parietal peritoneum are opposed. This potential space contains from 10–15 mL of fluid that is freely exchanged with the remaining extracellular space. The entire area of the peritoneal cavity approximates the total body surface area. Therefore, the irritative effects of secondary bacterial peritonitis can result in hemodynamic changes similar to those that occur following a major burn injury. It is the consequence of this imbalance of peritoneal homeostasis that poses the major threat to a patient with bacterial peritonitis and, if uncorrected, can lead to death from the ill effects of septic shock.

The compensatory response to peritonitis is a complex interaction resulting in activation of systemic and local host defense mechanisms that are meant to combat the invading bacterial pathogens. Initially there is an outpouring of extracellular fluid into the peritoneal cavity in response to the bacterial contamination. Opsonins and chemotactic substances are transported to the inflamed peritoneal cavity to promote the phagocytosis of bacteria by white blood cells. This fluid response dilutes the concentration of bacteria into a medium that is richly laden with both humoral and cellular components of the inflammatory response. This outpouring of fluid also enhances the transportation of bacteria to the stomata of the caudal surface of the diaphragm where they are absorbed into the lymphatic circulation. Diaphragmatic motion empties these lymphatics into the mediastinal lymphatic circulation. Bacteria will appear in the bloodstream within 15 minutes following intraperitoneal contamination.

Bacterial contamination also initiates an influx of leukocytes into the peritoneal cavity. Macrophages comprise the majority of resident white blood cells in the peritoneal cavity. However, neutrophils are rapidly mobilized into the peritoneum following bacterial contamination and become the predominant phagocytic cell within a few hours.[2] These white blood cells are important for the phagocytosis and killing of bacteria. Translymphatic absorption and both resident and recruited white blood cells serve as the principal mechanisms for the clearance of bacteria from the peritoneal cavity.[3]

Within the peritoneal cavity, fibrinogen is converted to fibrin that assists in localizing bacteria. Not surprisingly, attempts by the white blood cells to engulf and kill bacteria may be inhibited by excessive fibrin deposition. However, it seems logical that this response is moderated to optimize bacterial clearance and ensure the likelihood of host survival.

Microbiology of Peritonitis

The microbiology of secondary bacterial peritonitis is complex and there is a natural selection process that results in a reduction in the number of bacterial species eventually cultured compared to the large variety of bacteria that are present in the intestinal lumen. Bacteria can promote their own growth and that of other species by producing enzymes that facilitate their adherence to and invasion of body tissues. These microorganisms can synthesize nutrients that support the reproduction and survival of other bacteria. The metabolism of one species may create an environment in which host defenses are rendered less effective to eliminate other bacterial species. Adjuvants such as bile, hemoglobin, fibrin, intestinal contents, foreign bodies, and necrotic tissue can serve as nutrients for bacterial growth or these substances can inhibit the phagocytosis of bacteria by white blood cells. Clearly, decreases in pH and pO_2 within the inflamed peritoneal cavity may render some antimicrobial agents ineffective.

The response to peritonitis is related to the extent and duration of bacterial contamination, the virulence of the bacteria involved, the presence of adjuvant material, and the nature of the host response to infection. Survival following experimental bacterial peritonitis is related to the amount of the bacterial inoculum and a large inoculum can overcome usual effective therapy.[4] An important experiment in which experimental peritonitis was induced by injection of feces into the peritoneal cavity of rats, demonstrated that *Escherichia coli, Bacteroides fragilis,* and enterococci were the predominant species cultured from resultant intra-abdominal abscesses.[5] In a subsequent experiment using facultative and anaerobic bacteria to investigate peritoneal infection, Onderdonk et al.[6] demonstrated that mortality was directly related to the presence of *E. coli* in the inoculum and that in the absence of this bacterium survival following experimental peritonitis was nearly 100%. These authors also demonstrated that intra-abdominal abscess formation occurred only in the presence of both a facultative bacterium (eg, *E. coli* or enterococci) and an anaerobe. When *E. coli* and *B. fragilis* were given together, there was both a substantial lethality and intra-abdominal abscess formation occurred uniformly in the surviving animals. Because these observations were similar to the clinical situation in humans, this model has proven useful to investigate the pathogenesis of peritonitis.

Bacteria that comprise the infectious component of peritonitis are the specific targets of antimicrobial chemotherapy. Perforation of a hollow viscus presents an enormous number and variety of bacterial species into the peritoneum. Over time, the species of bacteria are reduced and modified to the point that when operative intervention is undertaken, culture of the infection grows a relatively sparse number of organisms compared to the multitude of bacteria present at the time of contamination. However, these surviving bacteria are of major concern since antimicrobial chemotherapy must be directed against these hearty pathogens in order to successfully treat this infection.

Human studies of the microbiology of peritonitis have demonstrated that as the techniques of specimen transport and processing have improved, a greater number of bacterial species can be recovered from patients with secondary bacterial peritonitis.[7] In particular, improvement in anaerobic culturing methods and a broadened taxonomic classification of anaerobes has resulted in an enhanced recovery of these species from patients with bacterial peritonitis. Studies of the microbiology of human peritonitis over the last two decades have consistently demonstrated the cultures from patients with peritonitis grow multiple organisms and that anaerobic bacterial species outnumber facultative and aerobic bacteria at least 2:1 (Table 1).[8-10]

The normal gastrointestinal ecology illustrates that a symbiotic relationship of bacterial species normally exists. This relationship changes to a pathologic one when there is contamination of the peritoneal cavity. Drasar and Hill[11] have studied the microflora of the gastrointestinal tract unaffected by disease. While the oropharynx contains large numbers of bacteria, the unfavorable acidic environment of the normal stomach inhibits bacterial growth. There is a progressive increase in the number of bacteria recovered from the gastrointestinal tract from the duodenum to the colon (Table 2). Importantly, there is also a change in the predominant species of bacteria that inhabit the gut as it progresses distally.

The flora of the oropharynx, esophagus, stomach, duodenum, and upper jejunum are comparable. Colonization of these areas occurs mainly from swallowed bacteria of the mouth and pharynx. The major species recovered from these areas of the gastrointestinal tract include

Table 1
Microbiology of Peritonitis

	Total	
	No. of Species	*% of Cultures*
Aerobic and Facultative Bacteria		
E. coli	235	60
Streptococci	108	28
Enterobacter/Klebsiella	101	26
Proteus	87	22
Enterococci	66	17
Pseudomonas	30	8
Staphylococci	29	7
Candida	6	2
Anaerobic Bacteria		
Bacteroides	288	72
B. fragilis	153	38
Eubacteria	94	24
Clostridia	67	17
Peptostreptococci	55	14
Peptococci	42	11
Propionibacteria	36	9
Fusobacteria	34	8

Data from references 8–10.

facultative and anaerobic streptococci and staphylococci, *E. coli*, and anaerobic gram-negative bacilli that usually do not include the *B. fragilis* group bacteria. While the bacterial content of the stomach is usually quite low, increases in gastric pH due to disease or inhibition of acid are accompanied by an increase in the absolute concentration of bacteria and a change in the species encountered. In a less acidic environment, enterococci and increased numbers and species of gram-negative enteric bacilli as well as fungi can be recovered from the stomach.[12]

The concentration of bacteria begins to increase in the proximal small intestine. However, in the absence of disease, an important increase in the concentration of organisms does not occur until the ileum is reached. The bacterial content in the ileum increases as the ileocecal valve is approached where the content of bacteria is about 10^8 organisms per gram of effluent. Bacterial concentrations within the appendix and

Table 2
Numbers of Bacteria Recovered from Areas of the Normal Gastrointestinal Tract

Oropharynx	10^9
Stomach and duodenum	10^2
Jejunum	10^4
Ileum	10^5–10^8
Colon	10^{10}–10^{12}

colon are identical for practical purposes and commonly approach 10^{11} organisms per gram of feces.

E. coli is the dominant facultative organism within the distal small intestine and colon. However, *Klebsiella* and *Proteus* species, enterococci and occasional streptococci are also found. Although *B. fragilis* group organisms are the most prevalent anaerobic bacteria in the colon, anaerobic streptococci and staphylococci, *Clostridia* and *Eubacteria* are also found. On occasion, peritonitis can also originate from the biliary tract. When it does, the bacteria involved are usually *E. coli*, *Klebsiella*, enterococci, or *Clostridia*. Bacteria actually comprise one third of the total stool mass. The content and recovery of bacterial species within the normal gastrointestinal tract can be affected by diet, disease, and the administration of antibiotics as well as a variety of other factors.

Recovery of *E. coli* and *B. fragilis* from a high percentage of intraperitoneal cultures of patients with secondary bacterial peritonitis and demonstration that these organisms reproduced peritonitis in experimental model have led to common acceptance that choices for antimicrobial chemotherapy must be effective against these bacteria.

Many species of bacteria recovered from intraperitoneal cultures of patients with intra-abdominal infections may not be true pathogens and will be eradicated during a process of selection in which only a bacteria survive. Obviously, it is futile to attempt to treat all organisms recovered from a culture of peritonitis. It has not been demonstrated that any organisms initially present within the intestine but later eliminated through this selection process require effective antimicrobial chemotherapy. Malangoni et al.[13] reported that recovery of bacteria resistant to the antimicrobial regimen used is more frequently associated with treatment failure. This concept has recently been reinforced by another study.[14] Although laboratory models of secondary bacterial peritonitis attempt to duplicate the human situation, all are subject to inherent bias that affect their usefulness. Despite this caveat, these models have proven effective to evaluate the usefulness of antimicrobial agents for the treatment of this disease.

Using a model of experimental peritonitis, Weinstein et al.[15] demonstrated that treatment against both *E. coli* and *B. fragilis* not only decreased mortality but also resulted in a lower incidence of intra-abdominal abscess formation. Failure to provide an antibiotic effective against gram-negative enteric bacteria resulted in a substantial increase in mortality and failure to treat anaerobes led to an increase in the incidence of intra-abdominal abscess formation in survivors. Treatment of both the facultative and anaerobic components of infection in this model resulted in optimal survival with the lowest frequency of abscess formation and therefore it generally has been accepted that antimicrobial chemotherapy must be effective against both of these components of infection in order to be successful. Hau et al.[16] have reported a laboratory model of peritonitis in which operation and intraperitoneal saline lavage were incorporated into the treatment regimen 24 hours following the intra-abdominal infection. This model, which mimics the treatment of human peritonitis, confirms that maximum survival occurs among animals treated with antibiotics effective against both the facultative and anaerobic bacterial components of the infection. Therefore, it seems prudent that we apply the principles learned in these laboratory models of peritonitis to guide the selection of antimicrobial agents.

Systemic Response to Peritonitis

In addition to the local response within the peritoneal cavity, the systemic response of the patient also affects the ability to successfully combat an intra-abdominal infection. The extremes of age and the presence of significant comorbid diseases are associated with a higher mortality from secondary bacterial peritonitis. The ability to stratify patients according to the magnitude of the disturbance of normal physiology has been proven to be important. Although a variety of systems has been developed to measure parameters that are associated with a poor outcome following intra-abdominal infection, the APACHE II score has been demonstrated to correlate with mortality due to peritonitis.[17] The APACHE II score is a compilation of the acute physiology score (a summation of parameters that demonstrate important aspects of normal physiology) such as age and chronic health status (Table 3).[18] A joint working party of the Surgical Infection Society of North America and Europe has shown that the APACHE II score is useful to determine the probability of death following intra-abdominal infection.[19]

An earlier study of patients with generalized peritonitis suggested that prognosis was also related to site of contamination.[20] A subsequent evaluation of more than 180 patients with peritonitis and intra-abdominal abscess has demonstrated that mortality following these diseases is similar regardless of the site of origin of intra-abdominal infection, except for infections emanating from the appendix that have a lower associated mortality.[21] This suggests that the response to peritonitis rather than the site of contamination is the most important factor determining outcome. There is a great variability in mortality of patients with intra-abdominal infections, reflecting the heterogenous population of patients with this disorder. Stratification of patients based upon an accurate physiologic scoring system is important not only to assist in the prediction of mortality but also to evaluate the usefulness of various therapies in intra-abdominal infection.

Pitcher and Musher[22] have demonstrated that a delay in the definitive treatment of intra-abdominal infections correlates with an increased mortality and an increased rate of complications. The prognosis of patients with intra-abdominal abscess has been shown to be adversely

Table 3
Parameters Evaluated in the Acute Physiology Scope

(Apache II)[19]

Temperature
Mean arterial pressure
Ventricular heart rate
Respiratory rate
Oxygenation ($A\text{-}aDO_2$ or PaO_2)
Arterial pH (serum CO_2)
Serum sodium
Serum potassium
Serum creatinine
Hematocrit
White blood cell count
Glasgow coma score

affected by a higher frequency of failed organ systems, positive blood cultures, increasing age, the presence of multiple abscesses, failure of initial antimicrobial therapy and the presence of abscesses in the lesser sac and subhepatic spaces, two areas associated with a delay in the diagnosis of infection.[23] Deveney et al.[24] have recently shown that improvements in technology, such as abdominal computed tomographic scanning, have resulted in more rapid diagnosis of intra-abdominal abscess and have led to a decrease in mortality.

The final factor affecting the overall response to peritonitis is the appropriateness of the initial therapy. Delays in institution of treatment as well as inappropriate treatment courses can significantly reduce survival. The proper administration of intravenous fluids and appropriate use of monitoring devices and vasoactive agents are an important part of the overall treatment of the infected patient. Errors of omission in these areas can have dramatic impact upon survival from intra-abdominal infection.

Selection of Antimicrobial Chemotherapy

Antimicrobial agents selected to treat any serious infection should have demonstrated effectiveness against the infection at hand, be relatively free of significant side effects or toxic reactions, achieve an appropriate concentration at the site of infection, should be simple to administer, and should be relatively inexpensive. Unfortunately, there is not a single drug that is uniformly effective against all infections. Thus, familiarity with the selection and proper use of antimicrobials in general is imperative in order to successfully treat patients with intra-abdominal infections.

Due to the critical nature of bacterial peritonitis, antimicrobial therapy is frequently indicated on an empiric basis, that is without documentation of the exact site of origin of infection or of the pathogens responsible for the infection. The choice of antibiotics is based upon knowledge of which bacteria are responsible for intra-abdominal infections (Table 1) as well as studies that have demonstrated which antibiotics are efficacious for treatment. Aspiration of the peritoneal cavity to obtain material for culture prior to initiation of therapy is difficult and often unrewarding. Intra-abdominal infections are predictably polymicrobial in nature and usually are caused by a combination of facultative and anaerobic bacteria. When the source of peritoneal contamination is unknown prior to definitive treatment, antibiotic administration should be instituted with the worst possible source for infection in mind, that is a presumption of contamination from the colon. Blood cultures should be done prior to beginning antibiotics in the febrile patient. However these cultures will be positive in only 10–15% of cases.

At operation, the first purulent material encountered should be collected for culture. The specimen should be collected in an anaerobic transport vial or alternatively in a syringe from which air had been evacuated. The culture must be collected properly and transported and processed expediently to assure that it represents the infection encountered. Hill[7] has demonstrated that the composition of a mixed bacterial infection can change over time as conditions in the transport medium favor the growth of selected bacteria. The specimen should also be processed for Gram's stain. The Gram's stain is of critical importance to confirm that the initial antibiotic selection is appropriate. While demonstration of pleomorphic bacteria that stain both gram-positive and gram-negative usually confirms the suspicion of a mixed bacterial infection, on occasion, the Gram's stain may demonstrate a single bacterial species and in this situation the antimicrobial spectrum can be adjusted.

It has been observed for some time that anaerobic bacteria produce certain gaseous by-products that give a characteristic odor to infections involved with these organisms. Spiegel and colleagues[25] have shown that delineation of the characteristic volatile acids produced by anaerobic bacteria using gas liquid chromatography provides an accurate means to identify the involvement of anaerobes in an intra-abdominal infection. These methods may be most useful to exclude the presence of anaerobic bacteria and therefore allow the use of an antimicrobial regimen with a more narrow spectrum of antibacterial activity.

In addition to procuring a specimen for culture, it is appropriate to obtain antimicrobial susceptibility studies of the bacteria recovered. This is useful to determine whether the antibiotic therapy selected is effective and whether other agents are potentially useful. This information is important since patients who grow bacteria resistant to the antimicrobial regimen selected are at greater risk for treatment failure.[13,14]

Antimicrobial chemotherapy should be initiated at the time that peritonitis is diagnosed. The intravenous administration of antibiotics provides the most rapid delivery of high concentrations of drug into the bloodstream and the peritoneal cavity. There is no place for intramuscular or oral antibiotic administration in this serious disorder.

While a variety of antibiotics may have demonstrated in vitro antibacterial activity against the pathogens of peritonitis, a smaller number have been shown to be efficacious in clinical trials. The therapeutic effectiveness of an antibiotic is usually tested first in an animal model and then the antibiotic or combination of drugs is evaluated in humans with intra-abdominal infections. Although a number of antibiotic regimens have been demonstrated to be effective in the treatment of intra-abdominal infections, most comparative clinical trials have failed to show superiority of a single drug or combination of agents. The defects in study design and reporting of comparative antibiotic trials for intra-abdominal infections that account for some of the difficulty in drawing conclusions about minor differences in outcome has been summarized by Solomkin et al.[26] The Scientific Studies Committee of the Surgical Infection Society has recently outlined guidelines to standardize the construction and conduct of antibiotic trials so that different reports can be compared.[27]

Early studies have established the combined use of an aminoglycoside antibiotic and an agent effective against *B. fragilis* group organisms, usually clindamycin or metronidazole, as the standard regimen to which other drug treatments have been compared. No single agent among the aminoglycosides has proven to be superior to the other drugs in this class. A large number of other antimicrobial agents have been compared to this standard of therapy in clinical trials. The Surgical Infection Society has recently published a position paper that evaluates the various antimicrobial regimens that have proven to be effective for the treatment of intra-abdominal infections.[28] This report also denotes drugs that have not been shown to be effective for the treatment of secondary bacterial peritonitis. The authors point out that early appendicitis, simple cholecystitis without perforation or gangrene, necrotic bowel without established peritonitis or intra-abdominal abscess, gastroduodenal ulcer perforation operated upon within 24 hours of onset, and traumatic intestinal perforation operated on within 12 hours of injury do not require prolonged antibiotic therapy. The recommended antibiotics from this study are shown in Table 4. Each of these drugs or drug regimens has various deficiencies in antimicrobial activity. The prescriber should be familiar with these deficiencies in order to anticipate bacteria that may possibly be resistant to therapy.

Although most comparative antibiotic trials have shown no difference between the drug regimens used to treat intra-abdominal infections, one such report has demonstrated superior efficacy for a single

Table 4
Antimicrobial Regimens Recommended for the Treatment of Intra-Abdominal Infections

Single drugs
    cefmetazole
    cefotetan
    cefoxitin
    imipenem-cilastatin
    ticarcillin-clavulanate
Drug Combinations
    aminoglycoside plus clindamycin or metronidazole
    aztreonam plus clindamycin
    cefotaxime or ceftizoxime plus clindamycin or metronidazole

Data from reference 28.

agent and is worthy of comment. In a multicenter study of 162 patients with serious intra-abdominal infection, Solomkin et al.[29] demonstrated that imipenem/cilastatin was more effective than tobramycin and clindamycin. Patients were stratified by APACHE II score and both treatment groups had similar characteristics. Patients receiving imipenem/cilastatin had a significantly lower treatment failure rate and a lower incidence of necrotizing fascitis. There was no difference in overall mortality. Not surprisingly, patients who failed treatment had a higher APACHE II score than those treated successfully in both antibiotic groups. Analysis of treatment failures showed there was a higher incidence of persistent, initially sensitive gram-negative rods in the tobramycin/clindamycin-treated patients. Patients in the aminoglycoside treatment group were determined to have sufficient peak serum aminoglycoside concentrations and there was no difference in the peak serum concentration between patients who failed therapy and those treated successfully. This unique study suggests that imipenem/cilastatin may be the preferred antibiotic for treatment of intra-abdominal infections, particularly when the risk of necrotizing infection is high.

When possible, a single drug is preferred for treatment of intra-abdominal infections. There are a number of cephalosporins that are efficacious and serve as preferred therapy. These include cefoxitin, cefmetazole, and cefotetan. The major reason to use combination therapy for the treatment of intra-abdominal infections is when patients have serious penicillin or cephalosporin allergy, or in patients who are profoundly immunosuppressed and may have unusual bacteria causing peritonitis.

The use of any antimicrobial regimen can be criticized because it will not be uniformly effective against the multitude of bacteria that can be cultured from intra-abdominal infections. Mosdell et al.[14] have shown no difference in the outcome of patients with intra-abdominal infections who were treated with a variety of effective drug regimens. In particular, this study demonstrated no advantage to the use of combination drug therapy.

The recovery of enterococci from the intraperitoneal culture of patients with intra-abdominal infections has stirred considerable debate as to whether these bacteria are true pathogens deserving of antibiotic therapy. This is of interest since most of the antimicrobial regimens recommended in Table 4 are not effective against enterococci. Barie and colleagues[30] have demonstrated that although enterococci are frequently cultured from intra-abdominal infections, the use of antimicrobial agents that are ineffective against these organisms is not associated with a greater risk of treatment failure. Patients who have valvular heart disease should receive antibiotic therapy effective against enterococci since the complications of enterococcal endocarditis far outweigh the risk of additional antibiotics. Enterococcal infections should be treated when this organism has been recovered from a previous intra-abdominal infection, is present on blood culture, or is demonstrated at another site of infection.[30] The use of high-dose ampicillin (6–8 g/day), a ureidopenicillin, or vancomycin are acceptable for treatment. Patients with severe immunological compromise who are excessively susceptible to opportunistic pathogens should also receive treatment against enterococci.

Occasionally, *Candida* and other fungal species are isolated on cultures from patients with secondary bacterial peritonitis. There is no indication to treat these organisms unless they are cultured from an additional site outside of the abdomen or prove to be the only microorganism isolated from the intraperitoneal infection.[31] When necessary, amphotericin B or fluconazole are effective drugs.

Initiation and Duration of Antimicrobial Use

Antibiotics should be given intravenously to achieve the most rapid and effective blood and tissue levels prior to surgery and these agents should always be used at a dose suggested for serious infections. The serum half-life of an agent is a pharmacokinetic parameter useful in selecting the proper dosage interval. As a general rule, antibiotics should be redosed approximately every four half-lives.

Some drugs will require an adjustment in dosage if there is physiologic compromise of the system by which the drug is excreted. This is true particularly for patients with chronic renal failure in whom a dose or dosage interval of aminoglycosides and many other antibiotics needs to be adjusted. Patients with hepatic failure need dosage adjustments if they are treated with metronidazole or clindamycin. It is frequently helpful to monitor serum antibiotic concentrations when organ failure is present in order to assure proper antimicrobial dosing. The presence of subtherapeutic antimicrobial concentrations is associated with higher frequency of treatment failure.[32] Ongoing continuous monitoring of antimicrobial serum drug levels is usually not done except when aminoglycosides are used.

Serum levels of aminoglycosides should be evaluated frequently because of the narrow therapeutic-to-toxic ratio of these drugs and the many variables that affect serum concentrations. Aminoglycoside antibiotics are metabolized and cleared by the kidneys and renal function due to intrinsic disease, concomitant diuretic use, hypovolemia, and age can lead to excessive serum concentration of these drugs and result in either nephrotoxicity or ototoxicity. While a number of formulas have been developed to predict the appropriate dose of these drugs, all have their drawbacks and may be unreliable for any particular patient. Aminoglycosides dose adjustment should be delayed until three doses of drug have been given to allow for sufficient equilibration of the volume of distribution of drug and to provide for a more reliable dose scheduling.

Examination of the urinary sediment is the most sensitive indicator of nephrotoxicity and the appearance of granular casts serves as an early indicator of dysfunction. Changes in blood urea nitrogen and serum creatinine levels and urinary creatinine clearance are later indicators of nephrotoxicity.

Two methods of monitoring of peak and trough serum aminoglycoside levels have been purported to be helpful to avoid toxic side effects. The peak serum concentration is measured 60 minutes following the start of an intravenous dose given over a 30-minute time period. Peak values of 4 to 10 µg/mL are considered optimal for therapy. Peak aminoglycoside levels in excess of 12 µg/mL are associated with nephrotoxicity. The trough concentration is measured within 1 hour prior to the administration of the next drug dose and should be less than 2 µg/mL in order to avoid serious side effects. Once the proper dosage is established, monitoring should be repeated at least two to three times per week in patients without evidence of renal dysfunction and more frequently in patients with preexisting renal disease. Recommendations to avoid ototoxicity are less well defined.

Zaske et al.[33] have suggested that pharmacokinetic dosing of aminoglycosides is more appropriate. This method involves measurement of repeated serum drug concentrations following a single dose, the results of which are used to calculate the proper dose and interval of administration based upon the volume of drug distribution and the serum half-life. This method is more involved than the other one mentioned previously, and often requires assistance from someone skilled in its interpretation such as a clinical pharmacist. It remains to be demonstrated which of these two methods of monitoring is more beneficial. Flint et al.[34] have shown a reduction in the incidence of toxic side effects by the routine monitoring of serum aminoglycoside concentrations.

There is a paucity of data concerning the importance of antibiotic concentration within the inflamed peritoneal cavity. Gerding et al.[35] have measured peritoneal fluid antibiotic concentrations in patients with ascites. They have demonstrated that aminoglycosides and clindamycin are found in lower concentrations in the peritoneal fluid than in the serum. Despite this reduction in antibiotic concentration within the peritoneal cavity, drug levels remained in the therapeutic range necessary to effectively eliminate most pathogens. The acidic environment and low oxygen tension within the peritoneal cavity in the presence of bacterial peritonitis have been postulated to potentially impair the antibacterial activity of the aminoglycosides, which require oxygen-dependent cellular transport mechanisms in order to be effective.

Patients with recurrent or persistant intra-abdominal infections may be exposed to pathogens that are resistant to antimicrobial agents usually selected for initial empiric therapy. In this situation, treatment should be individualized and previous culture results as well as local antimicrobial susceptibility patterns should be used to guide decisions about appropriate antimicrobial chemotherapy. Patients who develop recurrent intra-abdominal infection should have antibiotic therapy altered to include drugs active against the microorganisms grown on the previous culture. If all organisms appear to be sensitive, it is appropriate to change antimicrobial agents.

The exact duration of antibiotic administration necessary to eradicate peritonitis is controversial. The best guide to the proper duration of antimicrobial use is the clinical course of the patient. Antibiotics are generally continued until the patient is afebrile, gastrointestinal function has returned, and the white blood cell count is decreasing to normal. Anti-infective agents are ususally given for a minimum of 5 to 7 days. Failure of the temperature and white blood cell count to return to normal is associated with a high rate of treatment failure.[36] If there is no clinical improvement within 72 hours of the initial treatment or if fever and leukocytosis persist following therapy, persistent intra-abdominal infection or another site of infection should be suspected and sought. The return of intestinal function is an important indicator that the acute inflammatory response of peritonitis has subsided and that antimicrobial therapy can be stopped. Antibiotic treatment should not be prolonged beyond 14 days without investigation for persistent intra-abdominal infection or a new focus of infection. Minimizing the dose and duration of antibiotic use decreases the incidence of side effects.[37]

References

1. Malangoni MA, Shumate CR, Thomas HA, Richardson JD: Factors influencing the treatment of intraabdominal abscesses. *Am J Surg* 159:167-171, 1990.
2. Dunn DL, Barke RA, Knight NB, et al: Role of resident macrophages, peripheral neutrophils, and translymphatic absorption in bacterial clearance from the peritoneal cavity. *Infect Immun* 49:257-264, 1985.
3. Dunn DL, Barke RA, Eward DC, Simmons RL: Macrophages and translymphatic absorption represent the first line of host defense of the peritoneai cavity. *Arch Surg* 122:105-110, 1987.
4. Nichols RL, Smith JW, Fossedal EW, Condon RE: Efficacy of parenteral antibiotics in the treatment of experimentally induced intraabdominal sepsis. *Rev Infect Dis* 1:302-309, 1979.
5. Onderdonk AB, Weinstein WM, Sullivan NM, et al: Experimental intraabdominal abscess in rats: quantitative bacteriology of infected animals. *Infect Immun* 10:1256-1259, 1974.
6. Onderdonk AB, Bartlett JG, Louie T, et al: Microbial synergy in experimental intraabdominal abscess. *Infect Immun* 13:22-26, 1976.
7. Hill GB: Effects of storage in an anaerobic transport system on bacteria in known polymicrobial mixtures and in clinical specimens. *J Clin Microbiol* 8:680-688, 1978.

8. Gorbach SL, Thadepalli H, Norsen J: Anaerobic microorganisms in intraabdominal infections. In: Balows A, DeHann RH, Dowell VR, Guze LB, eds. *Anaerobic Bacteria: Role in Disease.* Springfield, IL: Thomas; 1974:339.
9. Lorber B, Swenson RM: The bacteriology of intraabdominal infections. *Surg Clin North Am* 55:1349, 1975.
10. Stone HH, Kolb LD, Geheber CE: Incidence and significance of intraperitoneal anaerobic bacteria. *Ann Surg* 181:705, 1975.
11. Drasar MS, Hill MJ: *Human Intestinal Flora.* London: Academic Press; 1974.
12. Muscroft TJ, Deane SA, Youngs D, et al: The microflora of the postoperative stomach. *Br J Surg* 68:560-564, 1981.
13. Malangoni MA, Condon RE, Spiegel CA: Treatment of intraabdominal infections is appropriate with single agent or combination antibiotic therapy. *Surgery* 98:648-655, 1985.
14. Mosdell DM, Morris DM, Voltura A, et al: What's new in general surgery: antibiotic treatment for surgical peritonitis. *Ann Surg* 214:543-549, 1991.
15. Weinstein WM, Onderdonk AB, Bartlett JG, et al: Antimicrobial treatment of experimental intraabdominal sepsis. *J Infect Dis* 132:282-286, 1975.
16. Hau T, Nishikawa R, Phuangsab A: Irrigation of the peritoneal cavity and local antibiotics in the treatment of peritonitis. *Surg Gynecol Obstet* 156:25-30, 1983.
17. Bohnen JMA, Mustard RA, Oxhold SE, et al: APACHE II score and abdominal sepsis: a prospective study. *Arch Surg* 123:225, 1988.
18. Knaus WA, Draper EA, Wagner DP, Zimmerman JE: APACHE II: A severity of disease classification system for acutely ill patients. *Crit Care Med* 13:818, 1985.
19. Nystrom PO, Bax RB, Dellinger EP, et al: Proposed definitions for diagnosis, severity scoring, stratification, and outcome for trials on intraabdominal infection. *World J Surg* 14:148-158, 1990.
20. Bohnen JMA, Boulanger M, Meakins JL, McLean APH: Prognosis in generalized peritonitis. *Arch Surg* 118:285-290, 1983.
21. Dellinger EP, Wertz MJ, Meakins JL, et al: Surgical infection stratification system for intraabdominal infection. *Arch Surg* 120:21-29, 1985.
22. Pitcher WD, Musher DM: Critical importance of early diagnosis and treatment of intraabdominal infection. *Arch Surg* 117:328-333, 1982.
23. Fry DE, Garrison RN, Heitsch RC, et al: Determinants of death in patients with intraabdominal abscess. *Surgery* 88:517-523, 1980.
24. Deveney CW, Lurie K, Deveney KE: Improved treatment of intraabdominal abscess. *Arch Surg* 123:1126-1130, 1988.
25. Spiegel CA, Malangoni MA, Condon RE: Gas-liquid chromatography for rapid diagnosis of intraabdominal infection. *Arch Surg* 119:28-32, 1984.
26. Solomkin JS, Meakins JL, Allo MD, et al: Antibiotic trials in intraabdominal infections: a critical evaluation of study design and outcome reporting. *Ann Surg* 200:29-39, 1984.
27. Solomkin JS, Dellinger EP, Christou NV, Mason AD: Design and conduct of antibiotic trials. *Arch Surg* 122:158-164, 1987.
28. Bohnen JMA, Solomkin JS, Dellinger EP, et al: Guidelines for clinical care: anti-infective agents for intraabdominal infection. *Arch Surg* 127:83-89, 1992.
29. Solomkin JS, Dellinger EP, Christou NV, Busuttil RW: Results of a multicenter

trial comparing imipenem/cilastatin to tobramycin/clindamycin for intraabdominal infections. *Ann Surg* 212:581-591, 1990.

30. Barie PS, Christou NV, Dellinger EP, et al: Pathogenicity of the enterococcus in surgical infections. *Ann Surg* 212:155-159, 1990.

31. Solomkin JS, Flohr AB, Quie PG, Simmons RL: The role of *Candida* in intraperitoneal infections. *Surgery* 88:524-530, 1980.

32. Drusano GL: Role of pharmacokinetics in the outcome of infections. *Antimicrob Agents Chemother* 32:289-297, 1988.

33. Zaske DE, Cipolle RJ, Strate RJ: Gentamicin dosage requirements: Wide interpatient variations in 242 surgery patients with normal renal function. *Surgery* 87:164-169, 1980.

34. Flint LM, Gott J, Short L, et al: Serum level monitoring of aminoglycoside antibiotics. Limitations in intensive care unit-related bacterial pneumonia. *Arch Surg* 120:99-102, 1985.

35. Gerding DN, Hall WH, Schierle EA: Antibiotic concentrations in ascitic fluid of patients with ascites and bacterial peritonitis. *Ann Intern Med* 86:708, 1977.

36. Lennard ES, Dellinger EP, Wertz MJ, Minshew BH: Implications of leukocytosis and fever at conclusion of antibiotic therapy for intraabdominal sepsis. *Ann Surg* 195:19-24, 1982.

37. Fry DE, Harbrecht PJ, Polk HC Jr: Systemic prophylactic antibiotics. *Arch Surg* 116:466-469, 1981.

6

Antibiotic Pharmacokinetics in Peritonitis

David E. Pitcher, MD and Donald E. Fry, MD

The use of antibiotics has become an important aspect of the treatment for patients with peritonitis. The selection of antibiotics for treatment has primarily focused upon the antimicrobial spectrum of the drug that is chosen. Toxicity of the agent has been a secondary, but important consideration. However, as is illustrated by the prevalent use of aminoglycoside antibiotics, physicians have accepted increased risks of toxicity in the interest of achieving a comprehensive coverage profile.

One area of antibiotic use that has received little attention has been antibiotic pharmacology.[1] Antibiotics are customarily administered in a manner consistent with recommended dosing schedules. Unfortunately, these dosing schedules are determined by the pharmacological profile of the drug in healthy volunteers or in minimally-ill patients.[2,3] The critically-ill patient with peritonitis is not used as a study subject.

It is the fundamental premise of this presentation that the failure to study antibiotics in the septic surgical patient with peritonitis may result in inappropriate treatment of patients. Inappropriate antibiotic regimens potentially result in the greater risk of inadequate therapy rather than the general fear of antibiotic toxicity.[1,2,4] Indeed, failure of antibiotic therapy in the peritonitis patient may be more commonly related to pharmacologic considerations rather than inadequate spectrum.

From Fry DE, (ed): *Peritonitis.* Mount Kisco NY, Futura Publishing Co., Inc., © 1993.

The Multicompartment Model of Pharmacokinetics

Clinical pharmacologists have found it desirable to develop methods to quantitatively define the degree of drug distribution throughout the body. These quantitative methods provide both the scientist of pharmaceuticals and the clinician using the drugs in patients with a means to compare antibiotics and other drug agents with each other.

Traditional teaching in drug pharmacology has used the one-compartment model to describe the distribution and clearance of pharmaceutical agents. The one-compartment model has basically used the concept that the distribution of a given drug occurs universally across the water volume to which it is accessible. Drugs may have access to the intracellular water volume or they may not, but distribution is uniform within the water volume to which it has access. In the one-compartment model, descriptions of measured drug clearance from the plasma would be representative of clearance from all water in which the drug is distributed. While a simplified concept that may actually apply for some small number of drugs, it suffers from the fundamental flaw that most drugs have a more complex distribution.[1,2,5-9] A more appropriate theoretical framework for understanding drug distribution is the two-compartment model. The two-compartment model identifies that plasma distribution and clearance may occur in an independent fashion from tissue concentrations. Drug concentrations may be greater or less in the tissue compartment than concomitant concentrations within the plasma.[1,2]

Figure 1 illustrates the relationship between the plasma and peripheral compartments. Absorption or uptake of the drug following administration results in increasing plasma, or central pool, concentration of the drug. The drug is then distributed from the central pool into the peripheral tissues at a rate that is described as K_1. As drug concentration within the tissues increases, then equilibration between the two compartments will occur. The rate of efflux from the tissues back into the central pool is described as K_2. The relationship between K_1 and K_2 determines whether net drug is moving into the tissues or net drug is moving out of the tissues and back into the central pool. In general terms, net drug moves from the central pool and into the tissues when the central pool concentration is greater than the tissue concentration. When metabolism or excretion of the drug from the central pool results in lower

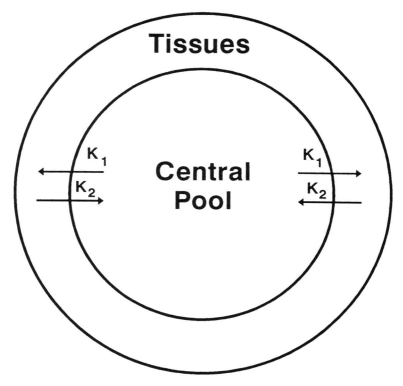

Figure 1: Illustrates the two-compartment model of drug distribution. Movement of the drug from the central pool into the tissues is governed by the constant K_1 while the return movement back into the central pool is governed by the constant K_2.

central pool concentrations, then movement of drug is away from the tissue and back into the central pool.

In reality, the tissue distribution of a drug in the two-compartment model is the biological summation of drug uptake by the multiple different tissues, each of which may have separate distribution constants. Thus, a given drug may have much greater access to one tissue, but is quite effectively excluded from another.[2,5-7] In essence, the two-compartment model is actually a multicompartment model. The multicompartment model is illustrated in Figure 2.

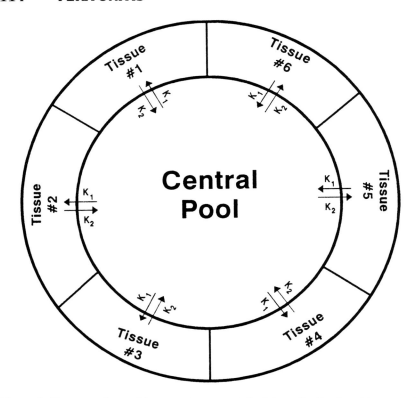

Figure 2: Illustrates the multicompartment model of drug distribution. Movement of the drug into each separate tissue compartment is governed by separate K-values.

An example of the different distribution characteristics of a given drug among different tissues is best illustrated by examining the cephalosporin antibiotic cefazolin. It is a highly protein-bound drug and is principally distributed within the extracellular water of the body. It is concentrated many times over its serum concentration within the bile, obviously reflecting an active transport mechanism by the hepatocytes in excreting the antibiotic. There are essentially no concentrations of the drug that are achieved within the cerebrospinal fluid of the central nervous system. Concentrations within the subcutaneous tissue fluids are less than serum concentrations, but do have a linear relationship with the central pool, albeit at a lesser degree of magnitude. The summed movements among all tissues can be expressed as a single tissue concentration, but actually repesent the multiply different contributions from each tissue.[1,10]

Numerous variables are responsible for the different distributions of a given antibiotic among different tissues.[1,2,5-9] The electrical charge and the size of the antibiotic molecule itself will influence tissue penetration.[5-7] The intrinsic lipophilic or lipophobic character of the molecule will clearly affect fat penetration and will likewise affect the equilibration of a drug with the central pool when a given tissue has a high fat content.[5,6] The quantitative blood supply considerations will be important since well vascularized organs will have a more rapid distribution of the drug and will generally have an equilibration that mimics the one-compartment model of drug distribution.[5,6] Poorly vascularized tissues such as mature human bone will take up the antibiotic from the central pool very slowly.[5-7] Accordingly, significant excretion of the administered antibiotic will have occurred from the central pool for many drugs, and peak concentrations within the bony tissue will not be achieved. Finally, the degree of protein binding of the drug will be quite important since a high degree of protein binding restricts the drug to the extracellular water and particularly to the intravascular water volume.[1,2,5-9,11]

Pharmacokinetics

It is important to understand that the relationship between the central pool concentration and the concentration of the antibiotic within the tissues is a constantly changing and dynamic process.[2,7] The process is constantly changing because the excretion or elimination of the drug is in a dynamic flux with the central pool concentration that is changing the tissue concentration. To understand the complex circumstances of peritonitis, it is essential to understand drug clearance or elimination under normal circumstances.

From the minute that an administered antibiotic dose arrives within the central pool, the elimination phase of the drug begins. Drug elimination is achieved by either hepatic metabolism, hepatic elimination into the bile but without transformation or metabolism of the drug, or by renal clearance.[2,5-9] Most antibiotics have a solitary mechanism for excretion. The drug may be metabolized by the liver or excreted by the kidney without any metabolism. Some drugs may actually have mixed elimination routes. For example, cefotaxime is metabolized by the liver, but is also excreted by the kidney.

The pharmacokinetics of drugs in the central pool are generally described in terms of the peak serum concentration, the biological elimination half-life, and the volume of distribution.[1,2,5-9] The peak serum concentration is dictated by the rapidity of drug administration into the central pool (Figure 3). Thus, orally administered drugs have low peak concentrations, intramuscularly administered drugs have somewhat higher peak concentrations, and intravenously administered antibiotics will have very high peak concentrations. Drugs given by a rapid intravenous push will have the highest peak concentration of all.[5,6]

When antibiotics are given intravenously, the peak serum concen-

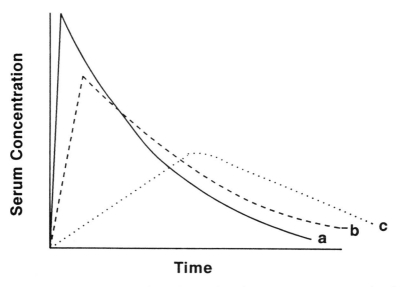

Figure 3: Demonstrates a nonlogarithmic plot of serum concentrations after the administration of the same drug via different routes. Curve a is an intravenous administration that has a higher peak concentration, but is cleared from the serum faster. Curve b is an intramuscularly administered dose, which takes longer to reach the peak concentration, but the drug persists within the serum for a longer period of time than the intravenously administered drug. Curve c is an orally administered dose. The peak concentration is lower and requires a longer period of time to be reached. The drug persists for a longer period of time in serum.

tration rapidly declines over the ensuing several minutes as equilibration into the various tissue compartments occurs. After this equilibration, an equilibrated peak concentration is achieved. This equilibrated peak concentration then leads to the clearance phase of the drug. The clearance phase reflects the reduction in serum concentration as a reflection of drug elimination or metabolism.[1,5,6]

The clearance of antibiotics from the central pool is best described by the biological elimination half-life ($T_{1/2}$). The $T_{1/2}$ is that period of time necessary for the serum concentration to decline by 50%. By plotting the serum clearance as a function of the $\log_{10}$ of the serum concentration against time, the resultant plot assumes a linear relationship. Thus, the clearance curve data for intravenous administration that is identified in Figure 3, become a straight line in the semilogarithmic plot of Figure 4. A reduction by 50% of any concentration on this linear plot occurs at the rate of $T_{1/2}$ regardless of the concentration point selected. Thus, the period of time necessary for a serum concentration to decline from 50 µg/mL to 25 µg/mL of a given antibiotic is the same time for the decline from 4 µg/mL to 2 µg/mL. An understanding of $T_{1/2}$ becomes very important with respect to future discussions of selecting dosing intervals.

By using the linear semilogarithmic plot of antibiotic clearance from the serum, the volume of distribution (V_d) of an antibiotic can be calculated. The volume of distribution is an estimate of how the drug is distributed throughout the body. The volume of distribution is that volume of body water in which an antibiotic would be present at the maximum equilibrated peak concentration assuming no metabolism and no excretion. As is illustrated in Figure 4, the linear clearance of the drug from the serum is extrapolated to time 0. This time 0 extrapolated concentration when combined with the known total amount of drug that was administered to the patient permits calculation of the V_d.[2,5-7]

For example, if a 1-gram (1000 mg) dose of an antibiotic is administered and the extrapolated time 0 concentration is 50 mg/L (50 µg/mL), then the V_d can be calculated by

> Administered dose/Time-zero concentration
> =1000 mg/50 mg/liter
> =20 liters

If the theoretical patient who received the antibiotic had a body weight of 70 kg, such a person would have an estimated total body water of 42

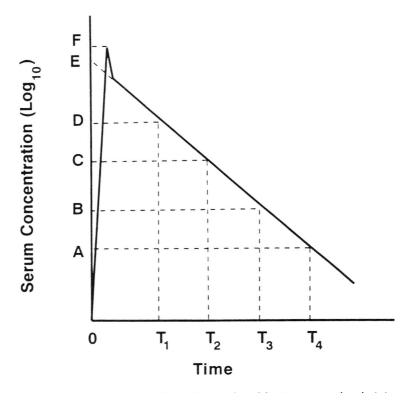

Figure 4: Demonstrates the semilogarithmic plot of the intravenously administered drug from Figure 3. After equilibration following the peak concentration (point F), clearance assumes a linear configuration. Point E is the time 0 extrapolated concentration and is the concentration that is used to compute the V_d. Concentration C is one half of concentration D. The time for the concentration to decline from D to C is T_2-T_1. Thus, the time interval from T_1 to T_2 is the $T_{1/2}$. The $T_{1/2}$ is constant along the linear clearance portion of the curve. Concentration A is one half of B, and T_4-T_3 is again the $T_{1/2}$.

L and an estimated extracellular water volume of 14 L. Thus, a V_d for a given antibiotic that is 20 L probably has a degree of penetration into the intracellular water compartment.

V_d is a theoretical calculation and must be interpreted carefully. The V_d can actually be calculated as a volume that is larger than the patient's entire water volume. Binding of an antibiotic to receptors within cells or within tissues will result in the time 0 extrapolated concentration being less than if the drug were totally dissolved in body water. Despite some of the special problems of V_d, it is a useful calculation that becomes very important in the determination of what dose of a drug can be used in a patient to achieve adequate, but not excessive serum and tissue concentrations for desired therapeutic effects. When one examines the pathological pharmacokinetic changes that attend peritonitis, changes in V_d are significant but are seldom considered by the clinician in adjusting dosing schedules of antibiotics or other pharmaceutical agents.[1,2,11-14]

A final consideration in antibiotic pharmacokinetics is protein binding.[2,15] Antibiotics are bound to serum proteins in varying degrees. Some drugs are highly protein bound to a level of 90% or more of administered drug. Others are minimally bound. As noted earlier, protein binding obviously affects the V_d of an antibiotic in that highly bound drugs are restricted to the water domain of the serum proteins.[5-7] Another important consideration in protein binding is whether antibiotic activity is attenuated by binding. This is a complex question and obviously depends upon the affinity of protein binding versus the affinity of target receptor binding upon the pathogenic bacteria. The clinical effectiveness of the highly protein-bound antibiotics would imply that dissociation of the drug from the serum protein to achieve drug effect is what occurs in the clinical scenario. In general, antibiotic binding is not given much consideration in antibiotic selection, although that certainly does not mean that this is an unimportant issue.

In summary, the design of the dosage regimen for a given antibiotic is to give sufficient drug so that therapeutic concentrations can be maintained for a defined period of time prior to the administration of the next dose. The amount of drug that is given is dictated by the V_d and is sufficiently great to achieve the maximum possible concentration without reaching toxic concentrations of the drug. The $T_{1/2}$ of the drug then dictates the total time necessary for the drug to be eliminated and for concentrations to drop below the minimum therapeutic concentration required for drug effect. Thus, the V_d and toxicity considerations dictate drug dose, and peak achievable concentrations and the $T_{1/2}$ govern the dosage interval.

Pharmacology of Peritonitis

As has been emphasized previously, enormous changes in the patient's circulatory dynamics attend severe peritonitis. Pertinent physiologic and biochemical changes include increased cardiac output, reduced total systemic vascular resistance, altered capillary permeability, and "third spacing" of total body water. These pathophysiologic changes mean that the pharmacology of therapeutic drugs must be significantly altered.[2,3]

Previous studies have demonstrated that the V_d of the critically ill,[3,11-13] the trauma patient,[13] and patients with peritonitis[12,13] is dramatically expanded for most drugs that have been studied. The expanded water volume necessary for the resuscitation and support of the peritonitis patient means that V_d must be increased. The impact of doubling the V_d is illustrated in Figure 5. For a given dose of drug, the peak equilibrated concentration will be reduced by 50%. If one assumes that the $T_{1/2}$ is constant (which may not be true), the reduced peak equilibrated concentration means that serum concentration will drop below the critical therapeutic threshold at one $T_{1/2}$ earlier than would have otherwise been the case.

Considerable evidence also suggests that the $T_{1/2}$ changes with the stress and septic response.[2,11] The hyperdynamic response and potential hyperperfusion of the excretory mechanism may accelerate drug elimination and actually reduce the $T_{1/2}$. A corticomedullary redistribution of blood flow within the kidney has been postulated in the septic response, and results in the paradox of a relatively reduced flow to the cortex of the kidney, but hyperperfusion of the medullary portion. With juxtamedullary and medullary portions of the kidney being responsible for drug secretion, secreted drugs (eg, gentamicin) may have secretion accelerated and the $T_{1/2}$ reduced.[16-19]

Gentamicin has been the antibiotic that has been most frequently studied under conditions of critical illness and the septic response.[4,11-13,16-21] These data have demonstrated enormous variation in the pharmacokinetics of gentamicin. These data indeed have shown that the V_d is expanded, but that the $T_{1/2}$ is highly variable. It would appear that younger patients with high cardiac output and normal renal function are capable of very rapid excretion of the administered dose such that 3–5 times the recommended dose of gentamicin are necessary to achieve therapeutic concentrations. The hyperperfusion of the medullary portion of the kidney in the hyperdynamic septic state likely reduces the $T_{1/2}$ in the younger patient with normal renal function. In contrast, older patients with compromised renal function and a limited hyperdynamic response may require less than one half of the 3–4 mg/kg per day of gentamicin dosing.[21]

7

Adjunctive Surgical Treatment in the Management of Severe Peritonitis

J. David Richardson, MD

The surgical treatment of peritonitis remains as the foundation of all therapeutic modalities for this problem. While an increasing number of conditions that once were the domain of the surgeon are now treated by medical or other nonsurgical means, the diagnosis and treatment of peritonitis remains essentially always surgical (except in those relatively unusual cases of "primary peritonitis"). If one examines the results of treatment of peritonitis over the past 50 years on a "disease-for-disease" or "operation-for-operation" basis, the results have been extraordinary. Appendicitis, which frequently caused deaths until the middle of this century, now has a dramatically lower mortality and morbidity. The majority of the deaths from appendicitis today occur in the very elderly or the immunocompromised patient. Similarly, the reported mortality for diverticulitis has decreased dramatically even while "more radical" therapy such as one or two-staged operations have largely supplanted the older three-stage procedure. Despite the unquestioned improvement in many of the once potentially lethal causes of peritonitis such as appendicitis, diverticulitis, acute cholecystitis, or perforated ulcer, the morbidity and mortality from peritonitis remains quite high.[1] While it is often difficult to garner good mortality rates for conditions causing peritonitis (simply because few reports on "peritonitis" per se are writ-

From Fry DE, (ed): *Peritonitis.* Mount Kisco NY, Futura Publishing Co., Inc., © 1993.

ten) it seems clear that the mortality for this condition is high even as the 21st century approaches.

The reasons for this continued high mortality are several. Most countries with modern systems of medical care have an advancing population age that often renders patients poor candidates for treatment of complicated problems such as peritonitis. In the United States, the most rapidly growing segment of our population is that group aged 80 and older. These patients generally tolerate elective operations quite well, but often do not tolerate prolonged illnesses as may be engendered by severe peritonitis whatever the cause. Secondly, a variety of difficult operations are now frequently undertaken that would not have been contemplated one or two decades ago. The pancreatico-duodenectomy, once regarded as a rare tour de force for the tertiary teaching institution, is commonly performed in community hospitals. Although gastric operations have dramatically declined, operations for inflammatory bowel disease utilizing techniques such as ileo-anal pouches have burgeoned in frequency and are the cause for an occasional postoperative problem. Thirdly, we see patients who are victims of injury who now die of or with peritonitis, who would not have survived their initial surgery in the past. Better resuscitation, improved operative technique, better ventilatory care, and overall improved intensive care have created a patient population of patients with peritonitis that did not exist several decades ago. Thus, the focus of this chapter will be on these difficult problems in which adjunctive procedures might be helpful rather than on the patient with straightforward peritonitis that can be treated by standard surgical means.

Diagnosis

The diagnosis and treatment of peritonitis remains one of the primary tasks of the surgeon and despite the development of a myriad of technological advances, the principle tools used are long-standing and relatively straightforward. Physical examination remains the keystone of diagnosis of peritonitis although other diagnostic modalities have gained acceptance, particularly in the evaluation of complicated patients such as the young, the elderly, patients with altered consciousness, or those who are immunocompromised. The diagnosis of peritonitis is not the thrust of this chapter, but the role of diagnostic peritoneal lavage (DPL) in diagnosing peritonitis will be discussed because of its important adjunctive use in the patient who may not be able to be evaluated by traditional physical examination.

The majority of patients with suspected peritonitis, who have not undergone previous operation can be diagnosed by the traditional methods of physical examination with or without the use of standard plain radiological views of the abdomen and basic laboratory tests. In an awake, alert patient who is able to cooperate with a physical examination, the presence of abdominal tenderness, muscle guarding or rigidity, and rebound tenderness usually will be diagnostic of peritoneal irritation. Auscultation for bowel sounds is generally not helpful, although the absence of intestinal activity might further heighten the suspicion of peritonitis. Plain abdominal films may be used in a correlative fashion in patients in whom the diagnosis is in doubt, but are not generally required if the patient has unequivocal signs of peritoneal irritation. The presence of extravisceral gas or "free air" is a classic plain radiological sign that would prompt urgent operation, but most patients with this finding have an impressive abdominal examination as well. Other radiological signs such as a distended loop of intestine ("sentinel loop"), obscure psoas shadow, gas in the biliary tree or along the psoas muscle, or the presence of a "ground glass" appearance suggesting excess fluid, or the presence of an appendiceal fecalith may be useful adjunctive radiological signs in the evaluation of peritonitis.

Routine laboratory studies should include a complete blood count with a differential leukocyte determination, a urinalysis, and an amylase. Other tests such as electrolyte determination may be needed depending on the clinical situation but are not helpful in the diagnostic evaluation of peritonitis. The use of more sophisticated tests such as a computed tomography (CT) scan is generally not required in the initial evaluation of patients with peritonitis who are admitted in an ambulatory setting. However, in the complicated patient who has an equivocal diagnosis or has suspected peritonitis following a perineal abdominal operation, the CT scan may be invaluable. The use of CT scans in this context is discussed elsewhere.

As mentioned previously, the diagnosis of peritonitis is generally straightforward. However, as the population ages and patients are treated with new modalities, situations now commonly arise where peritonitis is suspected but cannot be diagnosed by traditional means such as physical examination and basic laboratory tests. Patients who are particularly difficult to examine may fall into one of several categories as shown in Table 1.

Table 1
Diagnostic Dilemma in Peritonitis

Patient Category	Comment
• Extreme advanced age (nursing home patient patient found unresponsive from unknown cause)	May be unable to cooperate with examination; peritoneal signs may be diminished even with established peritonitis
• Neurologic impairment -previous stroke or head injury -severe mental retardation -drug overdose, heavy medication, or sedation -mental illness -previous paraplegia	Abdomen often unable to be evaluated. These patients may have fever, abdominal distension, positive blood cultures suggesting peritonitis. Particularly prone to other confounding problems such as pneumonia, urosepsis, infected decubitus ulcer, etc.
• Severely ill from other cause -ICU patient with suspected problem -renal, lung, or cardiac transplant patient -post-open cardiac surgery with complications	Peritonitis from a variety of causes common in critically-ill patients. May be difficult to diagnose due to need for sedation, pain medication, or ventilator that hampers communication, etc.

Patients may be difficult if not impossible to evaluate regarding the potential for peritonitis for a variety of reasons. Not uncommonly, our general surgical unit is called to evaluate patients who are elderly who have some abdominal findings worrisome for an intra-abdominal inflammatory problem. These patients may have come from other institutions such as nursing homes and have been referred simply because they are critically ill without a readily obtained diagnosis. On other occasions, the patient may have a nonspecific abdominal finding such as distension which prompts a surgical evaluation. The diminished inflammatory response often seen with the elderly may lead to a normal leukocyte count even with established peritonitis.

A second group of patients who are difficult to evaluate are those with previous neurologic impairment. This neurologic impairment may occur as a result of various problems all of which renders abdominal examination difficult at best. These patients also are prone to other problems such as fever, leukocytosis, abdominal distension due to urosepsis, or pneumonia that may confound the diagnosis. A third subset of patients who are difficult to evaluate are those who are critically ill from other causes. The patient who has undergone a coronary artery bypass grafting 2 weeks previously but has suffered complications and is still on the ventilator when he develops questionable abdominal signs of peritonitis is a major problem in diagnosis. This patient may not be able to communicate adequately, may have multiple reasons to explain the findings that prompted the evaluation, and certainly would represent a poor candidate for a negative or nontherapeutic exploratory laparotomy. In such a patient, we have found the use of DPL to be an extremely useful adjunct in the diagnosis or exclusion of peritonitis.

Our unit previously reported on the value of DPL in the evaluation of peritonitis.[2] Our personal experience with this technique for peritonitis now exceeds 500 cases and has been extremely reliable. The indications for the procedure would be in patients who present diagnostic dilemmas as outlined in Table 1 who have sufficient concern that they might have peritonitis to warrant consideration of operation. Contraindications to the procedure might include previous abdominal operations (particularly with a full midline or bilateral subcostal incision); findings sufficiently diagnostic of peritonitis to warrant surgery; and the presence of other problems or situations that would preclude definitive operation or make it unwise. The technique of DPL is the same as that used in the routine trauma patient, ie, the use of an infraumbilical approach with either the open or closed technique. The closed technique using the Seldinger principle has been shown to provide results equal to that of the open DPL in a randomized trial[3] and it is particularly useful in evaluating critically-ill patients. We infuse nearly a liter of fluid in the average-size adult and send the effluent for cell count. Patients with intestinal necrosis often have a dark, bloody fluid that is present immediately upon catheter insertion. The majority of the "positive" tests have leukocytosis present in the effluent. We have used 500 leukocytes per cubic millimeter as a "positive test" and have recommended surgery as we would for a trauma patient. The rate of positive DPL has continued fairly constant in the total series of over 500 patients as it did in our previous report. Approximately 30% of these examinations are positive. The findings causing the positive DPL include the commonly diagnosed reasons for peritonitis including perforated viscera at all levels, appendicitis, diverticulitis, acute cholecystitis, and intestinal infarction or necrosis. This latter problem is particularly common in the elderly. An occasional patient is encountered with a positive DPL who has a nontherapeutic operation. Pancreatitis is the most common cause of this problem in our hands. Similar findings have been noted in cirrhosis with ascites or in patients with nonperforated diverticulitis that did not warrant resection.

"False negative" examinations (patients with major inflammatory problems in the abdomen without an elevated leukocyte count) have rarely occurred in our experience. We have encountered three patients who had a negative lavage and subsequently had a positive operation. In two of these patients the interval between the DPL and subsequent operation was many days. Ultrasonic evaluation of the gallbladder should be performed if calculous or acalculous disease is suspected. However, in most patients with cholecystitis who underwent a DPL, the test has been positive. Based on our extensive experience, our surgical group feels very comfortable that a patient with a negative DPL has a very small likelihood of having peritonitis.

Operative Strategies in Treatment of Peritonitis

Polk[4] has outlined the important elements of treatment of peritonitis. These are control of the infectious focus, proper resuscitation, and systemic antibiotics. Several others[5,6] have nicely outlined the principles of treatment strategies that we have found useful. These are outlined in Table 2.

Regardless of the diagnosis responsible for peritonitis, the most crucial element of treatment is elimination or effective control of the primary focus initiating the peritoneal infection or inflammation. One of the critical errors that our unit encounters in review of complicated cases of peritonitis is a failure to accomplish this basic tenet of therapy. Extreme care should be taken in cases of perforation present more than a few hours in having good tissue to close. The use of buttressing patches of omentum or other viable tissue should be considered when feasible. Any situation that results in a loss of integrity of the colon wall that leads to established peritonitis should cause strong consideration for a colostomy. While the use of primary colon repair has gained popularity following colon trauma, colostomy should be strongly considered if active inflammation is present, if the wound edges are not healthy appearing, or if there is any concern about the integrity of the colonic wound closure.

Table 2
Operative Strategies for Treatment of Peritonitis

Initial Operation
- Eliminate source of primary contamination
  - Close perforations, resect necrotic tissue, divert as indicated, etc.
- Remove sources of secondary contamination
  - Thoroughly explore the abdomen, treat interloops, pelvic, lateral gutter, and subdiaphragmatic collections
  - Debride loose collections of purulence that are readily removable
- Drain established abscess or potential spaces only
- Thoroughly irrigate the abdominal cavity
- Primary fascial closure (provided fascia is healthy)
- Open treatment of skin and subcutaneous tissue

Secondary Operation(s)
- Verify source of primary contamination eliminated. If not, close, resect, divert, etc. (caveat: secondary closure of an intestinal perforation or failed anastomoses rarely succeeds)
- Establish drainage in areas of fistulae, anastomotic failure, or sources of ongoing contamination
- Avoid secondary injury to bowel or solid viscera (eg, spleen) Balance the need for complete exploration against the risk of secondary injury
- Consider open or semi-open management of the abdomen. Semi-open method uses mesh closure with material such as Marlex, PTFE, polyglycolic acid, etc.

At the time of the initial operation, a thorough and extensive evaluation of the abdomen must be performed. The surgeon must be as confident as possible when he/she leaves the operating suite that all problems have been detected or excluded and dealt with as completely as technically possible. Particularly in trauma cases, multiple sources of contamination must be considered. In nontrauma situations, the abdomen should be thoroughly explored if the source of peritonitis is not readily apparent. For example, periappendicitis must not be confused for the actual disease while failing to recognize a perforated ulcer with drainage into the right paracolic gutter.

After the primary problem has been treated, care should be taken to eliminate sources of secondary contamination. Areas of the abdomen that are prone to collection of purulent material should be investigated. Depending on the circumstances, the bowel may need to be evaluated for interloop abscess, but generally the infradiaphragmatic areas, pelvis, and pericolic gutters should routinely be at least manually explored to exclude an abscess.

Since the classic studies of Yates[7] reported in 1905, it has been recognized that the peritoneal cavity itself vigorously resists efforts at drainage. Within a few hours, the drain has usually been isolated from the generalized peritoneal cavity. However, if a defined abscess is present under the diaphragm or in the pelvis, this should be drained. Drainage of a potential space for a day or two even though no definite infection is present may also be beneficial. In this situation, elimination of blood or serum may be helpful in preventing a secondary infection. Few of the opinions held by individual surgeons regarding drainage are based on hard, scientific data or good clinical trials. Most of the experimental studies on drainage are highly contrived and bear little relevance to the clinical situation. Therefore, there is little justification for dogmatic statements regarding drainage. It is my opinion that drains should be used for a relatively short duration unless they continue to drain purulent material. Care should be taken to keep drains open as well. Studies have indicated that active drains are more effective than passive drains of the Penrose type. The use of passive drains and sump drains has the restricted disadvantage of promoting secondary contamination, but also the creation of a negative pressure that promotes bacterial ingress. Hard suction drains have the advantage of not being collapsed by surrounding tissue but are prone to erosion into viscera after a few days. If firm drains are used, the duration of drainage should be particularly short. Based on these aforementioned considerations, relatively brief use of drains of the soft, closed-suction type is preferred.

The use of irrigation of the peritoneal cavity is another frequently performed maneuver for which there is relatively "soft" scientific evidence. Rosato[8] found that the mortality from experimental peritonitis created by rendering a segment of bowel ischemic could be reduced from 100% to 35% with use of peritoneal irrigation. Additional studies[9,10] in murine and canine models demonstrated that peritoneal lavage at the time of operation decreased the mortality in treated animals. On the other hand, studies from Hau[11] and associates showed no improvement with peritoneal lavage in experimental murine peritonitis. The theoretic basis for irrigation in peritonitis was to dilute the number of bacteria present. In residency training, the dictum was, "Dilution is the solution to pollution." Clearly, bacterial dilution does occur with large volume irrigation. In addition to the dilution of bacteria, irrigation may well dilute inflammatory mediators. However, it is not clear whether this effect would be beneficial or harmful. Experimental work from Simmons' laboratory[12] has indicated that inflammatory cells which combat peritonitis function less effectively in a liquid milieu. No clinical data are available to determine whether this is true in human peritonitis. An additional theoretical concern regarding drainage is that purulence that is localized may be disseminated throughout the peritoneal cavity. In this regard, gravity and diaphragmatic motion probably disseminate bacteria more widely than irrigation.

Based on these considerations, I have relied less on copious irrigation recently than in the past. I attempt to thoroughly remove all purulence and necrotic material. I remove the fibrinous material that is easily removed and do not attempt to perform radical peritoneal debridement which will be discussed later. I am extremely careful when irrigating a confined abscess or infected collection, to not permit the irrigant to disseminate to other portions of the abdomen. I rarely use antibiotic irrigation which will be discussed later in the chapter.

Irrigation of the Abdomen With and Without Antibiotics in Peritonitis

The concept of improving the mortality of peritonitis by thorough irrigation and mechanical cleansing of the peritoneum is nearly a century old. In 1893, Nolan published a report on a single case of appendicitis with peritonitis in which irrigation was associated with eventual recovery. In 1905, Price reported a series of cases of peritonitis treated with irrigation. Since that time various experimental and clinical studies have explored and argued the relative merits of irrigation of the abdominal cavity in the treatment of peritonitis. A great deal of confusion has arisen in this field because of differing experimental models used to produce peritonitis, a variety of antibiotics have been used in the irrigants and often systemically as well, and because results from one type of model were often incorrectly extrapolated as producing benefit in a different clinical situation. In addition to simple intraoperative irrigation, there are at least three different adjunctive techniques concerning irrigation that have been proposed for the treatment of peritonitis. These include: (1) intraoperative irrigation of the peritoneum with antibiotics; (2) intraoperative irrigation of the peritoneal cavity with antiseptic solution; and (3) continuous postoperative lavage with antibiotic-containing solutions. Each of these adjunctive techniques will be discussed.

Intraoperative Antibiotic Irrigation
of the Peritoneal Lavage

If peritoneal irrigation improved results with peritonitis it seems logical that the addition of antibiotics might further improve results. Studies on the antibiotic irrigation of the peritoneal cavity can be divided into laboratory studies and clinical investigations. Both types of studies have inherent difficulties in comparing one report to another. With laboratory studies, differences in models and antibiotic regimens have varied widely, while clinical studies have rarely stratified patients according to their severity of illness.

Laboratory studies on antibiotic irrigation have yielded variable results. Smith[13] reported in 1973 that the addition of intraperitoneal cephalothin decreased the mortality from 100% to 10% in a canine model. Schumer[14] noted an identical improvement in mortality in a model using kanamycin irrigation. Our laboratory used a 1% cephalothin solution to treat peritonitis established in a rat model and found a reduction in mortality from 78% to 14%.[15] On the other hand, other investigators[11] could not improve on the results with the addition of cephalothin irrigation versus saline alone or with the addition of antibiotic irrigation versus systemic therapy alone.[8] Undoubtedly, many of their differences in results must depend on the level of inoculum used in the model. Other studies have questioned the safety of topical irrigation with povidone-iodine.

There have been a large number of papers written about the use of various lavage solutions in models of experimental peritonitis.[8-28] It is accurate to say that the results have been highly variable depending on the model used. There are clearly no "absolute truths" to be gleaned from the literature for despite the preponderance of data that appears to favor one approach, there is always at least one report that will contradict the positive findings of others. A summary of several frequently cited papers is presented in Tables 3 and 4. Despite the fact that the negative or contradictory papers are always present, there do seem to be several patterns or trends that emerge from the literature relating to lavage therapy for experimental peritonitis. These general trends which represent my personal interpretation of the literature in this field are listed in Table 5. Many of these general trends seem to mesh well with our clinical observations about the treatment of peritonitis. Saline lavage probably could be expected to be effective in situations where it could be used early to dilute the inoculum, but would be less effective when

Table 3
Value of Peritoneal Lavage in Experimental Peritonitis

Author	Animal Studied	Peritonitis Model Used	Lavage Solution Used	Method	Results
Hau[11]	Rat	Feces (gelatin capsule)	Saline and Cephalothin	Postimplantation isolated lavage	Both ineffective
Sleeman[20]	Mouse	E. coli and Hemoglobin	Saline and antibiotics	Postimplantation isolated lavage (8 + 12 hours)	Both improved outcome over control at 8 hours. Not effective at 12 hours.
Lally[9]	Rat	Feces (gelatin capsule)	Parenteral & antibiotic lavage (clindamycin & gentamicin)	Single lavage	Antibiotics better than control; however, lavage did not improve results over parenteral therapy
Rosato[8]	Dog	Isolated ischemic ileum	Saline alone no parenteral antibiotics	Large volume single lavage	Mortality reduced from 100% to 65%
Artz[23]	Dog	Fecal suspension	Saline and antibiotics	Early lavage (15 minutes)	Saline increased survival compared to antibiotics alone
Glover[18]	Dog	Fecal suspension	Saline	Late lavage	Ineffective
Schumer[14]	Guinea pig	Fecal suspension	Saline & kanamycin	Late lavage	Saline ineffective; kanamycin decreased mortality dramatically
Dobrin[34]	Rabbit	Fecal suspension	Systemic & local antibiotics in lavage (clindamycin & gentamicin)	Continuous 72-hour lavage	Lavage without antibiotics increased mortality; lavage with antibiotics reduced mortality in severe peritonitis
Perkash[21]	Rat	Fecal suspension	Saline & antibiotics	Intraoperative lavage	Antibiotics improved outcome
Stewart[22]	Rat	Fecal suspension	Saline & antibiotics with parenteral antibiotics	Intraoperative lavage	Lavage with antibiotics better than systemic antibiotics
Flint[15]	Rat	Feces (gelatin capsule)	Saline, cephalothin, & povidone-iodine	Intraoperative lavage	Combination of antiseptic and antibiotic most effective

135

Table 4
Value of Peritoneal Lavage in Clinical Reports

Author	# Patients. Studied	Anecdotal or Controlled	Cause of Peritonitis	Lavage Solution Used	Method	Results
Peloso[32A]	20	Anecdotal	Multiple	Saline & cephalothin	Operative & postop lavage	90% survival
Uden[35]	181 lavage; 188 nonlavage	Non-randomized trial in two hospitals	Perforated appendicitis	Balanced electrolyte solution & ampicillin	Postop lavage for 24 hours	No improvement with dialysis. Results were excellent in nonlavage so improvement would be difficult
Nomikos[10]	101	Randomized	Multiple	Saline vs. saline and chloramphen-icol	Intraoperative	No mortality difference but fewer septic complications in antibiotic group

Author	N	Study type	Condition	Lavage solution	Timing	Outcome
Stewart[16]	179	Surgeon preference; three groups	Appendicitis	No lavage; tetracycline lavage; noxythiolin lavage	Intraoperative	No significant difference but fewer intraabdominal septic processes in tetracycline group
Krukowski[17]	40	Trial (randomized)	Multiple	Saline alone or saline & tetracycline	Intraoperative	Saline decreased bacterial counts by dilution. Local antibiotics completely inhibited bacterial growth. Clinical correlates in outcome not reported
McKenna[31]	25	Anecdotal; compared results to historical controls	Multiple	Saline & kanamycin & penicillin	Postoperative continuous lavage	Improved mortality compared to historical controls
Stephen[32]	27	Anecdotal; compared to historical control	Multiple	Saline containing gentamicin, cephalothin & lincomycin	Postoperative lavage	Marked improvement compared to historical controls

137

Table 5
Lavage Therapy for Experimental Peritonitis: Possible Trends

1. Saline lavage as sole therapy appears to be beneficial in some models if used early, appears ineffective if used late.
2. Continuous lavage with saline alone appears not to be beneficial and may be harmful.
3. Antibiotic lavage appears in numerous studies to reduce mortality from peritonitis, particularly if systemic antibiotics have not been used.
4. The type of antibiotic appeared to make almost no difference in its beneficial effect.
5. If systemic antibiotics were used it was generally difficult for the antibiotic lavage to improve the outcome over systemic antibiotics.
6. Even in studies where mortality was improved by antibiotics or saline, abscesses were often present in the peritoneal cavity.

---

used in established peritonitis. Antibiotics used in a lavage solution were clearly beneficial in many models of peritonitis and often rendered dramatic improvements. However, when compared to animals receiving parenteral therapy, their effects were often less impressive. Finally, in some studies abscesses were present even in animals who survived the early insult which mimics the clinical experience. Thus, it may be that the value of antibiotic lavage lies not in its ability to mechanically or locally treat infection, but rather in the fact that this allows for systemic absorption of the drug.

In trying to assimilate these principles into clinical practice, there seem to be several lessons that appear reasonable. Intraoperative irrigation may be useful particularly in early peritonitis, but of lesser value in advanced disease. Antibiotics in the lavage are not likely to add much to therapy in patients with parenteral antibiotics administered.

Clinical studies on the use of antibiotic lavage during operation have been performed in several centers over the last thirty years. Artz and associates[23] compared the results of local irrigation with antibiotics including penicillin, kanamycin or chloramphenicol with systemic antibiotic therapy and could discern no difference in outcome. Other studies[26] showed that systemic antibiotics were more effective than those used locally with peritoneal irrigation. Noon and associates[27] performed a randomized study using kanamycin and bacitracin irrigation in 1967. While they were able to halve the wound infection rate, there was no difference between the rate of intra-abdominal abscess or mortality in the treated versus the control group. Later studies have produced similar findings.

There have been few studies on the use of peritoneal irrigation with the newer generation of antibiotics that are currently in use. There are numerous reasons for this fact. It appears that it is difficult to improve upon tissue levels of antibiotics over standard parenteral administration and additionally, there have been concerns about systemic toxicity from the rapid systemic absorption of drugs that have known toxicity. With the possible exception of treatment of peritonitis related to peritoneal dialysis catheters, antibiotic irrigation of the peritoneum is difficult to justify in our present treatment schemes.

Irrigation of the Peritoneum with Antiseptic Solution

The availability of safe and effective antiseptic solutions such as povidone-iodine stimulated an interest in the use of these agents for the treatment of peritonitis particularly during the decade of the 1970s. Several studies were conducted using povidone-iodine in experimental studies that purported to show a beneficial effect. Our laboratory examined the impact of irrigation with povidone-iodine on a model of peritonitis in rodents.[15] We compared saline controls with povidone-iodine with and without saline and with antibiotics. Povidone-iodine alone was not beneficial in improving mortality over the control group. Whereas the combination of intraperitoneal saline and povidone-iodine reduced mortality from 74% to 50% ($p < 0.05$), intraperitoneal cephalothin was much more effective in this model. In our model, povidone-iodine alone provided the greatest bacterial suppression at 3 hours, but rapid recurrence of intraperitoneal bacterial proliferation was noted by 6 hours. This is not surprising given the known mechanism of action of this antiseptic.

An additional study[28A] from that era confirmed the beneficial effects of povidone-iodine on experimental peritonitis with results that were similar to ours. However, one group reported that animals treated with povidone-iodine following cecal ligation had a higher mortality than untreated controls or animals subjected to lavage with a kanamycin solution.[29]

Anecdotal mention was sporadically made about the use of povidone-iodine as an adjunctive treatment measure in patients with peritonitis. The lack of overwhelming experimental benefit, concerns about toxicity, and the phenomenon of rapid bacterial proliferation after several hours have limited the use of this technique.

Continuous Postoperative Lavage With Antibiotics for the Treatment of Peritonitis

Just as antibiotic irrigation arose as a logical extension of saline lavage, the use of postoperative continuous peritoneal lavage has been studied in an attempt to mechanically remove bacteria, endotoxin and other mediators of the inflammatory response to peritonitis.[30] One of the first reports on the use of this technique was reported in Canada in 1970. McKenna and associates[31] studied the effects of continuous postoperative irrigation with saline plus antibiotics in 25 patients who were historically compared to a "matched" group of patients. These authors constructed drains with multiple perforations and inserted them into each upper quadrant for the instillation of fluid and into each lower quadrant for its removal. Penicillin and kanamycin were added to the solution being infused. They noted a reduction in mortality of 40% in the antibiotic treated group. These authors commented on the removal of "vasoactive amines" (long before they could be reliably measured) and postulated that their removal seemed to stabilize some of their septic patients. The use of continuous peritoneal lavage without antibiotics in the treatment of severe pancreatitis has been shown to have a similar ameliorating effect of hemodynamics in stability even through eventual outcome may not be improved. One could speculate that the beneficial effects of such therapy, if they are real, might be due more to the lavage itself removing inflammatory mediators than to the antibiotics which have been added.

In 1979, Stephen and Loewenthal[32] reported on a series of 27 patients treated in Australia for peritonitis using continuous peritoneal lavage. These authors treated a group of patients at high risk of death from peritonitis, ie, hypotension less than 100 mm Hg; multisystem organ failure with peritonitis; the presence of intraperitoneal feces, or anastomotic dehiscence causing peritonitis. Their patients had standard operative therapy followed by continuous, postoperative lavage with an antibiotic-containing solution through large drains placed at operation. The drains were placed in the hepatorenal pouch, subsplenic area, and the pelvis. The patients were treated with parenteral gentamicin sulfate, cephalothin sodium, and lincomycin; these same antibiotics were also administered by lavage for 72 hours. The authors compared their results to a larger historical control group that were treated within the same decade. The mortality in the control group was 48% (33 of 68) while the death rate in 27 lavage treated patients was 22% (6 of 27). Unfortunately, neither of the aforementioned reports had concurrent controls and no real details are presented that would allow for a stratification of patients according to the severity of their disease. Equally, unfortunately no large series of randomized patients has been studied since these reports.

In an excellent review article, Leiboff and Soroff[33] reviewed the world's literature dealing with the treatment of generalized peritonitis by closed postoperative peritoneal lavage (CPPL).[16,34-36] The authors reviewed 39 studies on the subject including 4 randomized, prospective studies; 8 nonrandomized comparative studies; and 27 noncomparative studies. Two of the four randomized studies involved treatment of peritonitis arising from appendicitis and obstetrical/gynecological origin. There were 2,746 patients in the collected series treated with CPPL who had a combined mortality of 13.4%. In the 648 patients not receiving CPPL (gleaned from various comparative trials) the mortality was 22.1%. The authors correctly noted that the patients would have to be similarly stratified for this difference to be meaningful. When the authors examined randomized trials there appeared to be a mortality difference favoring the use of CPPL—13.7% mortality in CPPL group versus 23.1% death rate in the nonlavage group. However, when only patients stratified for severity of illness were included, this difference in mortality decreases to 4.4% between the treated and the untreated groups. To put the value of CPPL even further into question, when the patients with appendicitis were eliminated from comparison, the difference in mortality between CPPL patients and those receiving "standard" therapy was 22.6% versus 23.3%.

Leiboff and Soroff[33] further evaluated the conclusion of the various authors about the value of CPPL with the type of study conducted. In papers conducted along nonrandomized comparative lines, 6 of 8 papers were favorable to CPPL, 1 was unfavorable, and 1 was inconclusive. In noncomparative studies, 25 were favorable and 2 were inconclusive. These authors concluded that "it is unlikely that further noncomparative or nonrandomized studies will yield useful information. There remains a need for a large-scale, prospective, randomized study to evaluate closed postoperative peritoneal lavage."

It would appear results are dramatic enough in some anecdotal or noncomparative series that further trials using current antibiotics in a well-stratified population of critically-ill patients seem justified. The primary objection to this technique seems to rest in the observation that most attempts to drain the peritoneal cavity are futile after 24 hours. Compartmentalization of the abdomen and plugging of the drains occurs very early and certainly would appear to limit the effectiveness of this technique. Individual practitioners with a desperately ill patient could reasonably use this technique, but the lack of a well-controlled series should diminish great enthusiasm for this method. Hopefully, multi-institutional trials may study this mode of therapy more adequately.

Radical Peritoneal Debridement

The elimination or reduction of bacteria by the use of solute lavage, antibiotics, or an antiseptic were tried in an attempt to decrease the degree of contamination within the peritoneal cavity. Logically, it followed that the excision of bacteria-laden detritus might be beneficial. Although Hudspeth[37] states he began practicing "debridement" of the peritoneal cavity in 1963 based on his empiric observations, scientific rationale for this technique was developed during a series of experiments performed in the 1970s primarily at the University of Minnesota.[12] These studies indicated that fibrin initially trapped bacteria as a protective mechanism to allow them to be managed by intraperitoneal host defense mechanisms. However, like many other protective mechanisms in biological systems, this bacterial trapping may have a potential downside in that bacteria may proliferate within this fibrin lattice. This phenomenon could theoretically lead to the development of abscesses or ongoing diffuse peritonitis. Thus, radical peritoneal debridement represented a logical maneuver to mechanically remove the fibrin, exudate, and trapped bacteria responsible for ongoing peritonitis.

As previously mentioned, Hudspeth[37] began to study the benefits of radical surgical debridement on patients with generalized peritonitis. He used a long midline incision from xiphoid to pubic and attempted to locate and control the source of peritonitis. Additionally, he placed a long tube to decompress the small bowel. This tube remained in place until at least 8 days after surgery. All abscess cavities were entered and purulent material was suctioned until removed. Peritoneal detritus, pseudomembranes, and exudates were then removed by suction, forceps or sponge debridement, or by gentle dissection. The peritoneal cavity was then irrigated with 1–10 L of saline. Hudspeth noted that this operation could be tedious and time-consuming with the average operation taking 3 hours. During the 11 years preceding his report in 1975, he treated 92 patients with this protocol. The source of peritonitis was varied; 32 of these patients had appendicitis and the remainder had a myriad of causes of peritoneal contamination. He noted that 92% of his patients had mechanical intestinal obstruction. Remarkably, all patients survived and few postoperative abdominal problems were reported.

Polk and Fry[38] performed a randomized trial comparing radical peritoneal debridement and standard operative therapy for peritonitis. The operative treatment outlined appeared similar to the technique used by Hudspeth, with the exception of the use of long intestinal tubes. Sixty patients were entered into the trial and 14 were excluded (usually because diffuse peritonitis was not encountered). These authors could detect no difference in outcome between patients undergoing peritoneal debridement and those who did not. There were seven deaths in each comparably sized group; five and six died from peritonitis in the debridement group and standard therapy group, respectively. Reoperations for peritonitis were virtually identical in the two groups. The outcome in the radical peritoneal debridement group was particularly poor in patients over 60 years of age in whom the mortality was 100%.

Thus, the concept of peritoneal debridement while theoretically attractive, does not appear to be able in all surgeons' hands to improve survival. Whether or not this operation is useful in selected patients is debatable, but based on its lack of efficacy in the only randomized trial of its use, it seems difficult to strongly advocate the use of radical peritoneal debridement.

Reoperation for Peritonitis

Treatment strategies that have been designed to be an adjunct to standard therapy for peritonitis include the use of reoperation or "relaparotomy". When reoperation is referred to in this section, it will be meant to construe a repeat exploration of the peritoneal cavity. There have been numerous papers written in the past two decades on the necessity for reoperation following abdominal exploration. From our institution, Harbrecht and associates[39] reported on the necessity for "early urgent relaparotomy" in 113 patients. Indications for early reoperation included infection (41 patients), anastomotic or organ disruption (17), dehiscence (14), bleeding (14), obstruction (13), and ischemia (6). This paper served to show that while reoperation for infection is the most common cause for reoperation, it is not the only one by any means and, in fact, constituted the indication for repeat laparotomy in far less than half of the patients so treated. Therefore, when reading the literature on the role of relaparotomy it is important to clearly delineate the precise indication for operation.

Reoperation for intra-abdominal infectious complications can take one of at least three forms, or roles, in treatment. Reoperation may be indicated by complications of operations, such as anastomotic disruption that may result in peritonitis but the operation itself is not done for peritonitis but for the complication itself. Obviously, these operations must be done to prevent further spillage of intestinal contents, to remove non viable organs or ischemic intestine, etc. The other indication for reoperation for peritonitis is to aid in infection control with the hope that multiple organ failure can be prevented or treated. In this context, reoperation may take the form of directed laparotomy or a nondirected reoperation. Directed relaparotomy is an operation that is generally clearly indicated. The patient generally has signs of infection and usually has positive signs that "direct" the need for operation and often provide a clue as to the source or site of the infection. Positive physical examination of the abdomen or diagnostic radiological evaluations are the common elements that lead to a directed relaparotomy. If a patient has fever and leukocytosis after an abdominal procedure, abdominal tenderness, and a positive CT scan consistent with an abscess, then reoperation should be performed rapidly. In this circumstance, there should be a high cure rate even though an abscess is present. In contradistinction to the above illustrated straightforward case, the other use of reoperation for potential abscess or diffuse peritonitis is the nondirected relaparotomy. The nondirected operation is usually performed in patients who appear septic or have organ failure. In this instance, there are often no positive indicators of peritonitis, ie, the abdominal examination is negative or equivocal, the CT scan is nondiagnostic, and the operation is driven by the desire to remove a septic focus that may be triggering the sepsis syndrome. Another variant of the nondirected laparotomy is in the patient who indeed has peritonitis but of the diffuse type where mechanical measures seem to offer little for its control. In the patient who does not have a drainable abscess or nonviable tissue to debride, the role of reoperation is of unproven benefit when applied to a large series of patients.

While the use of directed relaparotomy constitutes standard surgical therapy, the nondirected operation is controversial. One has only to review the results of reoperation for intra-abdominal infection presented by Bunt[40] on the two uses of reoperation to quickly discern the differences in the two approaches. Bunt referred to relaparotomy as "the high-risk, no-choice operation" and differentiated his institutional results into two groups: operation for (1) localized, intra-abdominal infection and for (2) nonlocalized systemic infection. The mortality for localized infection was 13% while that for diffuse peritonitis or systemic sepsis was 87%. Thus, while the issue favoring operation is clear for patients with a localized process, there are many surgeons who feel nondirected reoperations have no role in current practice. A historical perspective over the past 20 years is critical in understanding the rationale for the potentially beneficial role of the nondirected relaparotomy. In the mid 1970s, several reports[41-43] indicated that infection appeared to be the precipitating or proximate cause of remote organ failure that had burst on the intensive care unit scene with a vengeance. A review of these papers showed that infections from a variety of sources (eg, peritonitis, pneumonia, decubitus ulcers, and urosepsis) could cause multiple organ failure. However, the most commonly recognized inciting event appeared to be intra-abdominal infection.[44]

The importance of uncontrolled intra-abdominal infection as the potential "trigger" for the development of multiple organ failure was rapidly, and appropriately promulgated in the surgical literature. Polk and Shields[44] from our institution presented a small group of patients whose initial problem was organ failure that occurred as a result of "occult intra-abdominal infection." The notion that organ failure—whether of the single or multiple organ variety—results from unrecognized intra-abdominal infection has been an outstanding contribution from our department. Yet, the judgment of how to apply this very valid notion is often difficult. For several years in the late 1970s, our unit used nondirected laparotomy on practically all patients (with any chance of having peritonitis) who presented with organ failure. Occasional dramatic results were readily tempered by the continued high mortality in patients with diffuse peritonitis. Additionally, the risk of iatrogenic intestinal damage must be assessed when determining the risk:reward ratio for nondirected operations. Harbrecht, Garrison, and Fry[39] examined this issue in 42 patients who underwent relaparotomy for infection. The mortality was 51% and of the 20 survivors, 19 were felt to have benefitted from operation. Of the 22 nonsurvivors, 16 were felt not to have been harmed by operation. Six patients suffered some type of adverse technical outcome from operation and 5 of these died. Sinanan and associates[45] reviewed 100 laparotomies performed in 71 patients with a diagnosis intra-abdominal sepsis who were ill enough to be confined to the intensive care unit. These authors noted several trends that have confirmed our experience and that of others. First, they found that positive findings were encountered in a high percentage of patients whether the operation was a directed laparotomy or performed for the "sepsis syndrome" in a nondirected fashion. The positive findings were 89% and 80%, respectively. In this regard, it should be noted that this included patients who were undergoing initial operation as well as relaparotomy. Secondly, the authors reviewed the deleterious effects of septic shock on outcome and emphasized the importance of operation before systemic sepsis was apparent. If the sepsis syndrome was present, 90% of patients died, whereas the mortality was 55% when it was absent. In this regard, the mortality did not vary greatly between the directed and the nondirected group. Thirdly, the authors noted a 52% mortality for patients with a single abscess and 50% for multiple abscesses. This indicated that patients who could contain abscesses still had a meaningful salvage. However, all seven patients with diffuse peritonitis died.

Is there a role for nondirected relaparotomy at the present time? A review of the literature[39,45-55] on this subject consisting of over a 1,000 cases disclosed several trends that are outlined in Table 6. There are several situations in which nondirected laparotomy appears indicated. This approach would be particularly appropriate in the younger patient especially if he/she were a trauma victim. Schein[53] reviewed 551 collected cases of patients treated by planned relaparotomy with or without the abdomen being left open. He noted a mortality of 33% and felt the results were probably no better than those obtained by standard therapy. However, many of the patients reviewed were being treated for diverse conditions such as pancreatitis. In older patients with multiple organ failure or septic shock, the mortality is very high (about 60% to 80%) and no convincing case can be made that repeated planned relaparotomies improved outcome in this group. While there have been appeals[49] for randomized prospective trials to determine the utility of nondirected laparotomy, it is doubtful that therapeutic benefit would ever be conclusively demonstrated in any of these critically-ill subsets. However, the

Table 6
Role of Nondirected Relaparotomy: Current Trends

- The mortality from this procedure will be very high in patients over age 50 (with or without operation). Cumulative mortality greater than 80% as compared to overall mortality rates of 40% (range 20%–60%).
- Single abscess, when encountered, has a mortality of about 50% as opposed to the high mortality.
- Although performed less frequently in younger patients, (perhaps because they localize their disease better?) the yield is better and appears to be indicated in this subset of patients.
- Risk factors ↑ in addition to age and multiple organ failure include technical misadventures, intestinal ischemia, and cirrhosis.
- The detection of peritonitis even in the form of mechanically treated disease did not improve survival as much as might be expected. In several series, if bacteremia, septic shock, or multiple organ failure were present, the results were virtually identical in those with a positive (treatable) situation as with a negative or untreatable situation.
- The elimination of intraperitoneal bacteria by relaparotomy does not eliminate the continuation of the sepsis syndrome or necessarily decrease mortality.

fact that mortality may be high in this group does not obviate the need to diligently pursue treatable causes of peritonitis. Our unit continues to treat several patients annually who present with organ failure caused by occult abdominal sepsis, similar to those patients reported from Harborview in Seattle.[45] Our practice has been to be vigorous in pursuing initial laparotomy or even first relaparotomy in patients at risk for harboring occult intra-abdominal infection. However, multiple reoperations have generally proved futile unless the patient is collecting localized, drainable abscesses. Thus, our unit has used planned relaparotomy with much less frequency over the past decade.

Management of Peritonitis by the Open Abdomen Approach

Just as antibiotic irrigation of the abdomen arose as a logical extension of routine saline irrigation, the "open abdomen" approach arose as a logical extension of the multiple relaparotomy approach to the treatment of peritonitis. In essence, the logic was "why close the abdomen at all?"; "why not leave the abdomen open where we can even do dressing changes in the intensive care unit?" Several reports[54-68] dealing with this type of treatment were published in the late 1970s and numerous surgical units have now published their results with this technique (Table 7).

While the indications for open peritoneal drainage may have varied somewhat, in general, it was used for diffuse peritonitis that did not appear amenable to treatment with standard techniques. Matani and Tobe[59] outlined their indications for this procedure as being: (1) severe systemic manifestations of peritonitis; (2) ineffective drainage with the use of conventional procedures; and (3) extensive suppuration or necrosis of the deep layers of the abdominal incision. The majority of patients treated with this procedure in all series had either severe abdominal trauma, perforation of the gastrointestinal tract or anastomotic disruption.

The technique used for open peritoneal drainage has varied widely. Clearly the majority of these patients are treated in an intensive care unit and most required mechanical ventilation. If evisceration was possible, several authors used paralysis to allow the intestines to become adherent to surrounding structures to prevent evisceration. Generally, the abdomen was opened widely and thoroughly irrigated. Most investigators felt that diversion was a useful technique particularly for colon fistulae. However, several investigators have used enterostomies to divert small bowel fistulae as well. These ostomies are usually laterally placed away from the midline wound. If fistulae are present in the base of the wound, frequent dressing changes or suction drainage have been used to control the pooling of enteric contents. The method of managing the abdominal contents varied greatly. Some surgeons frequently returned their patients to the operating room for "more formal" exploration of the abdomen, while others treated the wound in the intensive care unit. The use of irrigation techniques with saline or povidone-iodine has been reported while others preferred to pack the wound with moist gauze.

A variety of techniques has been used to manage the wound itself. Basically, these techniques could be grouped into two types: those that packed the wound edges with gauze (either regular or lubricated) and those that use a more elaborate system for bowel protection (while leaving the abdomen readily available for irrigation and/or packing). Bradley and associates[63] reported on the use of a plastic intestinal bag or glove that was packed with gauze. This gauze edge was then exteriorized and the wound partially closed. Wound protectors have also been used. If closure was not feasible at all, then silastic was sewn to the wound edges.

Table 7
Open Abdomen Treatment of Peritonitis

Author	# of Patients	Specific Complications	% Mortality	Positive Results	Comments
Steinberg[61]	14	None	7	Yes	Very good results
Anderson[56]	20	Enteric fistula 25% Ventral hernia	60	No	Only half were rendered free of bacteria; results not better than historical control
Mastboom[60]	14	Spontaneous perforation of small bowel (not from mechanical injury)	64	No	Noted appearance of "perforations" that were not thought to be due to dressing changes, etc.
Metani[59]	13	Anastomosis disruption in one patient	7	Yes	Reoperation for abdominal wall reconstruction usually necessary
Duff[62]	18	Enteric fistula 27%	39	Yes	Skin graft eventually used to cover wound. All had abdominal hernias.
Bradley[63]	13	Enteric fistula 22%	23	Yes	Better results than closed drainage method with fewer complications & improved mortality

149

The results of open treatment have been difficult to assess (like many other adjunctive treatment measures) because careful stratification data have not been included. Most early reports on this technique were positive while more recent studies have been negative or noncommittal on its value. Reoperation has clearly been required in a large number of patients and has been facilitated by the open abdomen. Mortality figures have ranged from 7% to 60%, but clearly the patients in these two reports were not comparable. Steinberg[61] reported a 7% mortality but he placed wire sutures and "after 48 to 72 hours" . . . the previously placed wires are then tied, closing the abdominal wall." Clearly, the patients reported in most other series had fistula and severe peritonitis that would not have been amenable to this type of early abdominal wall closure.

In addition to the general complications typical of patients with severe peritonitis, there are several problems or complications that are inherent with the method of treatment. The early use of this technique may lead to evisceration that has prompted some surgeons to use paralysis early in the postoperative period. Concerns about abdominal wall integrity may also limit mobility of the patient. They may not move to a chair or ambulate as frequently as other patients with a closed abdomen. Obviously, some patients are so ill that sitting in a chair or walking is not feasible and this issue is moot. The major complication with the open drainage treatment is intestinal fistulization. The fistula rate in patients who have this method used for a significant period of time is 20% to 60%. The use of petroleum gauze, silastic sheets, or other types of protective dressings may limit or delay the fistula formation, but ordinarily this complication can be expected despite careful attention to the details of wound management. To the extent that the trade-off for the fistula is survival that would not otherwise be expected, then this complication can be accepted. However, in may cases the addition of a fistula (or commonly multiple fistulae) greatly escalates the nursing care involved, exponentially increases the projected recovery time, often obviates the use of the gastrointestinal tract for nutritional support, and decreases the chances for survival.

An additional problem with open treatment is that it may deprive the intestines of needed growth factors for healing and repair. The biological fact that intestinal wounds heal better in a "closed peritoneal environment" is often forgotten. Studies on healing intestinal anastomosis 40 years ago showed that wrapping the repair with a clear plastic wrap prevented healing. Presumably this wrapping prevented ingrowth of macrophages or limited exposure to growth factors necessary for healing. Virtually all reports on the open treatment note that anastomoses do not heal even when infection is controlled. Mastboom and colleagues[60] reported on the occurrence of 53 small bowel "perforations" in 14 patients treated by the open method. The authors stressed that these perforations were not believed to have occurred during operation. Although they felt these perforations could be caused by the mechanical trauma of dressing changes with gauze dressings, they believed other factors were related. This phenomenon has been noted in our unit and we have attributed the cause to mechanical injury with frequent dressing changes. However, it is my belief that the open method of treatment facilitates these spontaneous perforations because it does not allow for normal reparative processes of the intestinal wall to occur. Thus, we theorize that areas of bowel serosa which are dissected apart to treat the peritonitis develop areas of weakness that "perforate" when left open. If closure were feasible, healing of these areas might occur. Having treated large numbers of patients with both the open and the mesh closure method of closure of the abdomen, it is my belief that the use of mesh decreases the incidence of fistula formation and often allows for anastomotic healing.

Recovery following the use of the open method usually leaves the patient with a large wound hernia. As we have followed these patients, such wound hernias often become major problems and usually must be repaired. This is a reasonable price to pay for a living patient who would not otherwise have survived, but must be factored into the negative side of the equation when using the open treatment method. Because of the problems encountered many units have moved to the use of some type of semi-closed (or semi-open) method of treatment.

Treatment of Peritonitis by the Semi-Open or Mesh Method

The drawbacks of the "open" method including evisceration, intestinal fistula formation, need for ventilatory support, hinderance of mobilization, and large hernia formation. This leads to consideration of methods that preserved the advantages of the open method while controlling some of its problems. The unifying concept in this form of treatment is that some type of material is used to ensure abdominal wall integrity while allowing for relatively easy access into the peritoneal cavity. The most commonly used type of material has been polypropylene mesh Marlex® (C.R. Bard, Billerica, MA, USA). Marlex® provides excellent strength to the abdominal wall with prevention of evisceration and improved patient mobility. It can be surgically opened in the center of the mesh for ready access to the peritoneal cavity[48]. This defect can then be reapproximated with a running polypropylene suture. The use of Marlex® can be combined with a zipper[47,57] that allows for even easier access to the peritoneal cavity particularly if daily irrigations are performed in the intensive care unit. The use of zippers sutured directly to the abdominal wall has been reported as well. Wittman and associates[54] have reported extensively on the use of "etappenlavage" in which patients are returned to the operating room daily for wound exploration and generous lavage. The abdomen is closed between trips to the operating room by a Velcro[005] mechanism consisting of a hook and loop system that allows for variable tension on the wound as edema subsides and the wound contracts. A summary of several papers from different countries is included in Table 8.

Various authors report different methods of controlling intraperitoneal sepsis—irrigation versus packing either in the intensive care unit or the operating room. As indicated in the mortality data that cluster between 20% and 30%, it appears difficult to recommend one method of wound management to another. However, several reports on this semi-open or semi-closed method have scored or stratified patients and report a lower than predicted mortality. Garcia-Sabrio and associates[58] reported an actual survival of 22% instead of the expected 45%, while Wittman[57] had a mortality rate of 24% including an expected mortality that was much higher.

The problem with the use of Marlex® mesh occurs as the patient's abdominal situation is improved. Once granulation tissue becomes luxuriant, the mesh is frequently engulfed and fistula formation occurs if one attempts to remove the mesh from the granulating wound surface. While many authors discuss removal of the mesh with primary closure of the abdominal wall prior to this granulation phase, this is often very difficult.

With experience our unit has learned a great deal about the use of Marlex® in the management of severely contaminated abdominal wounds. First, it is not necessary to ever remove the Marlex® mesh as long as certain principles are followed. As the edema from the bowel subsides, the mesh should be tightened by trimming away the mesh in the center and suturing it taut over the viscera. If this is not done,

Table 8
Semi-Open or Mesh Techniques for Treatment of Peritonitis

Author	Means of Abdominal Closure	Means of Access	Peritonitis Treatment Technique	%Mortality	Comment
Voyles[48]	Marlex®	Opening in mesh (suture closed)	Return to operating room for wound exploration	14	Lowered rate of intestinal fistulae and hernias from that with closed technique
Hedderich[64]	Marlex®	Zipper	Daily treatment in ICU	20	Facilitated wound care
Gardia-Sabrido[58]	Zipper alone or zipper with Marlex®	Zipper	Daily treatment in ICU	22	Authors felt expected mortality should be 45% instead of observed 22%
Wouters[47]	Marlex®	Opening created in mesh	Re-exploration	20	Stressed use of drains as well
Wittmann[54]	Velcro slider ± Marlex® mesh	Velcro is opened	Return to operating room every 24 hours until improvement	24	"Etappenlavage" performed on 116 patients Predicted mortality (by APACHE/SIS scoring of 34%–93% decreased to 24%

wound contraction will cause a "buckling" of the mesh with ridges in it. Trimming of these ridges should never be done because of the high likelihood that intestinal fistula will occur. As the wound contracts and granulation tissue occurs, there is a temptation to skin graft the tissue over the Marlex®. This should be avoided because late problems of mesh extrusion can occur through the skin graft that can be difficult to manage. It is imperative that definitive wound closure be done with full thickness tissue such as mobilized skin flaps. If the abdomen needs to be reentered (for colostomy closure or other reasons), this should be delayed for many months and preferably for a year or more. Clinical clues can be used to guide reexploration as well. The wound should be stable, edema and inflammation of the wound edges should have long subsided, and the wound itself should have contracted significantly. Although Marlex[005] is frequently adherent to the bowel, the abdominal cavity itself may be relatively free of dense adhesions if the operation is properly timed.

Closure of the wound over Marlex® can be accomplished by ensuring that the wound is clean. Our unit utilized culture of wound biopsies to ensure that the wound is not heavily colonized. Topical antibiotics are frequently used in preparation for wound closure. Mobilization of thick skin flaps above the fascial level lateral to the wound will usually allow for tension-free skin closure. Myocutaneous flaps are not necessary. Once adequate mobilization of skin flaps has occurred, the wound is closed over large suction drains. The wound may appear erythematous but should not be opened unless definite signs of infection are present. If infection does occur, the wound should be minimally opened and packed. In this manner, the wound can then heal over the Marlex® in the depths of the wound.

Summary

Since the beginning of this century with Yates' studies[7] on peritoneal drainage there has been intense interest in adjunctive surgical measures to treat peritonitis. While simple irrigation of the peritoneal cavity is probably beneficial, antibiotic irrigation has been of questionable benefit. Numerous nonrandomized, noncomparative studies have claimed benefit but randomized trials are few and demonstrate questionable value. Postoperative peritoneal lavage has shown intriguing promise in several studies but has not been effectively randomized for serious disease. This is one area where a randomized, clinical trial might be in order.

Radical peritoneal debridement seems to have been ineffective in a randomized prospective series[38] and is not indicated except in special circumstances (eg, extensive fibrinopurulent material in a young, good-risk patient).

Planned relaparotomy has yielded conflicting results but like many other modalities, its initial promise has dimmed somewhat with broad application. It seems clear that directed relaparotomy is indicated and that initial consideration of the abdomen as the source of sepsis in a patient who presents with organ failure is clearly justified. The role of nondirected relaparotomy for multiple organ failure is not warranted when broadly applied.

The use of the open method of peritoneal drainage allowed for peritonitis control in many patients but was accompanied by many management problems and complications. The addition of a means of providing abdominal continuity although the use of Marlex® with frequent lavages or abdominal explorations seems to have decreased mortality and may be indicated for the most critically-ill patients suffering from peritonitis.

References

1. Sawyer RG, Rosenlof LK, Adams RB, et al: Peritonitis into the 1990s: changing pathogens and changing strategies in the critically ill. *Am Surg* 58:82, 1992.
2. Richardson JD, Flint LM, Polk HC Jr: Peritoneal lavage: a useful diagnostic adjunct for peritonitis. *Surgery* 94:826-829, 1983.
3. Cue JI, Miller FB, Cryer HM, et al: A prospective, randomized comparison between open and closed peritoneal lavage techniques. *J Trauma* 30(7):880-883, 1990.
4. Polk, HC Jr: Generalized peritonitis: a continuing challenge. *Surgery* 86:777, 1979.
5. Shuck JM: Newer concepts in intra-abdominal infection. *Am Surg* 51:304, 1985.
6. Farthmann EH, Schoffel U: Principles and limitations of operative management of intra-abdominal infection. *World J Surg* 14:210, 1990.
7. Yates JL: An experimental study of the local effects of peritoneal drainage. *Surg Gynecol Obstet* 1:473, 1905.
8. Rosato EF, Oram-Smith JC, Mullis WF, et al: Peritoneal lavage treatment in experimental peritonitis. *Ann Surg* 175(3):384-387, 1972.
9. Lally KP, Trettin JC, Torma MJ: Adjunctive antibiotic lavage in experimental peritonitis. *Surg Gynecol Obstet* 156:605-608, 1983.

10. Nomikos IN, Katsouyanni K, Pappaioannou A: Washing with or without chloramphenicol in the treatment of peritonitis: a prospective clinical trial. *Surgery* 99:20-25, 1986.
11. Hau T, Nishikawa R, Phaungsab A: Irrigation of the peritoneal cavity and local antibiotics in the treatment of peritonitis. *Surg Gynecol Obstet* 156:25-30, 1983.
12. Hau T, Ahrenholz DH, Simmons RL: Secondary bacterial peritonitis: the biologic basis of treatment. *Curr Prob Surg* 16:1, 1979.
13. Smith EB: Adjuvant therapy of generalized peritonitis with intraperitoneally administered cephalothine. *Surg Gynecol Obstet* 136:441, 1973.
14. Schumer W, Lee DK, Jones B: Peritoneal lavage in postoperative therapy of late peritoneal sepsis: preliminary report. *Surgery* 55:841, 1964.
15. Flint LM, Beasley DJ, Richardson JD, et al: Topical povidone-iodine reduces mortality from bacterial peritonitis. *J Surg Res* 26:280-284, 1979.
16. Stewart DJ, Matheson NA: Peritoneal lavage in appendicular peritonitis. *Br J Surg* 65:54-56, 1978.
17. Krukowski Z, Al-Sayer HM, Reid TM, et al: Effect of topical and systemic antibiotics on bacterial growth kinesis in generalized peritonitis in man. *Br J Surg* 74:303-306, 1987.
18. Glover JL, Atkins P, Lumpke RE: Evaluation of peritoneal lavage therapy for peritonitis. *J Surg Res* 9:531, 1969.
19. Dalton AC, Courtney RA, Miller HH: Peritonitis treated with prolonged, intermittent peritoneal lavage. *JAMA* 207:1345, 1969.
20. Sleeman HK, Diggs JW, Hayes DK, et al: Value of antibiotics, corticosteroids, and peritoneal lavage in the treatment of experimental peritonitis. *Surgery* 66:1060, 1969.
21. Perkash I, Satpati P, Agarnal KC, et al: Prolonged peritoneal lavage in fecal peritonitis. *Surgery* 68:842, 1970.
22. Stewart DJ, Matheson NA: Peritoneal lavage in fecal peritonitis in the rat. *Br J Surg* 65:57, 1978.
23. Artz CP, Barnett WO, Grogan JB: Further studies concerning the pathogenesis and treatment of peritonitis. *Ann Surg* 155:756, 1962.
24. Jennings WC, Wood CD, Guernsey JM: Continuous postoperative lavage in the treatment of peritoneal sepsis. *Dis Colon Rectum* 25:641, 1982.
25. Kumars GV, Smile SR, Sibal RN: Postoperastive peritoneal lavage in generalized peritonitis: a prospective analysis. *Int Surg* 74:20, 1989.
26. Rambo WM: Irrigation of the peritoneal cavity with cephalothin. *Am J Surg* 123:192, 1972.
27. Noon GP, Beall AC Jr, Jordan GL Jr, et al: Clinical evaluation of peritoneal irrigation with antibiotic solution. *Surgery* 62:73, 1967.
28. Hunt JL: Generalized peritonitits: to irrigate or not to irrigate the peritoneal cavity? *Arch Surg* 117:209, 1982.
28A. Lavigne JE, Brown CS, Machiedo GW, et al: Treatment of experimental peritonitis with intraperitoneal betadine solution. *J Surg Res 16:307, 1974.*
29. LaGarde MC, Bolton JS, Cohn I: Intraperitoneal povidone-iodine in experimental peritonitis. *Ann Surg* 87:613, 1978.
30. Hau T: Bacteria, toxins and the peritoneum. *World J Surg* 14(2):167-174, 1990.
31. McKenna JP, Currie DJ, MacDonald JA, et al: The use of continuous postop-

erative peritoneal lavage in the management of diffuse peritonitis. *Surg Gynecol Obstet* 254-258, 1970.

32. Stephen M, Loewenthal J: Continuing peritoneal lavage in high-risk peritonitis. *Surgery* 85:604-606, 1979.

32A. Peloso OA, Floyd VT, Wilkinson LH: Treatment of peritonitis with continuous postoperative peritoneal lavage using cephalothin. *Am J Surg* 126:742-747, 1973.

33. Leiboff AR, Soroff HS: The treatment of generalized peritonitis by closed postoperative peritoneal lavage. *Arch Surg* 122:1005-1010, 1987.

34. Dobrin PB, O'Keefe P, Tatarowicz W, et al: The value of continuous 72-hour peritoneal lavage for peritonitis. *Am J Surg* 157:368-371, 1989.

35. Uden P, Eskilsson P, Brunes L, et al: A clinical evaluation of postoperative peritoneal lavage in the treatment of perforated appendicitis. *Br J Surg* 70:348-349, 1983.

36. Atkins RC, Scott DF, Holdsworth SR, et al: Prolonged antibiotic peritoneal lavage in the management of gross generalized peritonitis. *Med J Aust* 1:954, 1976.

37. Hudspeth AS: Radical surgical debridement in the treatment of advanced generalized bacterial peritonitis. *Arch Surg* 110:1233-1236, 1975.

38. Polk HC, Fry DE: Radical peritoneal debridement for established peritonitis. *Ann Surg* 192(3):350-355, 1980.

39. Harbrecht PJ, Garrison RN, Fry DE: Early urgent relaparotomy. *Arch Surg* 119:369-374, 1984.

40. Bunt TJ: Urgent relaparotomy: the high-risk, no-choice operation. *Surgery* 98:555, 1985.

41. Fulton RL, Jones CE: The course of post-traumatic pulmonary insufficiency in man. *Surg Gynecol Obstet* 140:179, 1975.

42. Richardson JD, Fry DE, Van Arsdall L, et al: Delayed pulmonary clearance of gram negative bacteria: the role of intraperitoneal sepsis. *J Surg Res* 26:499, 1979.

43. Eiseman B, Beart R, Norton L. Multiple organ failure. *Surg Gynecol Obstet* 144:323, 1977.

44. Polk HC Jr, Shields CL. Remote organ failure: a valid sign of occult intra-abdominal infection. *Surgery* 81:310, 1977.

45. Sinanan M, Maier RV, Carrico CJ. Laparotomy for intra-abdominal sepsis in patients in an intensive care unit. *Arch Surg* 119:652-658, 1984.

46. Pennick, FM, Karreman RP, Lauwers PM: Planned relaparotomies in the surgical treatment of severe generalized peritonitis from intestinal origin. *World J Surg* 7:762, 1983.

47. Wouters DB, Krom RAF, Slooff MJH, et al: The use of Marlex mesh in patients with generalized peritonitis and multiple organ system failure. *Surg Gynecol Obstet* 156:609, 1983.

48. Voyles CR, Richardson JD, Bland KI, et al: Emergency abdominal wall reconstruction with polypropylene mesh. *Ann Surg* 194:219, 1981.

49. Bohnen JMA, Mustard RA: A critical look at scheduled relaparotomy for secondary bacterial peritonitis. *Surg Gynecol Obstet* 172:25, 1991.

50. Ferraris VA: Exploratory laparotomy for potential abdominal sepsis in patients with multiple organ failure. *Arch Surg* 118:1130, 1983.

51. Hinsdale JG, Jaffe BM: Reoperation for intra-abdominal sepsis: indications and results in a modern critical setting. *Ann Surg* 191:1, 1984.
52. Schein M, Saadia R, Freinkel Z, et al: Aggressive treatment of severe diffuse peritonitis: a prospective study. *Br J Surg* 75:173-176, 1988.
53. Schein M: Planned reoperations and open management in critical intra-abdominal infections: prospective experience in 52 cases. *World J Surg* 15:532-537, 1991.
54. Wittmann DH, Aprahamian C, Bergstein JM: Etappenlavage: advanced diffuse peritonitis managed by planned multiple laparotomies utilizing zippers, slide fastener and Velcro analogue for temporary abdominal closure. *World J Surg* 14:218-226, 1990.
55. Malangoni MA, Richardson JD, Shallcross JC, et al: Factors contributing to fatal outcome after treatment of pancreatic abscess. *Ann Surg* 203:605, 1986.
56. Anderson ED, Mandelbaum DM, Elliso EC, et al: Open packing of the peritoneal cavity in generalized bacterial peritonitis. *Am J Surg* 145:131-135, 1983.
57. Bose SM, Kalra M, Sandhu PS. Open management of septic abdomen by Marlex mesh zipper. *Aust N Z J Surg* 61:385-388, 1991.
58. Garcia-Sabrido JL, Tallado JM, Christou NV, et al: Treatment of severe intra-abdominal sepsis and/or necrotic foci by an "open abdomen" approach. *Arch Surg* 123:152-156, 1988.
59. Maetani S, Takayoshi T: Open peritoneal drainage as effective treatment of advanced peritonitis. *Surgery* 90(5):804-809, 1981.
60. Mastboom W, Kuypers HC, Schoots FJ, et al: Open treatment of generalized peritonitis. *Arch Surg* 124:689-692, 1989.
61. Steinberg D: On leaving the peritoneal cavity open in acute generalized suppurative peritonitis. *Am J Surg* 137:216, 1979.
62. Duff JH, Moffat J: Abdominal sepsis managed by leaving abdomen open. *Surgery* 90:774, 1981.
63. Bradley SJ, Jurkovich GJ, Pearlman NW, et al: Controlled open drainage of severe intra-abdominal sepsis. *Arch Surg* 120:629, 1985.
64. Hedderich GS, Wexler MJ, McLean APH, et al: The septic abdomen: open management with Marlex mesh with a zipper. *Surgery* 99:399, 1986.
65. Broome A, Hansson L, Lundgren F, et al: Open treatment of abdominal septic catastrophies. *World J Surg* 7:792, 1983.
66. Richardson JD, Polk HC, Jr: Newer adjunctive treatments for peritonitis. *Surgery* 90:917, 1981.
67. Christou NV: Invited commentary on open management. *World J Surg* 15:537, 1991.
68. Maudauss MA, Simmons RL: Leave the abdomen open for peritonitis: yes, no, maybe? *Adv Surg* 21:1, 1987.

8

Management of Intra-Abdominal Fluid Collections by Percutaneous Drainage

Bruce S. Turlington, MD, Marie T. Boyd, MD, and Jerry N. King, MD

With the advancement of imaging techniques such as ultrasound and computed tomography (CT) over the past 10 to 15 years, percutaneous drainage of intra-abdominal fluid collections using catheter techniques has gained greater acceptance.[1-4] Percutaneous drainage techniques have developed in part as an extension of biopsy techniques. Abscess cavities are the most commonly drained collections. However, similar methods have been applied to the management of pancreatic pseudocysts, urinomas, lymphoceles, and bilomas.

In spite of the development of newer generation antibiotics, the undrained abdominal abscess has a mortality rate of approximately 80%.[5,6] Operative drainage of abscesses is associated with a mortality rate of 10% to 20%.[7,8] Percutaneous drainage compares quite favorably, with complication rates ranging from 10% to 15% and serious complications in less than 5% of procedures. In most series, mortality rates directly attributable to major procedure-related complications are under 1%.[1,3,4,7,9] Percutaneous drainage also compares favorably to surgical treatment in regard to overall clinical success, with many series reporting success rates of 80% to 90%.[3,7,8,9] In simplistic terms, the advantage of percutaneous over surgical drainage seems to stem largely from

From Fry DE, (ed): *Peritonitis.* Mount Kisco NY, Futura Publishing Co., Inc., © 1993.

minimizing manipulation and trauma of the abscess, which may in turn decrease septic complications. Other attractive features of percutaneous techniques include (1) avoiding the inherent risks of general anesthesia and surgery with their attendant respiratory complications and pain incurred by the patient; (2) increasing cost effectiveness by avoiding operating room and anesthesia charges and consistently decreasing duration of hospitalization;[8] and (3) ease of post-procedural care of the closed drainage system.

Imaging Modalities

The imaging methods most commonly used for detecting intra-abdominal abscesses and fluid collection include CT, ultrasound, radionuclide scanning, and plain film radiography with or without contrast media. Currently, magnetic resonance imaging (MRI), because of its limited availability, long examination times, and restrictive patient requirements (they must be cooperative and medically stable), plays a rather limited role. In addition, as with CT, the MRI appearance of intra-abdominal abscess is not specific enough to totally alleviate the need for diagnostic aspiration.

Computed Tomography

Computed tomography (CT) is an accurate method of diagnosing intra-abdominal abscess, with many series reporting approximately 95% accuracy.[10-12] Technique is critical for proper diagnosis. Adequate opacification of bowel loops with oral contrast is probably the single most important factor, with most false-positive diagnoses attributable to mistaking nonopacified bowel or fluid filled stomach for pathologic fluid collections. The abdomen and pelvis should be imaged in their entirety from the diaphragm to the pubic symphysis.[13] The principal advantage of CT over the other modalities is that it provides exquisite anatomic detail of the collection and surrounding normal structures, enabling planning of a safe access route for drainage. The CT characteristics of an abscess are quite variable and depend significantly upon maturity and location. Initially, the abscess will appear as a relatively homogeneous spherical or elliptical mass of soft-tissue density. With maturation, the abscess undergoes liquefactive necrosis centrally (depending on contents, attenuation values usually measure 0–25 Hounsfield units) and develops a rim of highly vascularized connective tissue that usually enhances with the administration of intravenous contrast.[10] Roughly 30% of abscesses contain visible gas, which may manifest itself either as a gas-fluid level or microbubbles.[10,13,14] If a long gas-fluid level is observed, this is suggestive of communication with the gastrointestinal tract.[14] Secondary signs of abscess include obliteration of fascial planes and increased streaky densities in the mesenteric fat. Although the above described findings are characteristic of abscesses, they are not pathognomonic. Other pathologic entities that demonstrate central low attenuation include necrotic neoplasm, pseudocyst, hematoma, biloma, and urinoma.[12,13] Gas may also be identified within necrotic noninfected neoplasms that communicate with the gastrointestinal tract.

Ultrasound

Advantages of ultrasound include safety (absence of ionizing radiation), availability, portability, and relative ease of operation. Ultrasound can be used in the intensive care unit on unstable patients for abscess detection as well as guidance of needle aspiration/percutaneous drainage procedures at the bedside.[15] Overall accuracy of detection generally varies from 90% to 95%.[13,16,17] However, an accuracy of as low as 44% has been reported.[18] With the liver, spleen, and distended bladder serving as acoustic windows, the upper abdomen and pelvis are the areas that are most amenable to ultrasound diagnosis. Examination of the midabdomen is often significantly limited due to mesenteric fat and bowel gas, particularly if the patient has an associated paralytic ileus. Other factors limiting evaluation by ultrasound include open wounds, overlying dressings and drains, and obesity.[13,19] As with CT, ultrasound lacks specificity. Frequently, an abscess cannot be distinguished from other fluid collections. The ultrasonographer should be aware of several potential diagnostic pitfalls. Ascitic fluid, particularly if loculated, may be misinterpreted as an abscess if the collection is not scanned in its entirety in orthogonal planes.[19] Scanning the patient in different positions may also allow the sonographer to demonstrate movement of fluid. In the pelvis, the fluid-filled rectosigmoid can be mistaken for an abnormal fluid collection. Differentiation can be achieved by the administration of a water enema during real-time ultrasound observation.[19] In the postoperative patient, the bladder may occasionally be displaced or distorted to the point where it may be confused with an abnormal fluid collection.

Repeating the scan after voiding or catheterization may allow differentiation in this instance.

Radionuclide Imaging

The radionuclide imaging agents commonly used for detecting and localizing intra-abdominal abscesses are gallium 67 citrate (67 Ga) and indium 111 labeled leukocytes. Various authors have published sensitivities of 80% to 90% for both agents.[17,20,21] One major advantage of radionuclide imaging over other modalities is that the entire body can be imaged with relative ease, occasionally allowing the detection of previously unsuspected sites of infection.[22] The principal disadvantages of gallium imaging include: (1) imaging may have to be carried out over 48 or even 72 hours to optimize target:nontarget ratios and reduce nonspecific background activity; (2) gallium is excreted by the colon (this can present considerable difficulty in differentiating an abscess from normal colonic activity); and (3) gallium is relatively nonspecific and may concentrate in neoplastic tissue or postsurgical and other areas of sterile inflammation.[17,20] The newer agent indium 111 has the advantages of shorter imaging times (usually ending at 24 hours), lack of bowel or renal excretion, and greater specificity.[11,21,23] The disadvantages of indium 111 are: (1) it is cyclotron produced, creating availability problems; (2) there is some question regarding its effectiveness in the case of chronic abscess and in patients treated with antibiotics; and (3) leukocytes function and migration may be impaired in the setting of splenectomy, hyperalimentation, hypoglycemia, and hemodialysis.[11,23]

An Integrated Imaging Approach

If right upper quadrant, left upper quadrant, or pelvic abscess is clinically suspected, ultrasound is a useful initial method of examination. This is probably not the case for suspected midabdominal or retroperitoneal processes, where if the ultrasound examination is negative, a follow-up CT should be obtained.

For many patients with acute illness and localizing signs, CT is the preferred initial imaging method for optimal detection and anatomic definition. If the CT scan can be interpreted as unequivocally normal, abscess if effectively excluded.[13]

Radionuclide imaging often provides information that is complementary to CT and ultrasound. If abnormalities are identified on CT or ultrasound, correlation with radionuclide imaging can be extremely helpful, provided the patient's condition allows some delay of therapeutic intervention. Radionuclide scanning can certainly be considered as an initial screening modality in patients who are not critically ill, as it is a very sensitive test. When the examination is positive, CT or ultrasound is usually needed to obtain more specific anatomic information, particularly if percutaneous drainage is a consideration. If the nuclear medicine study is negative, usually no additional radiologic examination is indicated.

A potential pitfall to be avoided in the work-up of the acutely-ill patient suspected of harboring an intra-abdominal abscess is the ordering of gastrointestinal contrast studies. Barium, and even water soluble contrast agents, used for conventional gastrointestinal studies often create extensive artifact on CT scans, resulting in a nondiagnostic study. An exception to this is the evaluation of possible anastomotic leaks in the immediate postoperative period, in which a conventional contrast study may be indicated.[19]

Patient Selection and Indications

Overall, 80% to 85% of intra-abdominal abscesses can be treated exclusively by percutaneous drainage.[4,9,14] In considering patient selection, factors favoring successful percutaneous drainage include: (1) unilocular collection; (2) well-defined margin; and (3) safe access via an extraperitoneal dependent route.[1,3,4,7,9,24] Although selection of such favorable patients will undoubtedly lead to more successful procedures, many patients present an unacceptably high surgical risk, with percutaneous drainage the only realistic therapeutic option. In some of these cases, percutaneous drainage may allow for improvement of the patient's condition to the point where definitive operative therapy may be implemented.[25] The only absolute contraindication to percutaneous drainage procedures is the inability to establish a safe access route, which is an infrequent occurrence when CT guidance is used.[26]

Preprocedural Care

The patient's prothrombin time, partial thromboplastin time, and platelet count should be obtained and corrected accordingly. Broad-spectrum antibiotic coverage is initiated before the procedure and sub-sequently altered in accordance with the results of the Gram's stain and cultures of the collection. Adequate analgesia is imperative before starting the procedure.[19]

Access Route: Anatomical Considerations

Directed by cross-sectional imaging, generally the shortest and straightest route to the fluid collection is selected. However, the path should avoid major vessels, bowel loops, the pleural space, and other vital structures. Bowel loops can usually be avoided in planning approaches to collections located in the subphrenic spaces, subhepatic spaces, paracolic gutters, and superior recess of the lesser sac. Planning an approach in which bowel is not traversed may be considerably more difficult for those collections located in the pelvis, inferior recess of the lesser sac and infracolic spaces.[19] However, successful drainage in the pelvis has been achieved with transsciatic notch, transrectal, and trans-vaginal approaches.[27,28] An innovative approach, using the injection of carbon dioxide has been used to "actively displace" normal structures and provide a more generous pathway for drainage procedures. This technique has proven successful in the pelvis and retroperitoneum. However, it has not been effective in the midabdomen or mediastinum, and is ineffective in displacing solid organs (eg, kidneys or spleen).[29]

Puncture Technique and Diagnostic Aspiration

Computed tomography guidance, ultrasound guidance, or a combined approach is most often used for the initial diagnostic aspiration. Real-time ultrasound has the advantage of enabling the radiologist to guide and observe the needle during the actual puncture procedure.[30] Specialized needles that are better visualized with ultrasound have recently been developed. Side-arm attachments for ultrasound transducers are available to aid in guiding the needle. Modified linear array biopsy transducers with a central canal for needle insertion may also be used.[19] Computed tomography is used for most cases in which there is concern that adjacent bowel or vital structures might be traversed. When using CT guidance, it is usually preferred to keep the needle directed perpendicular to the surface of the patient, simplifying placement and documentation of needle tip location. However, in certain instances, an angled approach is necessary to avoid pleura/lung or other vital structures. The use of a geometric approach for this purpose has been advocated by several authors.[31,32] The initial diagnostic aspiration is usually performed with a "skinny" needle (Chiba 22- or 23-gauge). Although inadvertent punctures of bowel, gallbladder, bladder, and even major vessels with 22- or 23-gauge needles rarely result in any complication, passage through bowel should definitely be avoided to prevent contamination of sterile collections.[4,26,33] Aspiration of viscous contents through a 22-gauge needle may prove impossible, and when necessary a larger needle (18- or 20-gauge) may be needed. The aspirated material is sent for immediate Gram's stain and culture. Electrolyte analysis, amylase, and cell count are obtained if appropriate, as they may help in differentiating the type of fluid collected.[19] If the material is grossly purulent, one may proceed with the drainage procedure. Conversely, if the collection is not obviously infected, the result of the Gram's stain may be used to determine if drainage is appropriate. In most instances, placement of drainage catheters into sterile collections is avoided for fear of contamination.[4,26,33] Some notable exceptions to this will be discussed later.

At the time of diagnostic aspiration the collection should not be entirely drained, as this may make the subsequent manipulation of catheter and guidewire difficult. In addition, displaced bowel may return to its original position and interfere with what was initially a safe access route. However, if the abscess cavity is small (less than 5 cm), treatment by complete aspiration without placement of a catheter is certainly an option, and several investigators have reported good results with complete needle evacuation.[19,33] In those cases in which it is not possible to find a safe route and the patient is not a surgical candidate, complete needle aspiration may be the only option. Some authors advocate the use of a Teflon® sheathed 20-gauge needle at the time of initial puncture, with the idea that the sheath be left in, in order to drain any fluid or pus that might reaccumulate. It is suggested that patients treated in this manner have a follow-up CT or ultrasound within 2 to 3 days. If the collection reaccumulates it may be reaspirated, though reaccumulation does not always imply reinfection.

Catheter Types

Two important requirements of catheters used for drainage procedures are: (1) a lumen of adequate size for free drainage of material and (2) multiple side holes to prevent catheter occlusion. Two main categories of catheters exist: sump and nonsump.

Nonsump catheters are available in sizes varying from 6 F to 14 F. The most commonly used types are the pigtail and Cope loop configurations.[34-36] Pigtail drainage catheters are similar to their angiographic counterparts. However, their side holes are located on the inner aspect of the curve. Theoretically, this placement of side holes enhances drainage when the collection becomes smaller by preventing tissue entrapment in the side holes. The pigtail configuration also reduces damage to the cavity wall and the possibility of perforation. Pigtail catheters are also somewhat self-retaining. However, the Cope loop catheter, with its loop maintained by internal string fixation, is better in this regard. The Malecot-type catheter, with its distal "mushroom" tip configuration, has also proven to be an effective self-retaining catheter design.[37] Nonsump catheters are usually limited to dependent drainage of relatively low viscosity collections. Unlike sump catheters, if suction is applied to the catheter it will often result in tissue encroachment upon the side holes and subsequent occlusion.[24] Sump catheters are available in 12 F and 14 F sizes. The van Sonnenberg sump catheter (Medical Information Technology, Inc., Westwood, MA, USA) uses a flexible double lumen design. The larger lumen has multiple large oval side holes at its distal end for drainage of viscous material. The smaller inner lumen provides circulation of air into the cavity, preventing collapse of the cavity when suction is applied. This design also provides for concurrent irrigation and drainage. The efficiency of this system may be 2 to 4 times that of conventional closed drainage. These catheters may also be introduced by standard guidance techniques or trocar technique.[24]

Catheter Management

Following placement of the catheter, the collection is completely evacuated. Sterile saline irrigation is then gently carried out until clear drainage is obtained. An abscessogram may then be obtained and correlated with the patient's CT or ultrasound to determine if the collection has been fully evacuated. Care should be taken not to overdistend the cavity during irrigation or contrast studies in order to decrease the possibility of inducing sepsis.[4,19,33] The abscessogram may potentially demonstrate an enteric fistula, though often a communication is not demonstrated on the initial study and is only seen on follow-up examinations. This may be related to the resolution of inflammatory debris and edema. Nonsump catheters are left to gravity drainage, while sump catheters may be left to low intermittent suction. The efficacy of daily irrigation has been debated, though many authors feel that frequent saline irrigation with relatively small volumes is helpful in maintaining catheter patency and reducing the viscosity of the material to be drained.[4] The use of proteolytic agents, such as 5% to 10% acetylcysteine is advocated by some to reduce catheter occlusion and promote clearance of necrotic debris and viscous pus. Other investigators argue that the clinical efficacy of acetylcysteine has not been proven, (citing studies that demonstrate that the agent is not particularly effective at a pH below 7.5), and that saline irrigation is equally effective.[38] Following successful percutaneous abscess drainage, clinical improvement is often quite remarkable. The patient usually defervesces within 24 to 48 hours. It should be emphasized that a complete course of appropriate antibiotic therapy should be completed. If the clinical response is not prompt, CT or ultrasound should be performed to determine if there is inadequate drainage or if a second abscess is present. When fever persists or drainage increases, a fistulous communication with either bowel or the biliary system should be suspected and a follow-up abscessogram/sinogram should be performed. If a fistulous tract is documented, percutaneous drainage should not automatically be discontinued, as it may still succeed. However, drainage may be considerably lengthened.[3,9] High-output fistulas may not respond solely to percutaneous drainage, requiring surgical intervention.[19] With uncomplicated percutaneous drainage the volume of drainage decreases markedly or ceases within 3 to 10 days.[7,19,33] At this point the catheter may be gradually withdrawn, approximately several centimeters per day. Prior to complete removal, a CT scan should be obtained to assure complete evacuation.

Drainage Techniques

If catheter drainage is planned following diagnostic aspiration, a guidewire is usually placed in the collection. The trocar technique is an exception to this, and is utilized when the collection is superficial and large, and there are no vital intervening structures. In this method, catheter, cannula, and trocar are advanced as a unit to a predetermined distance (usually in tandem with the diagnostic needle). The trocar is then removed, with the aspiration of pus confirming catheter location. The drainage catheter may then be advanced over the cannula and properly positioned in the cavity. Several methods are available for placement of guidewires.

Tandem Techniques

An 18-gauge needle is advanced to the same depth and at the same angle alongside the diagnostic needle. Fluid is aspirated to confirm its location and a 0.035- or 0.038-inch, J-tipped guidewire is coiled in the cavity. A scan is then obtained to assure the location of the wire within the cavity. At this point the needle is removed and the patient may be transferred to fluoroscopy for completion of the procedure, with passage of serial dilators (1 F or 2 F larger than the drainage catheter) and placement of the catheter. Fluoroscopic guidance during wire and catheter manipulations is emphasized by some authors in order to avoid complications such as backwall perforation, wire buckling and placement of catheter side holes outside the collection.[4,19,33] However, a creative approach using serial CT digital-scout radiographs to monitor guidewire and catheter placement and completion of evacuation has been successfully implemented in critically ill patients who are difficult to transport. These investigators emphasize that multilocular or otherwise complicated collections may not be amenable to this nonfluoroscopic technique.[34] A variation of the tandem technique involves defining the cavity initially with contrast medium, with a second puncture performed under fluoroscopy.

Cope's Method

This method is essentially the same as that adapted for nephrostomy tube placement. A 0.018-inch floppy-tipped guidewire is threaded through the diagnostic needle. The needle is removed and a curved 5 F Teflon® dilator is then advanced over the guidewire. This dilator has a sidehole allowing a 0.038-inch guidewire with a tight-J (3 mm) to exit.[35]

Recently, a straight dilator without a side hole has been developed which accepts both the 0.018- and 0.038-inch guidewires in a coaxial fashion, further simplifying the technique. In this manner, a small guidewire system can be replaced by a large one in a relatively atraumatic fashion. Catheter placement then proceeds as described above.

Hawkin's Method

A long (20-inch) 22-gauge needle with a back-loaded 5 F Teflon® accordion catheter is used for this technique. Following the diagnostic aspiration, a 0.018-inch guidewire is passed through the needle into the collection and the catheter is advanced over the needle and wire and placed in the cavity. The primary advantage of this method is that with one puncture and little manipulation a self-retaining catheter has been positioned.[36] The catheter's size (5 F) limits this method to relatively small collections of low viscosity.

Reasons for Therapeutic Failures

Success rates of 80% to 90% for percutaneous abscess drainage are widely quoted, and recurrence rates following successful drainage are on the order of 5%.[7-9,33] Some of the most frequent causes of failure include persistent high-output fistulas from the gastrointestinal tract; poorly defined abscesses, diffuse microabscesses and phlegmons; multiloculated abscesses; excessive viscosity of material to be drained; and abscesses that are simply too extensive. Necrotic tumors may simulate an abscess, but obviously do not respond well to drainage. It may be that fungal abscesses or pyogenic abscesses superinfected with fungi do not respond well to percutaneous drainage.[19] Whether this is related to the infectious agent or immunocompromised state of the patient is not entirely clear.

Complications

Complications resulting from percutaneous drainage are infrequent, with the occurrence of serious complications in fewer than 5% of procedures. Reported minor complications include transient septicemia, skin infection, and mild bleeding.[26] Major complications include septic shock, empyema, bowel perforation, fistula, and life-threatening hemorrhage. Deaths attributable to complications of the procedure occur in approximately 1% of cases.[19,26]

Specific Sites and Fluid Types

Subphrenic Space

The right and left subphrenic spaces are common locations for abscesses to develop following surgery. These are usually readily treated by percutaneous drainage.[39] In fact, it has been reported that subphrenic abscesses are more likely to be successfully treated by percutaneous drainage than those in other locations.[14] However, additional planning for a safe access route is needed to avoid traversing the pleural space, as this may result in empyema formation. An angled approach is often required. Pneumothorax is also a potential complication in the drainage of subphrenic abscesses.[39]

Pelvis

Abscess drainage in the pelvis by an anterior approach is often limited by intervening bladder, bowel, or bone. Alternative approaches, namely transgluteal, transrectal, and transvaginal, have proven successful.[27,28] Collections in the lower pelvis can often be managed by transrectal or transvaginal approaches. Collections high in the pelvis often require a transgluteal (via greater sciatic foramen) route. In one series by Butch et al.,[27] successful percutaneous drainage by the transgluteal route was obtained in 17 of 21 patients. The complication that was most often encountered with this approach was pain. However, this was usually transient, and resolved within 24 hours. In approximately one fifth of patients the pain persisted, presumably due to lumbosacral plexus irritation. However, there was no residual sensory or motor deficit in these patients. By traversing the inferior aspect of the greater sciatic foramen (through the sacrospinous ligament rather than the more superiorly located piriformis muscle) the sacral plexus and gluteal arteries may be avoided.[5]

Interloop and Potentially Complicated Abscesses

Due to their location, interloop abscesses can be more challenging to drain. Computed tomography is the guidance method of choice in order to avoid bowel perforation. Drainage of interloop abscesses secondary to Crohn's disease has been considerably successful.[40,41] Other potentially complicated abscesses, such as diverticular and periappendiceal, have been drained without complications. Percutaneous evacuation of diverticular abscesses may in certain cases convert two- or three-stage operative procedures to one-stage procedures, with decreased patient morbidity as a result.[42-44] Cases have been reported in which the percutaneous drainage of periappendiceal abscesses have been curative, eliminating the need for surgery.[45-50]

Lymphoceles

Lymphoceles are most often encountered in patients who have undergone renal transplantation or retroperitoneal lymph node dissection. Computed tomographic features of lymphoceles are often nonspecific, though the diagnosis may be suggested if negative Hounsfield numbers (due to the fat content of lymph) are obtained. Lymphoceles typically appear several weeks after surgery, usually later than seromas and urinomas.[13] The size of the lymphocele is a prognostic factor: small collections often spontaneously resorb, whereas large collections often require treatment.[51-53] Percutaneous drainage of lymphoceles may obviate the need for an often technically difficult reoperation. Indications for drainage include: symptoms, most commonly pain; signs of ureteral or venous obstruction; secondary infection; and continued enlargement.[51-53] Two series (van Sonnenberg et al.[52] and Cohan et al.[51]) report success rates of 70% to 80%. Drainage may be considerably longer (18 days average, up to 5 weeks) than that expected for abscess drainage (3 to 15 days). The use of sclerosing agents when there is no intraperitoneal communication may improve success rates and decrease the duration of drainage.[51]

Bilomas

Bilomas are most often iatrogenic or traumatic in etiology, though spontaneous rupture of the biliary tree has been reported. Small bilomas (several centimeters in diameter) may be observed. However, drainage is felt to be the appropriate treatment for larger bilomas. Most bilomas can be successfully managed by percutaneous drainage. Vazquez et al.[54] report a series of 15 percutaneous drainage procedures, all of which were successful and without complications. Many bilomas that are resolved by drainage do not require surgical repair of the bile leak.[54,55]

Pancreas

Pancreatic abscesses are often ill-defined and phlegmon-like, and their management by percutaneous drainage is controversial.[26] Moderate success has been reported by some investigators, with curative results in 50% of patients. However, multiple large diameter catheters are often required, along with frequent irrigation. If percutaneous drainage is attempted, clinical deterioration of the patient is usually an indication for surgical management.[5,56,57]

Percutaneous drainage of pseudocysts has shown promising results.[58-62] The most common indication for percutaneous intervention is suspected infection.[63-65] Other indications include pain, and biliary or gastric obstruction. Recently, transgastric drainage has been described. It is felt that this approach provides the advantages of the surgical cystogastrostomy, while avoiding the complications of external drainage.[57,60,62] It may allow a mature tract to develop from the cyst to the stomach, essentially eliminating the risk of pancreatico-cutaneous fistula. In two series this technique was successful in seven of eight (Nunez et al.[57]) and eight of twelve patients (Matzinger et al.[62]).

Summary

Effective and safe percutaneous drainage of intra-abdominal abscesses and other fluid collections has been made possible by the advancement of cross-sectional imaging and catheter techniques. Percutaneous methods adhere to such basic principles of surgical management as evacuation and maintenance of free drainage to prevent sepsis and other complications. Attractive features of percutaneous compared to operative management include:

1. Avoidance of the risks of major surgery, general anesthesia, and peri-operative complications

2. Decreased hospital stays
3. Improved patient tolerance
4. Simplification of nursing care.

Some key features regarding percutaneous drainage that deserve emphasis are listed below:

1. The procedure is most often successful when performed by a radiologist who is experienced in cross-sectional imaging and skilled in interventional techniques.
2. The vast majority of intra-abdominal abscesses can be successfully drained by percutaneous routes.
3. The extraperitoneal dependent route is preferred. However, the transperitoneal route may be safely used when CT is available to avoid the transgression of bowel loops.
4. Generally, drainage catheters should not be placed in sterile collections. These collections may be treated by diagnostic aspiration and evacuation if clinically warranted.
5. Percutaneous techniques and materials are relatively simple. Appropriate cross-sectional imaging methods are now widely available, enabling most community hospital radiology departments to perform such procedures.

References

1. Gerzof SG, Robbins AH, Johnson WC, et al: Percutaneous catheter drainage of abdominal abscesses. *N Engl J Med* 305:653-657, 1981.
2. Gerzof SG, Johnson WC, Robbins AH, Nabseth DC: Expanded criteria for percutaneous abscess drainage. *Arch Surg* 120:227-232, 1985.
3. Mueller PR, van Sonnenberg E, Ferrucci JT Jr: Percutaneous drainage of 250 abdominal abscesses and fluid collections. Part II. *Radiology* 151:343-347, 1984.
4. van Sonnenberg E, Ferrucci JT Jr, Mueller PR, et al: Percutaneous drainage of abscesses and fluid collections: techniques, results and applications. *Radiology* 142:1-10, 1982.
5. Karlson KB, Martin EC, Fankuchen EI, et al: Percutaneous drainage of pancreatic pseudocysts and abscesses. *Radiology* 142:619-624, 1982.
6. Karlson KB, Martin EC, Fankuchen EI, et al: Percutaneous abscess drainage. *Surg Gynecol Obstet* 154:44-48, 1982.
7. Aeder MI, Wellman JL, Haaga JR, Hau T: Role of surgical and percutaneous drainage in the treatment of abdominal abscesses. *Arch Surg* 118:273-280, 1983.

8. Brolin RE, Wosher JL, Leiman S, et al: Percutaneous catheter versus open surgical drainage in the treatment of abdominal abscesses. *Ann Surg* 50(21):102-108, 1984.

9. Lang EK, Springer RM, Glorioso LW, Cammarata CA: Abdominal abscess drainage under radiologic guidance: causes of failure. *Radiology* 159:329-336, 1986.

10. Aronberg DJ, Stanley RJ, Levitt RG, Sagel SS: Evaluation of abdominal abscess with computed tomography. *J Comput Assist Tomogr* 2:184-187, 1978.

11. Knochel JQ, Koehler PR, Lee TG, Welch DM: Diagnosis of abdominal abscesses with computerized tomography, ultrasound, and 111-indium leukocyte scans. *Radiology* 137:425-432, 1980.

12. Churchill RJ: CT of intra-abdominal fluid collections. *Radiol Clin North Am* 27:653-666, 1989.

13. Heiken JP: Abdominal wall and peritoneal cavity. In:Lee JK, ed. *Computed Body Tomography with MRI Correlation.* New York, NY: Raven Press; 1989:89-108.

14. Jacques P, Mauro M, Safrit N, et al: CT features of intra-abdominal abscess: prediction of successful percutaneous drainage. *AJR* 146:1041-1045, 1986.

15. McGahan JP, Anderson MW, Walter JP: Portable real-time sonographic and needle guidance systems for aspiration and drainage. *AJR* 147:1241-1246, 1986.

16. Gerzof SG: Ultrasound in the search for abdominal abscesses. *Clin Diagn Ultrasound* 7:101, 1981.

17. Korobkin M, Callen PW, Filly RA, et al: Comparison of computed tomography, ultrasonography, and gallium 67 scanning in the evaluation of suspected abdominal abscess. *Radiology* 129:89-93, 1978.

18. Landstedt C, Hederstrom E, Holmin T, et al: Radiologic diagnosis in proven intra-abdominal abscess formation. *Gastrointest Radiol* 9:213-217, 1984.

19. Tadavarthy SM, Letourneau JG, Elyaderani MK, et al: Drainage of abdominal abscesses. In: Castaneda-Zuniga WR, ed. *Interventional Radiology.* Baltimore, MD: Williams and Wilkins; 1988:814-855.

20. Levitt RG, Biello DR, Sagel SS, et al: Computed tomography and 67-Ga citrate radionuclide imaging for evaluating suspected abdominal abscess. *AJR* 132:529-534, 1979.

21. McDougall IR, Baumert JE, Lantiere RL: Evaluation of 111-In leukocyte whole body scanning. *AJR* 133:849-854, 1979.

22. Seabold JE, Wilson DG, Lieberman LM, Boyd CM: Unsuspected extra-abdominal sties of infection: scintigraphic detection with indium 111 labelled leukocytes. *Radiology* 151:213-217, 1984.

23. McAffe JG, Samin A: In-111 labelled leukocytes: a review of problems in image interpretation. *Radiology* 155:222-229, 1985.

24. van Sonnenberg E, Mueller PR, Ferrucci JT Jr, et al: Sump catheters for percutaneous abscess and fluid drainage by trocar or Seldinger technique. *AJR* 139:613-614, 1982.

25. van Sonnenberg E, Wing VW, Casola G, et al: Temporizing effect of percutaneous drainage of complicated abscesses in critically ill patients. *AJR* 142:821-826, 1984.

26. Picus D, Weyman PJ, Anderson DJ. Interventional computed tomography.

Management of Intra-Abdominal Fluid Collections · 175

In: Lee JK, ed. *Computed Body Tomography with MRI Correlation.* New York, NY: Raven Press; 1989:89-108.

27. Butch RJ, Mueller PR, Ferrucci JT Jr, et al. Drainage of pelvic abscesses through the greater sciatic foramen. *Radiology* 158:487-491, 1986.
28. Mauro MA, Jacques PF, Mandell VS, Mandel SR: Pelvic abscess drainage by the transrectal catheter approach in men. *AJR* 144:477-479, 1985.
29. Haaga JR, Beale SM: Use of CO_2 to move structures as an aid to percutaneous procedures. *Radiology* 161:829-830, 1986.
30. Gronvall S: Drainage of abdominal abscesses guided by sonography. *AJR* 138:527-529, 1982.
31. Gerzof SG: Triangulation: indirect CT guidance for abscess drainage. *AJR* 137:1080-1081, 1981.
32. van Sonnenberg E, Wittenberg J, Ferrucci JT Jr, et al: Triangulation method for percutaneous needle guidance: the angled approach to upper abdominal masses. *AJR* 137:757-761, 1981.
33. Gerzof SG: Guided percutaneous catheter drainage of abdominal abscesses. In: Anthanasoulis C, ed. *Interventional Radiology.* Philadelphia, PA: WB Saunders; 1982:557-567.
34. Wing VW, Jeffrey RB, Hightower DR, Federle MP: Digital scout radiograph assisted percutaneous abscess drainage. *AJR* 147:406-407, 1986.
35. Cope C: Conversion from small (0.018 inch) to large (0.038 inch) guidewires in percutaneous drainage procedures. *AJR* 138:170-171, 1982.
36. Hawkins IF: Single-step placement of a self-retaining "accordion" catheter. *Semin Intervent Radiol* 1:9, 1984.
37. Tadavarthy SM, Coleman C, Hunter D, et al: Dual stiffness Malecot catheter. *Radiology* 152:225, 1984.
38. Dawson SL, Mueller PR, Ferrucci JT Jr: Mucomyst for abscesses: a clinical comment. *Radiology* 151:342, 1984.
39. Mueller PR, Simeone JR, Butch RJ, et al: Percutaneous drainage of subphrenic abscess: a review of 62 patients. *AJR* 147:1237-1240, 1986.
40. Gore RM: CT of inflammatory bowel disease. *Radiol Clin North Am* 27:717-729, 1989.
41. Safrit ND, Mauro MA, Jacques PF: Percutaneous abscess drainage in Crohn's disease. *AJR* 148:859-862, 1987.
42. Neff CC, van Sonnenberg E, Casola G, et al: Diverticular abscesses: percutaneous drainage. *Radiology* 163:15-18, 1987.
43. Neff CC, van Sonnenberg E: CT of diverticulitis: diagnosis and treatment. *Radiol Clin North Am* 27:743-752, 1987.
44. Mueller PR, Saini S, Wittenberg J, et al: Sigmoid diverticular abscesses: percutaneous drainage as an adjunct to surgical resection in 24 cases. *Radiology* 164:321-325, 1987.
45. Jeffrey RB Jr, Federle MP, Tolentino CS: Periappendiceal inflammatory masses: CT directed management and clinical outcome in 70 patients. *Radiology* 167:13-16, 1988.
46. Shapiro MP, Elon Gale M, Gerzof SG: CT of appendicitis, diagnosis and treatment. *Radiol Clin North Am* 27:753-762, 1989.
47. van Sonnenberg E, Wittich GR, Casola G, et al: Periappendiceal abscesses: percutaneous drainage. *Radiology* 163:23-26, 1987.

48. Nunez D Jr, Huber JS, Yrizarry JM, et al: Non-surgical drainage of appendiceal abscess. *AJR* 146:587-589, 1986.
49. Jeffrey RB Jr, Tolentino CS, Federle MP, Laing FC: Percutaneous drainage of appendiceal abscess. *AJR* 146:587-589, 1986.
50. Barakos JA, Jeffrey RB Jr, Federle MP, et al: CT in the management of periappendiceal abscess. *AJR* 146:1161-1164, 1986.
51. Cohan RH, Saeed M, Sussman SK: Percutaneous drainage of pelvic lymphatic fluid collections in the renal transplant patient. *Invest Radiol* 22:864-867, 1987.
52. van Sonnenberg E, Wittich GR, Casola G, et al: Lymphoceles: imaging characteristics and percutaneous management. *Radiology* 161:593-196, 1986.
53. White M, Mueller PR, Ferrucci JT Jr, et al: Percutaneous drainage of postoperative abdominal and pelvic lymphoceles. *AJR* 145:1065-1069, 1985.
54. Vazquez JL, Thorsen MK, Dodds WJ, et al: Evaluation and treatment of intra-abdominal bilomas. *AJR* 144:933-938, 1985.
55. Mueller PR, Ferrucci JT Jr, Simeone JR, et al: Detection and drainage of bilomas: special considerations. *AJR* 140:715-720, 1983.
56. van Sonnenberg E, Wittich GR, Casola G, et al: Complicated pancreatic inflammatory disease: diagnostic and therapeutic role of interventional radiology. *Radiology* 155:335-340, 1985.
57. Nunez D, Yrizarry JM, Russell E, et al: Transgastric drainage of pancreatic fluid collections. *AJR* 145:815-818, 1985.
58. Freeny PC. Radiology of the pancreas: two decades of progress in imaging and intervention. *AJR* 150:975-981, 1988.
59. Sacks D, Robinson ML: Transgastric percutaneous drainage of pancreatic pseudocysts. *AJR* 151:303-306, 1988.
60. Ho CS, Taylor B: Percutaneous transgastric drainage for pancreatic pseudocyst. *AJR* 143:623-625, 1984.
61. Torres WE, Evert MB, Baumgartner BR, Behnardino ME: Percutaneous aspiration and drainage of pancreatic pseudocysts. *AJR* 147:1007-1009, 1986.
62. Matzinger FR, Ho CS, Yee AC, Gray RR: Pancreatic pseudocysts drained through a percutaneous transgastric approach: further experience. *Radiology* 167:431-434, 1988.
63. Lieberman RP, Hahn FJ, Imray TJ, Phalen JT. Loculated abscesses: management by percutaneous fracture of septations. *Radiology* 161:827-828, 1986.
64. Lang EK, Glorioso L: Management of urinomas by percutaneous drainage. *Radiol Clin North Am* 24:551-559, 1986.
65. Johnson RD, Mueller PR, Ferrucci JT Jr: Percutaneous drainage of pyogenic liver abscesses. *AJR* 144:463-467, 1985.

9

Laparoscopy in Peritonitis

Daniel T. Martin, MD, and Karl A. Zucker, MD

If laparoscopic cholecystectomy is now being regarded as the new "gold standard" therapy for the management of symptomatic cholelithiasis,[1] then what other avenues can be explored and conquered with laparoscopy? Since laparoscopy was first performed at the turn of the century by Kelling[2] and has been used for years in gynecology (pelviscopy), the advent of videolaparoscopy was part of the logical progression in technological development. The explosion of laparoscopic procedures and its impact on patient care has been phenomenal since Mouret performed his first laparoscopic cholecystectomy in 1987, which was then popularized by Dubois in Europe,[3,4] and Reddick and Olsen[5] in the United States. It was only a short period of time before the literature was beginning to publish reports of other laparoscopic endeavors. Today it is almost routine for surgeons to remove the appendix[6,7] or gallbladder,[3,4,5,] resect bowel,[8] perform anti-ulcer and anti-reflux procedures,[9] or even do nephrectomies,[10] splenectomies,[11] and lymph node dissections[12] laparoscopically. With all of this experience, the rigidity once applied to contraindications has all but disappeared and now more acute intraperitoneal pathology is being explored laparoscopically, and much of it can be treated in the same manner with minimally invasive surgery.

Lower abdominal pain was perhaps one of the first disease processes to stimulate the use of laparoscopy in patients with peritoneal signs, particularly in young females with questionable appendicitis. The ability to differentiate between pelvic inflammatory disease (PID), ectopic pregnancy, a ruptured ovarian cyst, or acute appendicitis by firmly

From Fry DE, (ed): *Peritonitis*. Mount Kisco NY, Futura Publishing Co., Inc., © 1993.

diagnosing and usually treating these problems laparoscopically has perhaps avoided numerous unnecessary laparotomies.[13] Added to this list more recently is laparoscopy for upper abdominal pain to differentiate between maladies such as a perforated ulcer, pancreatitis, acute cholecystitis, or mesenteric ischemia.[13] This technique has been used in blunt abdominal trauma patients[14,15] to further delineate who needs laparotomy, since diagnostic peritoneal lavage and computed tomography may occasionally lead to negative or unnecessary laparotomy.

In keeping with this surge in useful indications for laparoscopy, catalyzed by the evolution of more versatile instrumentation, some surgeons have added the truly acute abdomen to the list of possible indications for the insertion of a laparoscope.[16,17] Since the principles and tenets of surgery are closely followed in videolaparoscopic procedures, as in conventional surgery, it would follow that this tool could have a place in diagnosing and treating the etiology of peritonitis. In cases where the definitive diagnosis may elude the laparoscopist, open laparotomy remains a mainstay. If a diagnosis is established, often specific therapeutic intervention is possible using minimally invasive surgical techniques, and laparatomy may be averted.

Appendicitis

Acute appendicitis is perhaps the most frequent reason to operate on patients with peritonitis. As we all know, the diagnosis preoperatively can be difficult in some patients, particularly those with atypical symptoms, young women with the possibility of other pelvic (tubal or ovarian) pathology,[18] and children or elderly senescent individuals unable to give adequate historical information. The inflammation of the appendix may or may not be associated with perforation or abscess, but any of these can be safely treated laparoscopically.[6,7] The accepted removal of a normal appendix in 15% to 20% (or higher in young females) of those suspected of appendicitis in order to reduce the morbidity of perforation or abscess, may be able to be reduced if not eliminated utilizing laparoscopy.[16,19] In addition to eliminating unnecessary appendectomies, the ability to accurately make a diagnosis and the opportunity to intervene therapeutically, if necessary, make this a procedure that will surely establish itself in the surgical armamentarium.

Although few series are in the literature at present,[20,21] it is becoming clear that when the appendix is removed laparoscopically, fewer wound infections seem to occur. This can be accounted for by the fact that the specimen is never in contact with the skin or subcutaneous tissues, either being removed through the cannula or brought out in a specimen bag. The technique allows for visualization of the entire abdomen, and should there be any doubt about the diagnosis preoperatively, this should be resolved by the end of the procedure. Although an earlier report on laparoscopy for questionable appendicitis reported missing the diagnosis in two complex patients,[22] subsequent reports have not substantiated those findings.[16,23] With experience and good judgement, the appropriate definitive procedure will usually be determined, if not carried out, laparoscopically. Another benefit to women may be a reduction in tubal infertility related to ruptured appendicitis,[24] since almost 20% of appendectomies have been associated with perforation.[25] Perhaps this will spur surgeons to a more rapid intervention since the morbidity of a diagnostic or therapeutic laparoscopy is lower than that of a negative laparotomy.[26]

Diverticulitis and Intestinal Perforation

When operating on a patient with acute peritoneal findings, certainly diverticular rupture and inflammation enter the differential diagnosis in most adults from western cultures. While many surgeons may be reluctant to treat this disease process through the laparoscope, the diagnosis can be made with relative certainty, especially in those who may have other equivocal test results suggestive of extrinsic compression, possibly from ruptured appendicitis. In some instances the disease process may be amenable to minimal access surgery, while in others a laparotomy may be required.

Since the laparoscope can be used to visualize essentially the entire small bowel from the ligament of Treitz on distally, and the colon can be examined from cecum to rectum (with slight mobilization if necessary), other causes of perforation can be diagnosed and treated. Small bowel perforations can be repaired primarily, or resected and anastomosed through a small portal of evisceration if extracorporeal techniques must be used.[27] This can be beneficial in victims of blunt or penetrating trauma, foreign body perforation, or even diagnosing and treating Meckel's diverticulitis. Iatrogenic endoscopic perforations, although rare, may be treated similarly. In patients undergoing colonoscopy, the bowel prep is generally satisfactory to allow for primary closure of perforations. Duodenal perforations after esophagogastroduodenoscopy (EGD) or endoscopic retrograde cholangiopancreatography (ERCP) may also be closed primarily if the integrity of the tissues permits it.

Depending on the findings at laparoscopy, exploration can be aided by varying the table position, placing additional cannulas for exposure if necessary, and using endoscopic retractors and angled laparoscopes to visualize the anatomy. If there are adhesions present from previous surgery, these can be taken down and the abdominal survey completed. After completion of the diagnostic portion of the procedure, the decisions about intervention can be made and often the procedure may be undertaken laparoscopically, including bowel resection and creation of colostomies.[27]

Acute Cholecystitis

Acute cholecystitis accounts for approximately 20% of all cholecystectomies, some presenting as an acute abdomen[28] while others may have a more indolent course. Of those presenting with severe peritoneal signs, some will have a gangrenous, necrotic gallbladder with perforation, while others may have hydrops and severe edema of the gallbladder wall. The spectrum of disease presentation must be respected, and the surgeon must be prepared to deal with whatever is encountered, either laparoscopically or through conventional laparotomy.

Upon entering the abdominal cavity, one generally encounters peritoneal fluid that may be turbid, and cultures are usually taken to guide antibiotic coverage adjustment. Our preference in these cases is to use the Hassan[29] (open) technique for placement of the umbilical cannula, thereafter everything being done under videoscopic visualization. After placement of this initial 10-mm port and insufflation to 12–15 mm Hg of pressure, the abdominal cavity is surveyed in all four quadrants. If no fluid was encountered initially, any free fluid subsequently located is aspirated for laboratory analysis. Generally the omentum will be adherent to the gallbladder and liver, and standard placement of cannulas[5] will allow for adequate access. In some cases the hepatic flexure of the colon may be adherent to the gallbladder, as may the duodenum. There may even be a fistulous connection from one organ to the other. This can serve to clarify the point that meticu-

lous dissection must be carried out, looking for any perforations during the course of the operation.

When faced with this condition, we prefer to begin the dissection by gently peeling the omentum from the underlying viscera. Each anatomical structure is identified as it is encountered and as soon as the cystic duct is dissected out, a cholangiogram is obtained to assist further dissection and to ascertain the location of the common bile duct and common hepatic duct. This procedure is covered in more detail in the chapter on biliary peritonitis, and other surgeons may offer different methods of approaching the same problem. Our goal is patient safety, and if possible, completion of the procedure laparoscopically, remaining ever mindful that the election to proceed with laparotomy (if necessary) is not a complication.

Perforated Ulcer

Peritonitis secondary to ulcer perforation, either gastric or duodenal, is usually diagnosed based on history, clinical presentation, and free air on upright or decubitus abdominal radiographs. The history of abrupt onset abdominal pain may or may not have been preceded by chronic complaints referable to gastrointestinal hyperacidity. Many of these patients may have been on steroidal or nonsteroidal anti-inflammatory agents for another disease process. Occasionally patients will present with perforations, having long been known to have peptic ulcer disease, and being treated intermittently with acid suppressing medicines or antacids. In patients with a history of symptoms related to ulcers that have been present for more than 3 months, consideration should be given to performing a definitive anti-ulcer operation at the time of repairing the perforation. Other factors may preclude a definitive procedure in addition to closure of the hole. The risk factors appearing to be important in the decision process have been well documented[30] and will not be detailed here. Neither will we delve into a discussion of the alternative treatment methods. Suffice it to say that we are simply proposing that laparoscopic intervention be added to the list of available therapeutic modalities. As with any operation, the patient must first be considered a suitable candidate for repair, and be resuscitated and prepared accordingly. If the patient is in shock with a board-like abdomen, he or she needs to be stabilized and treated appropriately, but this probably is not laparoscopically. Referring to the risk factors, if the perforation is suspected of being less than 12 hours old and the patient has no severe concurrent medical problems and is not moribund, perhaps laparoscopy should be contemplated.

Before embarking on the venture of laparoscopic repair of perforations, appropriate skills must be acquired and advanced instrumentation available. The surgeon must be capable of placing and tying sutures intracorporeally using laparoscopic techniques in order to close any perforation. The method of open placement of blunt-tipped trocars (Hassan technique)[29] must be considered in these patients with severe inflammation, ileus and fibrinous adhesions making blind insertion of needles and trocars rather hazardous. The standard preoperative routines are observed, including the placement of a urinary catheter and a tube into the stomach for decompression throughout the case. Following insertion of the first cannula, videolaparoscopic exploration is carried out. Having insufflated to a a pressure of 12–15 mm Hg, the peritoneal cavity is systematically examined. Additional cannulas are placed under direct vision as needed and the patient is repositioned if necessary to complete the evaluation of all quadrants. The stomach, duodenum, jejunum, ileum, and colon are examined. The appendix is inspected. Peritoneal fluid samples are collected and sent for Gram's stain and culture as previously mentioned. If no etiology for the inflammation can be identified on the initial survey, the lesser sac should be entered through the gastrocolic ligament and a side-viewing (30' or 45') laparoscope inserted. This modification in angle is very useful if not mandatory in viewing this area, as well as the area up under the left lobe of the liver.

Suggested locations for cannula placement will vary. Generally, placing the laparoscope in the folds of the umbilicus and supplementing this with two 5-mm working ports, one in the midepigastrium caudad to the xyphoid and the other in the right upper quadrant, will allow for thorough exploration. Additional ports can then be placed as deemed necessary for retraction or additional instrumentation. An atraumatic grasper and an irrigating/aspirating probe are the most fundamental instruments necessary to explore the abdomen of a patient with peritonitis. If the above configuration of cannula placement is utilized, the grasper would be inserted through the lateral port and the irrigation/aspiration wand through the midepigastric port. Occassionally a larger trocar will need to be inserted for other instruments such as clip appliers, and this can be done by dilating a 5-mm port site and exchange of cannulas over a blunt probe. Finally, in women being explored for abdominal pain, a uterine probe allows for manipulation and more thorough examination of the pelvis.

Technical aspects of closing any encountered perforations of the gastrointestinal tract are similar to conventional methods, however the skills required to place and tie sutures with two needle holders within the confines of the abdomen must be mastered. If extracorporeal knot-tying methods are used, tension on the tissues is more variable and difficult to gauge, and likely to tear through such friable tissues. Sometimes a flexible endoscope, passed into the stomach or duodenum (using minimal insufflation), will allow better visualization of the repair and identify any other possible ulcers. A nasogastric tube is then left in place until bowel function resumes.

Following completion of the repair, peritoneal irrigation is carried out with copious amounts (6–8 L) of warmed saline. Our preferred irrigating system (Nezhat-Dorsey Hydro-Dissection Pump; Karl Storz Endoscopy-America, Inc., Culver City, CA, USA) will rapidly instill fluid, and at a pressure suitable for removing debris. The large (10 mm) pool-tip aspiration probes then effectively remove the irrigant and any other detritus. When irrigating or lavaging, all quadrants of the coelomic cavity are systematically washed out. Drains are selectively used, invoking the same criteria as we would in open surgery.

Several methods of treating chronic peptic ulcer disease that can be accomplished with laparoscopic assistance have been proposed.[9,31,32] The indications for definitive acid-reducing operations in the face of peritonitis that is not clearly of short duration are, in our estimation, tenuous. In those patients with perforation who present themselves for evaluation early in the course of events and who have a history compatible with protracted symptoms of peptic ulcer disease, the case for more aggressive surgical intervention coupled with an acid suppressing procedure is more tenable. Either way, the ability to approach either or both problems with the help of the laparoscope is an advance worthy of consideration and practice.

Summary

The diagnosis and treatment of peritonitis and the acute abdomen have been the domain of the general surgeon in the past, and should remain so into the future. This mandate will force us to be ever mindful of the latest technological advances and the techniques of using this progress to aid our patients. If we are to always be able to offer the most effective therapy, we must be willing to try new modalities prospectively, and when their efficacy is proven, adopt the best option for our patients. Likewise, we must be mindful that in the process of discovering and proposing new ways of approaching old problems, some of our old methods must not be cast aside without adequate assurance that a brighter horizon has been reached.

References

1. Soper NJ, Stockmann PT, Dunnegan DL, et al: Laparoscopic cholecystectomy: the new 'gold standard'? *Arch Surg* 127:917-923, 1992.
2. Kelling G: Zur Coelioskopie. *Arch Klin Chir* 126:226-229, 1923.
3. Dubois F, Icard P, Berthelot G, Levard H: Coelioscopic cholecystectomy: preliminary report of 36 cases. *Ann Surg* 211:60-62, 1990.
4. Dubois F, Berthelot G, Levard H: Cholecystectomy par Coelioscopie. *Presse Med* 18:980, 1989.
5. Reddick EJ, Olsen DO: Laparoscopic laser cholecystectomy: a comparison with mini-lap cholecystectomy. *Surg Endosc* 3:131-133, 1989.
6. Semm K: Endoscopic appendectomy. *Endoscopy* 15:59-64, 1983.
7. Gangal MT, Gangal MH: Laparoscopic appendectomy. *Endoscopy* 19:127-129, 1987.
8. Jacobs M, Verdeja JC, Goldstein HS: Laparoscopic assisted colonic surgery. In: Zucker KA, ed. *Surgical Laparoscopy—Update*. St. Louis, MO: Quality Medical Publishing; 1993:327-354.
9. Kathkouda N, Mouiel J: A new surgical technique of treatment of chronic duodenal ulcer without laparotomy by videocoelioscopy. *Am J Surg* 161:361-364, 1991.
10. Clayman RV, Kavoussi LR, McDougall EM, et al: Laparoscopic nephrectomy: a review of 16 cases. *Surg Laparoscopy Endoscopy* 2:29-34, 1992.
11. Tulman S, Reynhout J: Laparoscopic splenectomy. Program of the Society of American Gastrointestinal Endoscopic Surgeons, 1992. page 89 (video abstract).
12. Gershman A, Daykhovsky L, Chandra M, et al: Laparoscopic pelvic lymphadenectomy. *J Laparoendoscopic Surg* 1:63-68, 1990.
13. Berci G, Sackier JM, Paz-Partlow M: Emergency laparoscopy. *Am J Surg* 161:332-335, 1991.
14. Carnevale N, Baron N, Delany HN: Peritoneoscopy as an aid in the diagnosis of abdominal trauma: a preliminary report. *J Trauma* 17:634-641, 1977.
15. Berci G, Dunkelman D, Michel SL, et al: Emergency minilaparoscopy in abdominal trauma: an update. *Am J Surg* 146:261-265, 1983.
16. Paterson-Brown S, Eckersley JRT, Sim AJW: Laparoscopy as an adjunct to decision making in the "acute abdomen". *Br J Surg* 73:1022-1024, 1986.
17. Mouret P, Francois Y, Vignal J, et al: Laparoscopic treatment of perforated ulcer. *Br J Surg* 77:1006, 1990.

18. Nakhgevany KB, Clarke LE: Acute appendicitis in women of childbearing age. *Arch Surg* 121: 1053-1055, 1986.
19. Dunn EL, Moore EE, Elerding SC, Murphy JR: The unnecessary laparotomy for appendicitis—can it be decreased? *Am Surg* 48:320-323, 1982.
20. Schreiber J: Early experience with laparoscopic appendectomy in women. *Surg Endosc* 1:211-216, 1987.
21. Gotz F, Pier A, Bacher C: Modified laparoscopic appendectomy in surgery. *Surg Endosc* 4:6-9, 1990.
22. Leape LL, Romenofsky ML: Laparoscopy for questionable appendicitis: can it reduce the negative appendectomy rate? *Ann Surg* 191:410-413, 1980.
23. Whitworth CM, Whitworth PW, Sanfillipo J, Polk HC: Value of diagnostic laparoscopy in young women with possible appendicitis. *Surg Gynecol Obstet* 167:187-190, 1988.
24. Mueller BA, Daling JR, Moore DE, et al: Appendectomy and the risk of tubal infertility. *N Engl J Med* 315:1506-1508, 1986.
25. Koepsell TD, Inui TS, Farewell VR: Factors affecting perforation in acute appendicitis. *SG&O* 153:508-510, 1981.
26. Deutsch AA, Zelikovsky A, Reiss R: Laparoscopy in the prevention of unnecessary appendicectomies: a prospective study. *Br J Surg* 69:336-337, 1982.
27. Martin DT, Zucker KA: Laparoscopic Surgery of the Intestinal Tract in Endoscopic Surgery. Greene F, ed. (in press).
28. Sharp KW: Acute cholecystitis. *Surg Clin North Am* 68:269-279, 1988.
29. Hassan HM: Open Laparoscopy versus closed laparoscopy *Adv Plann Parent* 13:41-50, 1978.
30. Boey J, Choi SKY, Alagaratnam TT, Poon A: Risk stratification in perforated duodenal ulcers: a prospective validation of predictive factors. *Ann Surg* 205:22-26, 1987.
31. Oost Vogel HJM, Van Vroohoven TJMV: Anterior seromyotomy and posterior truncal vagotomy. technique and early results of a randomized trial. *Neth J Surg* 37:69-74, 1985.
32. Taylor TV, Lythgoe JP, McFarland JB, et al: Anterior lesser curve seromyotomy and posterior chronic duodenal ulcer. *Br J Surg* 77:1007-1009, 1990.

10

Special Problems in Peritonitis:
Primary Peritonitis and Peritonitis Associated with Continuous Ambulatory Peritoneal Dialysis

Donald E. Fry, MD

Primary Peritonitis

Peritonitis is generally a disease that is secondary to another pathologic process within the abdominal cavity. Perforation of a viscus occurs from malignancy (eg, colon cancer), or other inflammatory processes (eg, peptic ulcer disease, diverticulitis) of the gastrointestinal or biliary tract are the usual causes. The treatment of peritonitis that is secondary to another disease process requires surgical treatment of the primary disease. Thus, suture repair of the perforation, resection of a diseased segment of intestine, or exteriorization of colon become germane to the elimination of the bacterial source responsible for the peritoneal infection.

Primary peritonitis is a disease entity that is not associated with gastrointestinal or biliary tract disease as the source of the patient's infection. Commonly referred to as spontaneous bacterial peritonitis, primary peritonitis means that the bacterial contaminant has gained access to the peritoneal cavity from (1) hematogenous dissemination from a remote site, (2) lymphatic dissemination from the gastrointestinal

From Fry DE, (ed): *Peritonitis.* Mount Kisco NY, Futura Publishing Co., Inc., © 1993.

tract, or (3) direct transmural migration of microorganisms from the lumen of the gut without a mechanical perforation.

In general, the history and physical findings of patients with primary peritonitis are more subtle than may be found with the secondary peritonitis patient. However, differences between primary and secondary peritonitis can make the two clinical conditions initially identical. Since primary peritonitis does not require a surgical intervention, and because the patient with primary peritonitis usually has severe liver disease with ascites, surgeons must have a thorough understanding of peritonitis that is not associated with an intra-abdominal perforation.

Pathogenesis

The mesothelial cell lining of the peritoneal cavity forms a large sac. This lining may partially cover the surface of certain retroperitoneal structures such as the right and left colon, the duodenum, and the pancreas. Other structures have the mesothelial covering completely about their surface such as the jejunum and ileum.

The peritoneal sac normally contains a small amount of fluid. This fluid is a transudate that probably accumulates from increased hydrostatic pressure of the upright position. In the recumbent position at night, peritoneal fluid is probably not generated but rather is cleared by an intricate mechanism. The pressure gradients within the peritoneal cavity result in movement of peritoneal fluid toward the diaphragm, where it is absorbed into small fenestrations on the diaphragmatic surface.[1,2] These fenestrations lead directly to the thoracic duct. Normally, the volume of fluid is small and bacteria that may gain access to the peritoneal fluid are evacuated into the lymphatic system. In reality, the peritoneal cavity is a large lymphocele that directly communicates with the lymphatic system and is efficiently designed to eliminate an occasional bacterial contaminant.

The patient with severe liver disease and ascites is the prototypical patient to develop primary peritonitis.[3] These patients have multiple variables that result in the occasional systemic bacteremic event or the translocation of bacteria cells from the gastrointestinal tract, which become potential life-threatening sources of infection in the peritoneal cavity.

First, the volume of peritoneal fluid in the patient with ascites is measured in liters, instead of the milliliters of volume that are seen in the patient with normal peritoneal fluid at the time of an elective operative procedure within the abdomen. The ascites is the consequence of increased resistance to blood flow through the liver, increased mesenteric hydrostatic pressures because of portal hypertension, and the reduction of oncotic pressure secondary to the hypoalbuminemia of the cirrhotic patient.

Second, the stasis of fluid within the peritoneal cavity promotes the conversion of a small inoculum of bacteria into a clinically significant number. Peritoneal clearance mechanisms are clearly compromised, and the stagnant ascitic fluid becomes a medium for bacterial growth.

Finally, the peritoneal host defenses of the cirrhotic with ascites are compromised. Hepatic reticuloendothelial function is impaired both because of inefficient Kupffer cell function and because shunt flow through the liver bypasses these hepatic reticuloendothelial cells.[4] This loss of clearance function of bacteria from blood may enhance "seeding" of the peritoneum. Since alcoholic cirrhosis has been most commonly associated with primary peritonitis, acute and chronic alcoholism is associated with defective neutrophil function.[5,6] Macrophage phagocytic capacity appears to be impaired in the cirrhotic patient with ascites.[7] Complement proteins are of hepatic origin, and reduced complement components become another compromise to nonspecific host defense mechanisms.[8] It should be noted that antibody concentrations in alcoholic cirrhosis are not reduced, but then the antibody response plays a rather insignificant role in the host's acute response to bacterial infection.[9]

Bacterial contamination that gains access to the peritoneal cavity and results in primary peritonitis is from two general sources.[10-12] First, infections from anatomical areas that are adjacent to the peritoneal cavity or bacteremia from remote sources result in metastatic, bloodborne spread of small inocula of microorganisms. Bacterascites is thus created and with bacterial growth, clinical peritonitis is the outcome. Clinical sites of remote infection which have been implicated with causing primary peritonitis are listed in Table 1.

The gastrointestinal reservoir has become appreciated as a major source of bacteria for primary peritonitis. Portal venous bacteremia has been identified with intestinal manipulation by diagnostic endoscopy and with certain pathologic conditions.[13-16] Considerable basic science evidence would suggest that bacterial translocation from the gastrointestinal reservoir into the mesenteric lymphatic system and mesenteric lymph nodes is associated with numerous biologic insults.[17-28] With

Table 1

Source	Number of Cases
Urinary Tract Infection	19
Pulmonary Infection	15
"Local Infection"	14
Endoscopy	14
Gastric tubes (Linton tubes, Sengstaken tubes, NG tubes)	13
Biliary obstruction	11
Bowel obstruction	6
Abdominal abscess	6
Percutaneous catheter	5
Peritoneovenous shunt	3
Vasopressin	3
Recent Abdominal Surgery	2
Skin Infection	1
Total	112

Identifies the remote sites of infection that have been identified to result in primary peritonitis in a large review of 246 patients.[11] Obviously, not all patients have a high probability site that is responsible for the "seeding" of the peritoneal cavity. Thus, in this study only 112 sources are identified. There are clearly some arguable issues about what constitutes "primary" peritonitis versus "secondary" peritonitis.

lymph flow through the diaphragm in the ascites patient being impaired or overloaded, lymphatic-borne bacteria become sources for colonization of ascitic fluid. Finally, some evidence implicates transmural migration of microorganisms directly into the peritoneal fluid, perhaps actually being tranported into the ascitic fluid by the host's own macrophage cells.[29]

Bacterial contamination of the ascitic fluid results in bacterial proliferation. Some evidence supports that bacterascites can occur in the same way that bacteruria occurs, ie, there can be bacterial colonization of the fluid without frank infection being present.[30] However, when sufficient bacteria are present that the pathogens bind to the peritoneal mesothelial cells, then invasive infection is the result. Unlike secondary peritonitis, the relatively low inoculum of bacteria, the absence of anaerobes, and the ascitic volume results in primary peritonitis not having an abscess phase to the disease. The diffuse nature of the infection and the impaired defenses of the host commonly results in high mortality rates for primary peritonitis.

The bacterial pathogens of primary peritonitis are detailed in Table 2.[11,31] Gram-positive and gram-negative bacteria are identified pathogens. Infections were polymicrobial in the retrospective review of 1985,[11] but no polymicrobial infection was seen in the prospective study reported in 1991.[31] Anaerobes are seldom encountered probably because of the well-oxygenated environment of ascitic fluid.[32,33]

Diagnosis

The diagnosis of primary peritonitis is usually more difficult than secondary peritonitis. With secondary peritonitis, rebound tenderness or frank board-like rigidity of the abdomen on physical examination establishes the need for abdominal exploration. With primary peritonitis, history and physical examination findings may be quite overt, but more often are subtle and even occult. The diagnosis requires a high index of suspicion in the cirrhotic patient who is at risk for this infection.

Of 246 accumulated patients with primary peritonitis by Hoefs and Runyon,[11] clinical fever was identified at presentation in 67% and abdominal pain was present in 60%. Only 50% had abdominal tenderness

Table 2		
Organism	Review, 1985 (n = 246)	Prospective, 1991 (n = 100)
E. coli	131	22
Klebsiella pneumoniae	26	10
Streptococcus pneumoniae	24	9
Alpha-hemolytic streptococci	17	6
Group D Streptococci	17	6
Unclassified Streptococci	13	3
Beta-hemolytic Streptococci	12	2
Enterobacteriaceae	8	1
Pseudomonas sp.	6	1
Staphylococcus aureus	5	0
Others	48	1
Polymicrobial Infections	28	0

Identifies the bacterial isolates cultured from the peritoneal cavity of patients with primary peritonitis. The retrospective review[11] was from pooled data from several different clinical reports while the prospective data was accumulated in a randomized trial.[31]

on physical examination and only 42% had rebound tenderness. Twenty-seven percent had hypotension at presentation while 11% were hypothermic. In 81% of patients, clinical jaundice was present. Clearly, specific clinical findings are not dependable in this diagnosis.

Diagnostic paracentesis has become a useful method in the establishment of the diagnosis. The gross appearance of the ascitic fluid from patients with suspected primary peritonitis is not helpful in establishing the diagnosis. Ascitic fluid is commonly cloudy whether infection is present or not. The fluid is rarely bloody from infection. While glucose, protein, and other variables in the ascitic fluid have been studied, only the neutrophil count has been dependable. Thus, a diagnosis of primary peritonitis can be made when the polymorphonuclear cell count in the ascitic fluid is greater than 250 cells per cubic millimeter, the culture is positive, and the patient does not have another source of infection.[11] Others have suggested that polymorphonuclear cell counts greater than 500 cells per cubic millimeter are necessary for the diagnosis.[34,35] When counts exceed 1000 cells per cubic millimeter, then therapy is felt to be necessary for these patients even if the culture is negative for identification of a pathogen.[36]

The diagnostic dilemma of these patients is the differentiation of primary peritonitis from secondary peritonitis. A single study has compared primary peritonitis patients to patients with ascites who had gastrointestinal perforations.[37] No differences were identified between the primary and secondary peritonitis patients with respect to physical findings (Table 3). Secondary peritonitis patients were identified as having dramatic differences in ascitic fluid findings. Patients with a perforated viscus were statistically more likely to have low ascitic glucose concentrations, elevated lactate dehydrogenase (LDH) concentrations, and were more likely to have a polymicrobial infection (Table 3). White blood cell counts in the ascitic fluid were numerically higher in the secondary peritonitis patients, but did not reach statistical significance because of the large standard deviation. Mortality rates in both the primary and the secondary peritonitis groups of patients exceeded 70%, reflecting the poor outcome of peritonitis in patients with ascites regardless of cause.

Treatment

The current treatment of primary peritonitis has been less than satisfactory. The review of reported cases by Hoefs and Runyon[11] has

Table 3

	Primary Peritonitis *(n = 33)*	*Perforated Viscus* *(n = 6)*
Clinical Findings		
Abdominal pain	19 (58%)	4 (67%)
Fever	19 (58%)	2 (33%)
Ileus	13 (40%)	5 (83%)
Abdominal tenderness	14 (42%)	3 (50%)
Rebound tenderness	2 (6%)	1 (17%)
Confusion	24 (73%)	2 (33%)
Bacteremia	16 (48%)	1 (17%)
Multiorganism infection	4 (12%)	6 (100%)*
Deaths	23 (70%)	5 (83%)
Ascitic Fluid Findings		
Total protein (gm/dL)	0.8 ± 0.8	2.5 ± 1.1
Glucose (mg/dL)	128 ± 63	36 ± 47*
LDH (mU/mL)	173 ± 230	847 ± 594*
Total white count	6500 ± 6600	9400 ± 5600
Polymorphonuclear Cells	5200 ± 6000	8300 ± 6400

Identifies similarities and differences between the clinical findings and the ascitic fluid findings in patients with ascites that have a perforated viscus and those that have primary peritonitis

identified a 78% cumulative mortality rate. The poor success rate probably reflects the poor condition of the host to withstand the infection. It may also reflect a delay in diagnosis for those patients with subtle clinical findings. Several studies have failed to identify that antibiotics affected patient outcome whatsoever.

The systemic antibiotic selection should be targeted to cover the cultured pathogen. When a clinical diagnosis has been made, then antibiotic therapy should be initiated prior to culture results, particularly if the ascitic polymorphonuclear cell count is greater than 1,000 cells per cubic millimeter. Anticipated organisms listed in Table 2 should be covered until sensitivity data are available. Vancomycin is a commonly selected antibiotic when the Gram's stain of the ascitic fluid demonstrates a gram-positive organism. Vancomycin covers the possibility that a methicillin-resistant *Staphylococcus epidermidis* is the pathogen. When culture and sensitivity data are subsequently available, then more specific therapy may be chosen. For methicillin-sensitive staphylococcal pathogens, cefazolin is safe and inexpensive therapy. Several choices for gram-negative coverage are available. Numerous expanded-spectrum β-lactam antibiotics are potential choices and include cefotaxime, ceftazidime, and aztreonam. Ciprofloxacin is another potential choice. Anaerobic coverage is deliberately avoided with these choices. Because ascites represents a dramatic expansion of the volume of distribution for antibiotics, aggressive dosing should be entertained. Aggressive dosing means that antibiotics with a favorable therapeutic index are necessary to avoid toxicity problems. Thus, aminoglycosides are avoided. In general, hepatically cleared or metabolized antibiotics should be avoided.

Empirical anaerobic antibiotic coverage should be avoided in the management of these patients. As identified above, anaerobes do not appear to be pathogens of primary peritonitis, nor do they appear to be microorganisms that translocate from the intestinal tract. Furthermore, the normal anaerobic microflora of the gut represent a component part of the barrier function of the intestinal tract.[38-40] Elimination of the native anaerobic species will have potentially negative consequences.

Peritoneal Dialysis-Associated Peritonitis

Continuous ambulatory peritoneal dialysis (CAPD) is commonly used for renal failure patients. It has become an alternative to hemodialysis for many patients but it has also placed these patients at risk for catheter-associated peritontis.

Pathogenesis

Continuous ambulatory peritoneal dialysis (CAPD) associated peritontis arises when pathogenic microorganisms migrate along the pericatheter space of the in-dwelling dialysis catheter and into the peritoneal cavity. The peritoneal cavity with residual volumes of dialysis fluid essentially recreates the local environment of the cirrhotic patient with ascites. Peritoneal fluid appears to impair peritoneal clearance of microorganisms. Bacterial binding to the mesothelial lining of the peritoneum then occurs, and invasive infection is the result.[41]

Bacterial (or even fungal) access to the pericatheter space occurs by two mechanisms. First, normal skin flora of the patient proliferates around the site of catheter entrance through the skin. Normal flora of the skin becomes common pathogens of CAPD-associated peritonitis. Contamination of the peritoneal dialysis catheter when handled by the patient or health care provider becomes a second route of bacterial pathogens, which also tend to be skin flora from the perpetrator or pathogens carried from other patients.

The pathogens of CAPD-associated peritonitis are listed in Table 4.[42,43] *Staphylococcus aureus* and *Staphylococcus epidermidis* are the most common. However, when one reviews the literature on this subject, it can quickly be identified that nearly every bacterial or fungal pathogen known has been reported to cause CAPD-associated peritonitis.[44-46] Since these patients are frequently in the hospital environment and frequently receive antibiotics for other reasons, they may become colonized with or come into casual contact with all would be, hospital-acquired pathogens. The types of microorganisms are numerous and accurate culture information is important for treatment.

Diagnosis

The diagnosis of CAPD-associated peritonitis is similar to that of primary peritonitis. Overt history and physical findings are somewhat

Table 4

Isolated Microorganism	Valente[42]	Bint[43]	Saklayen[48]
Staphylococcus epidermidis	12 (25%)	112 (45%)	30%–45%
Staphylococcus aureus	5 (10%)	35 (14%)	10%–20%
Streptococcus sp.	2 (4%)	22 (9%)	10%–15%
E. coli	5 (10%)	20 (8%)	8%–12%
Pseudomonas sp.	9 (19%)	11 (4%)	5%–8%
Enterobacter sp.	9 (19%)	4 (2%)	2%–3%
Enterococcus sp.		9 (4%)	3%–5%
Klebsiella sp.		6 (2%)	2%–3%
Acetinobacter sp.		6 (2%)	2%–3%
Fungi	1 (2%)	5 (2%)	
Others	5 (10%)	20 (8%)	3%–5%

Identifies the bacterial isolates from one recent U.S. study,[42] a study from the United Kingdom,[43] and a review article.[48] The number of isolates from each report will exceed 100% of the patients because of the polymicrobial cases that are identified.

more helpful, although renal failure patients may still have occult evidence of peritonitis. In general, patient complaints of abdominal pain and physical findings of abdominal tenderness with rebound are more common than are identified in the cirrhotic with primary peritonitis.[47]

The evaluation of the peritonitis dialysate is of greatest value in the diagnosis of CAPD-associated peritonitis.[45,47] The dialysate return is usually cloudy. Positive Gram's stains are useful. Neutrophil counts greater than 100 cells per cubic millimeter are usually used as the threshold for diagnosis. Cultures are necessary to establish the pathogen responsible for the peritonitis. It is advisable to send 100–200 mL of the returned dialysate fluid to the laboratory for centrifugation, since cultures of the sediment increase the probability of a positive culture.[45] Anaerobes are not generally thought to be pathogens of CAPD-associated peritonitis. Some centers still culture the peritoneal dialysate for anaerobes, since a positive culture is significant evidence to indict a perforation of the gastrointestinal tract.[48]

Two additional diagnoses should be kept in mind in the patient with suspected CAPD-associated peritonitis. Eosinophilic peritonitis may be seen within the first few days following placement of the peritoneal dialysis catheter.[49] The dialysate return has a cloudy appearance similar to active bacterial infection, but has eosinophils on microscopic examination of the fluid. No bacteria can be identified. This inflammatory response is thought to be a reaction to the foreign body effect of the catheter within the peritoneal cavity. This is a self-limiting process and need not be cause for either changing the catheter nor for discontinuation of peritoneal dialysis. A second entity, known as sclerosing peritonitis, represents a vigorous peritoneal reaction to the dialysate solution itself.[50,51] The process provokes generalized adhesion formation. Inflammatory cells are seen in the dialysate but without bacteria. When a diagnosis of sclerosing peritonitis is made, peritoneal dialysis must be discontinued.

Treatment

Prompt recognition and initiation of treatment can avoid hospitalization for many patients with CAPD-associated peritonitis. Sensitization of patients and nursing personnel to recognize early evidence of infection can permit rapid initiation of treatment.

Intraperitoneal antibiotics are the preferred route of administration for the treatment of these patients.[52] These can be effectively administered through the dialysis catheter itself by adding antibiotics to the dialysis solution. Systemic absorption of the drug can maintain good systemic drug concentrations from the peritoneal reservoir without the need for systemically administered antibiotics. Peritonitis has actually been experimentally shown to increase antibiotic absorption from the peritoneal cavity.[53] Heparin is usually added to the dialysate to reduce fibrin formation since fibrin debris may occlude the dialysis catheter.

Since staphylococcal bacteria are the most common isolates from these infections, antistaphylococcal treatment is most commonly employed. A positive Gram's stain for gram-positive bacteria is sufficient to implement antibiotic therapy. Because *Staphylococcus epidermidis* is the most common pathogen, vancomycin is most commonly used for antibiotic therapy since this bacterial pathogen has a high frequency of being methicillin resistant.[48] When gram-negative infections are identified, aminoglycosides are generally avoided lest any residual renal function be compromised. Broad-spectrum cephalosporins, aztreonam, and quinolones are desirable agents to use for sensitive gram-negative CAPD-associated peritonitis, since they do not have anaerobic activity for all the reasons that have been previously identified.

Patients with CAPD-associated peritonitis rarely have bacteremia, but will occasionally become sufficiently ill to require hospitalization. Hospitalization may be required when infection is the consequence of unusual organisms such as *Pseudomonas sp.* or *Candida albicans*. In unusually difficult cases, removal of the catheter is required and alternative forms of dialysis need to be pursued until the infection is resolved.

References

1. Allen L, Weatherford T: Role of fenestrated basement membrane in lymphatic absorption from the peritoneal cavity. *Am J Physiol* 197:551-554, 1956.
2. Tsilibary EC, Wissig SL: Absorption from the peritoneal cavity: SEM study of the mesothelium covering the peritoneal surface of the muscular portion of the diaphragm. *Am J Anat* 149:127-132, 1977.
3. Conn HO: Spontaneous peritonitis and bacteremia in Laennec's cirrhosis caused by enteric organisms. *Ann Intern Med* 60:658-680, 1964.
4. Rimola A, Soto R, Bory F, et al: Reticuloendothelial system phagocytic activity in cirrhosis and its relation to bacterial infections and prognosis. *Hepatology* 4:53-58, 1984.
5. Klepser RG, Nengster WJ: The effect of alcohol upon the chemotactic response of leukocytes. *J Infect Dis* 65:196-199, 1939.

6. Marr JJ, Spilberg I: A mechanism for decreased resistance to infection by gram-negative organisms during acute alcoholic intoxication. *J Lab Clin Med* 86:253-258, 1975.
7. Hassner A, Kletter Y, Shlag D, et al: Impaired monocyte function in liver cirrhosis. *Br Med J* 282:1262-1263, 1981.
8. Runyon BA, Morrissey RL, Hoefs JC, et al: Opsonic activity of human ascitic fluid: a potentially important protective mechanism against spontaneous bacterial peritonitis. *Hepatology* 4:634-637, 1985.
9. Bjorneboe M, Jensen KB, Scheibel I, et al: Tetanus antitoxin production and gamma globulin levels in patients with cirrhosis of the liver. *Acta Med Scand* 188:541-546, 1970.
10. Correia JP, Conn HO: Spontaneous bacterial peritonitis in cirrhosis: endemic or epidemic? *Med Clin North Am* 59:963-981, 1975.
11. Hoefs JC, Runyon BA: Spontaneous bacterial peritonitis. *Dis Mon* 31:1-48, 1985.
12. Hallak A: Spontaneous bacterial peritonitis. *Am J Gastroenterol* 84:345-350, 1989.
13. Eade MN, Brooke BN: Portal bacteremia in cases of ulcerative colitis submitted to colectomy. *Lancet* 1:1008-1013, 1969.
14. Schatten WE, Despray JD, Holden WD: A bacteriologic study of portal vein blood in man. *Arch Surg* 71:404-409, 1955.
15. LeFrock JL, Ellis CA, Turchick JB, et al: Transient bacteremia associated with sigmoidoscopy. *N Engl J Med* 289:467-469, 1975.
16. Dickman MD, Farrell R, Higgs RH, et al: Colonscopy-associated bacteremia. *Surg Gynecol Obstet* 142:173-176, 1976.
17. Wolochow H, Hildebrand GH, Lamana C: Translocation of microorganisms across the intestinal wall of the rat: effect of microbial size and concentration. *J Infect Dis* 116:523-528, 1966.
18. Deitch E, Berg RB, Specian R: Endotoxin promotes the translocation of bacteria from the gut. *Arch Surg* 122:185-190, 1987.
19. Arnold L, Brody L: Passage of bacteria through the intact intestinal mucosa. *Proc Soc Exp Biol Med* 25:247-248, 1928.
20. Li M, Specian RD, Deitch EA: Effects of protein malnutrition and endotoxin on the intestinal mucosal barrier to the translocation of indigenous flora in mice. *JPEN* 13:572-578, 1989.
21. Schweinburg FB, Heimburg F: Effect of chemical irritation of the peritoneum on transmural migration of intestinal organisms. *Proc Soc Exp Biol Med* 71:146-150, 1949.
22. Schweinburg FB, Frank HA, Frank ED, et al: Transmural migration of intestinal bacteria during peritoneal irrigation in dogs. *Proc Soc Exp Biol Med* 71:150-153, 1949.
23. Berg RD, Garlington AW: Translocation of certain bacteria from gastrointestinal tract to the mesenteric lymph nodes and other organs in a gnotobiotic mouse model. *Infect Immun* 23:403-411, 1978.
24. Berg RD: Promotion of translocation of enteric bacteria from the gastrointestinal tract of mice by oral treatment with penicillin, clindamycin, or metronidazole. *Infect Immun* 33:854-861, 1981.

25. Deitch EA, Sittig K, Li M, et al: Obstructive jaundice promotes bacterial translocation from the gut. *Am J Surg* 159:79-84, 1990.
26. Bennion RS, Wilson SE, Williams RA: Early portal anaerobic bacteremia in mesenteric ischemia. *Arch Surg* 119:151-155, 1984.
27. Owen WE, Berg RD: Bacterial translocation from the gastrointestinal tract of athymic (nu/nu) mice. *Infect Immun* 27:461-467, 1980.
28. Alverdy JC, Chi HS, Sheldon GS: The effect of parenteral nutrition on gastrointestinal immunity, the importance of enteric stimulation. *Ann Surg* 202:681-684, 1985.
29. Wells CL, Maddaus MA, Simmons RL: Role of the macrophage in translocation of intestinal bacteria. *Arch Surg* 122:48-53, 1987.
30. Conn HO, Fessel JM: Spontaneous bacterial peritonitis in cirrhosis: variation on a theme. *Medicine* 50:161-197, 1971.
31. Runyon BA, McHutchison JG, Antillon MR, et al: Short-course versus long-course antibiotic treatment of spontaneous bacterial peritonitis. *Gastroenterology* 100:1737-1742, 1991.
32. Targan SR, Chow AW, Guze LB: Role of anaerobic bacteria in spontaneous peritonitis of cirrhosis. Report of two cases and review of the literature. *Am J Med* 62:397-403, 1977.
33. Sheckman P, Onderdonk AB, Bartlett JG: Anaerobes in spontaneous peritonitis. *Lancet* 2:1223, 1977.
34. Bar-Meir S, Lerner E, Conn HO: Analysis of ascitic fluid in cirrhosis. *Dig Dis Sci* 24:136-144, 1979.
35. Jones SR: The absolute granulocyte count in ascites fluid. An aid to the diagnosis of spontaneous bacterial peritonitis. *West J Med* 126:344-346, 1977.
36. Runyon BA, Hoefs JC: Culture-negative neutrocytic ascites: a variant of spontaneous bacterial peritonitis. *Hepatology* 4:1209-1211, 1984.
37. Runyon BA, Hoefs JC: Ascitic fluid analysis in the differentiation of spontaneous bacterial peritonitis from gastrointestinal tract perforation into ascitic fluid. *Hepatology* 4:447-450, 1984.
38. van der Waaij D, Berghuis-de Vries JM, Lekkerkerk-van der Wees JEC: Colonization resistance of the digestive tract in conventional and antibiotic treated mice. *J Hygiene* 69:405-411, 1971.
39. van der Waaij D, Berghuis-de Vries JM, Lekkerkerk-van der Wees JEC: Colonization resistance of the digestive tract and spread of bacteria to the lymphatic organs in mice. *J Hygiene* 70:335-342, 1972.
40. Wells CL, Maddaus MA, Reynolds CM, et al: Role of anaerobic flora in the translocation of aerobic and facultative anaerobic intestinal bacteria. *Infect Immun* 55:2689-2694, 1987.
41. Haagen IA, Heezius HC, Verkooyen RP, et al: Adherence of peritonitis-causing staphylococci to human peritoneal mesothelial cell monolayers. *J Infect Dis* 161:266-273, 1990.
42. Valente J, Rappaport W: Continuous ambulatory peritoneal dialysis associated with peritonitis in older patients. *Am J Surg* 159:579-581, 1990.
43. Bint AJ, Finch RG, Gokal R, et al: Diagnosis and management of peritonitis in continuous ambulatory peritoneal dialysis. *Lancet* 1:845-848, 1987.

44. Arfania D, Everett D, Nolph KD, et al: Uncommon causes of peritonitis in patients undergoing peritoneal dialysis. *Arch Intern Med* 141:61-64, 1981.
45. Vas SI: Microbiologic aspects of chronic ambulatory peritoneal dialysis. *Kidney Int* 23:83-92, 1983.
46. Young JB, Ahmed-Jushuf IH, Brownjohn AM, et al: Opportunistic peritonitis in continuous ambulatory peritoneal dialysis. *Clin Nephrol* 22:268-269, 1984.
47. Peterson PK, Matzke G, Keane WF: Current concepts in the management of peritonitis in patients undergoing continuous ambulatory peritoneal dialysis. *Rev Infect Dis* 9:604-612, 1987.
48. Saklayen MG: CAPD peritonitis: incidence, pathogens, diagnosis, and management. *Med Clin North Am* 74:997-1010, 1990.
49. Steiner R: Clinical observations on the pathogenesis of peritoneal dialysate eosinophilia. *Peritoneal Dial Bull* 2:118-119, 1982.
50. Bradley JA, Hamilton DNH, McWhinnie DL, et al: Sclerosing peritonitis after CAPD. *Lancet* 2:572, 1983.
51. Slingeneyer A, Canaud B, Mourad G, et al: Progressive sclerosing peritonitis: a late and severe complication of maintenance peritoneal dialysis. *Trans Am Soc Artif Intern Organs* 12:633, 1983.
52. Johnson CA, Zimmerman SW, Rogge M: The pharmacokinetics of antibiotics used to treat peritoneal dialysis associated peritonitis. *Am J Kidney Dis* 4:3-17, 1984.
53. Fry DE, Trachtenburg L, Polk HC Jr: Serum kinetics of intraperitoneal moxalactam. *Arch Surg* 121:282-284, 1986.

11

Special Problems in Peritonitis:
Peritonitis in the Pediatric Patient

Diller B. Groff, MD, Hirikati S. Nagaraj, MD, and John B. Pietsch, MD

Newborn infants and children have some specific causes of peritonitis not seen in adults and may frequently demonstrate a different response to peritonitis than the adult (Table 1).[1] The newborn female infant has a small immature pelvis with the bladder, uterus, ovaries and tubes, appendix, and sigmoid colon being intra-abdominal rather than pelvic as in older patients. This anatomical difference in organ location and the less bulky omentum means less localization of sepsis and earlier generalized peritonitis in many conditions. The newborn is more susceptible to gram-negative infections because only IgG crosses the placenta and the newborn must actively immunize himself against newly colonized gram-negative organisms. Given time, the newborn can produce IgM antibodies against coliforms. Low levels of complement for opsonization and relative deficits in white cell function also decrease the effectiveness of the newborn reaction to peritonitis

Evaluation of the whole newborn is paramount in peritonitis because the classic distended tender rigid abdomen is infrequently encountered. One third of newborns with peritonitis[2] will have an associated bacteremia (usually *Escherichia coli*) and rapidly show signs of systemic effects from peritonitis. Initially, a newborn has less generalized muscle

From Fry DE, (ed): *Peritonitis*. Mount Kisco NY, Futura Publishing Co., Inc., © 1993.

Table 1
Etiology of Neonatal Peritonitis

Perforative	Non-Perforative
Sterile	Primary peritonitis
Meconium peritonitis	Omphalitis
Bile peritonitis	Gastroschisis
Bacterial	Ruptured
Gastric Perforation	omphalocele
Spontaneous	Pyelonephritis
Distal obstruction of duodenum	Infected V-P shunt
Stress ulcer	Appendicitis
Duodenal Perforation	Meckel's
Distal obstruction	diverticulitis
Stress ulcer	
Intestinal Perforation	
Distal obstruction (atresia/stenosis)	
Volvulus	
Intussusception	
Appendicitis	
Meckel's diverticulitis	
Necrotizing enterocolitis	
Iatrogenic (instrumentation/drugs)	
Idiopathic	

tone, the Moro and grasp reflexes are less active, and the ability to maintain body temperature decreases. Regurgitation and vomiting occur early, along with abdominal distention, but abdominal pain and guarding are less pronounced than in older children. Seizures may signal the onset of meningitis, a common occurrence in peritonitis in the newborn and infants and a factor in choosing antibiotics that cross the blood-brain barrier. Respiratory function decreases early in peritonitis and increased ambient oxygen or intermittent bagging may be required; if the CO_2 increases and the pH falls, endotracheal intubation may become necessary. A fall in platelets signals worsening sepsis and is often accompanied by intracranial bleeding. Properly performed and accurately interpreted x-rays are indispensable in diagnosing and treating peritonitis in the newborn and infant. The tender distended abdomen, which is gasless on x-ray (Figure 1A), is shown to be due to a malrotation with volvulus by the upper gastrointestinal (GI) series (Figure 1B).

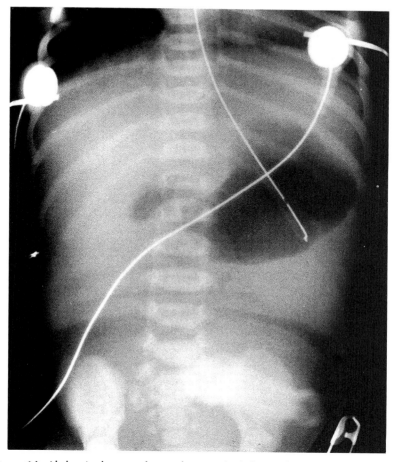

Figure 1A: Abdominal x-ray of a newborn with abdominal distention and tenderness showing a distended stomach and first portion of duodenum with a gasless abdomen beyond this point.

Bell, Ternberg, and Bower[2] carefully analyzed the peritoneal cultures taken at the time of celiotomy in 30 out of 31 newborns with peritonitis secondary to intestinal perforation from a variety of causes including volvulus, atresia, Hirschsprung's disease, necrotizing enterocolitis (NEC), and meconium ileus. Bacteria were grown from specimens in 30 patients and 26 of these patients grew one or more bacterial species. Multiple flora (2–5 species per patient) were grown in 57%, and 23%

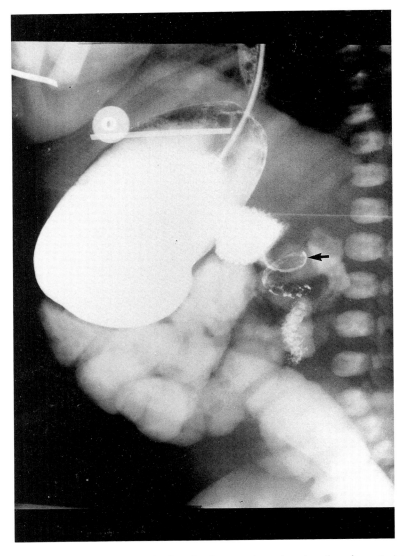

Figure 1B: Upper gastrointestinal series in a patient showing the characteristic "corkscrew" duodenum (arrow) confirming a malrotation with volvulus.

showed mixed aerobic and anaerobic peritoneal flora. The gram-negative organisms (usually *E. coli*) dominated the aerobic cultures, being grown 62% of the time. Group D *Streptococcus* was a common gram-positive aerobe. Bacteroides species composed 85% of the gram-negative cultures, and *C. perfringes* was cultured once. Only gentamycin was effective against all gram-negative aerobes, while all but one isolate of bacteroides was sensitive to clindamycin. Chloromycetin was also very effective against bacteroides in this study.

This study emphasizes that with proper collection and culture techniques, bacteria can be grown from the peritoneum in virtually all cases of neonatal peritonitis secondary to postnatal perforation of the gastrointestinal tract. Treatment with a combination of drugs, including gentamicin, ampicillin, clindamycin, and chloromycetin while awaiting species identification and antibiotic sensitivity is indicated. These antibiotics also provide protection against meningitis, a common complication of peritoneal sepsis in the newborn.

Meconium Peritonitis

Meconium is the product of swallowed amniotic fluid, sebaceous material, desquamated epithelial cells, bile salts, and pigments. Meconium starts to accumulate in the intestine of the 4-month-old fetus, reaches the ileocecal valve by the fourth fetal month, and the rectum by the fifth month. Normally, all newborns pass large amounts of meconium in the first 24 hours after birth. When meconium is released into the peritoneum (following intrauterine perforation of the gastrointestinal tract) it causes a severe peritonitis. If this occurs early in fetal life, the meconium causes intense inflammation and becomes calcified; occasionally, meconium can pass through the patent processus vaginalis and calcify in the scrotum, resulting in a hard scrotal tumor in the newborn. If the meconium enters the peritoneum late in gestation it does not have time to calcify and the newborn has signs of free peritoneal fluid which is brown-green and thick on paracentesis.

The clinical varieties of meconium peritonitis include: (1) meconium pseudocyst, which develops as a result of the organization of leaking meconium. The organized and fibrosing meconium results in encased loops of intestine in the area of perforation, but the rest of the peritoneum is free of adhesions; (2) adhesive meconium peritonitis developing after widespread prenatal meconium leak. Dense adhesions develop and if the infant is not obstructed immediately after delivery, later obstruction by these adhesions is common; (3) meconium ascites in which the peritoneal fluid is meconium stained as a result of late prenatal perforation. Calcium is usually not present; (4) infected meconium peritonitis as a result of continued postnatal contamination of the peritoneum from a perinatal perforation with meconium spill. These newborns need immediate surgery to stop the contamination of the peritoneum.[3]

The most common cause of meconium peritonitis is perforation of the intestine secondary to obstruction from intrauterine volvulus, atresia, idiopathic perforation (18%), or meconium ileus, which is almost always associated with cystic fibrosis (mucoviscidosis).[4] Although up to 50% of patients with meconium ileus from cystic fibrosis have associated meconium peritonitis, the finding of meconium peritonitis by itself does not mean that the newborn has cystic fibrosis.[4] Nevertheless, the surgeon must rule out cystic fibrosis in all patients with meconium peritonitis. The tenacious meconium and the inflamed bowel at surgery are signs suggestive of cystic fibrosis, but a properly performed sweat test is the definitive study, and this can only be performed many days after the emergency surgery. The surgeon must remember that a sweat chloride test must also be performed in all infants with intestinal atresia, with or without meconium peritonitis to rule out cystic fibrosis.

Diagnosis

Almost all meconium peritonitis is associated with newborn intestinal obstruction. Therefore, the baby is usually born with a distended abdomen and develops bilious vomiting. If the perforation and spillage of meconium have occurred late in fetal life, the abdomen may be very distended with a blue discoloration; masses can be seen and easily palpated through the abdominal wall. X-ray often shows calcification in the peritoneum (Figure 2) plus the signs of intestinal obstruction or the classic ground-glass appearance of the thick meconium-filled small bowel seen with mucoviscidosis. Those patients with meconium peritonitis will always need exploration in the newborn period and only a contrast enema (Figure 3) to demonstrate the unused colon (misnamed a microcolon in the literature) is helpful to complete the diagnostic studies because occasionally a patient with Hirschsprung's disease will present with intestinal obstruction and signs of meconium peritonitis on

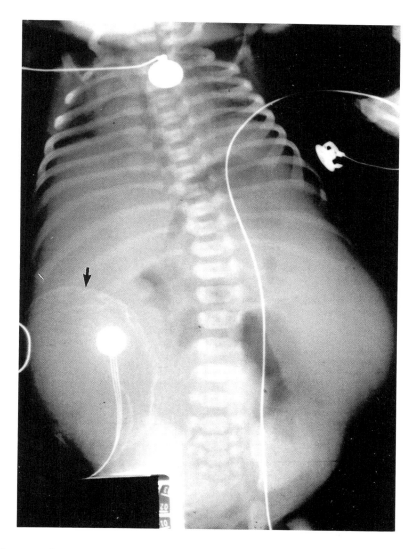

Figure 2: Plain film showing abdominal distention by masses, very little bowel gas, and calcification on the right side (arrow).

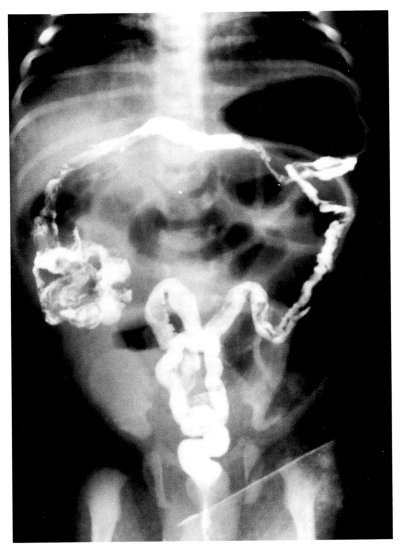

Figure 3: Contrast enema in a newborn showing the small unused colon. Strong support for the diagnosis of meconium ileus or small bowel atresia.

x-ray. In this situation, the contrast enema will demonstrate a dilated colon if it is Hirschsprung's disease.

Treatment

Treatment of meconium peritonitis requires correction of the under-lying cause. Atresia, volvulus, and idiopathic perforations are treated by resection and primary anastomosis or exteriorization as in ileostomy or colostomy. When prolonged intestinal dysfunction is expected, a gas-trostomy should be performed. Meconium ileus with meconium perito-nitis (complicated meconium ileus) can be treated by laparotomy and irrigation of the bowel to remove abnormal meconium followed by resection of the proximal dilated inflamed bowel at the site of perfora-tion. Primary repair can be performed, but exteriorization by a Bishop-Koop type enterostomy is safe and technically expedient.[5]

Survival in complicated meconium ileus with meconium peritonitis can be as high as 93% in the immediate postoperative period.[6] Meconium peritonitis associated with atresias, intrauterine volvulus, and simple perforation lowers survival, but with modern neonatal intensive care support and total parenteral nutrition even most of these complicated newborns survive. Mortality is related more to gestational age, birth weight, and the presence of other major congenital anomalies.[7,8]

Primary Peritonitis in Infancy

Primary peritonitis is now a rare condition, accounting for fewer than 1% to 2% of all pediatric abdominal emergencies. However, this condition still occurs frequently in underdeveloped countries.[9] The de-crease in this condition is undoubtedly due to better antiseptic care of the umbilical stump in the newborn and early use of antibiotics in the septic child of any age. McDougal, Izant, and Zollinger[10] reviewed 84,000 pediatric admissions over 10 years and analyzed 183 cases of peritonitis. They found that, if only diffuse peritonitis in which no specific etiology such as intestinal perforation or appendicitis was considered, primary peritonitis accounted for 17% of the infants and 13.4% of the children above 2 years of age.

The cause of primary peritonitis is usually obscure, but many of these children have urinary tract infections and the close relationship of the urinary system to the peritoneum may allow cross-contamination.

Other theories of origin include bacteremia, transdiaphragmatic lymphatic migration of bacteria, or bacterial migration through the intestinal wall.

The infant with primary peritonitis usually presents with a rapidly progressing septic course. In approximately 50% of these infants, a radiologically proved pneumonia precedes the peritoneal signs. The infants are lethargic or irritable, apneic and anorexic, but the smaller patients do not initially show abdominal rigidity, distention, or other signs of peritonitis. The older child almost always has a short period from the onset of symptoms to the development of diffuse peritoneal signs. The older child does develop abdominal tenderness, rectal spasm, abdominal rigidity, rebound tenderness, and diffuse rectal tenderness, as does a child with peritonitis from other causes.

Patients with known cirrhosis or nephrosis in whom primary peritonitis is suspected usually have a more insidious progression of symptoms. Unfortunately, there are few distinguishing characteristics that separate primary peritonitis from peritonitis that is secondary to other intra-abdominal disease. The presence of peritoneal signs with an essentially normal abdominal x-ray suggests primary peritonitis. An infected urine should signal the physician to look for primary peritonitis first before considering other causes. The temperature, white count, and electrolytes do not differ in the various forms of peritonitis.

Most infants and older children who have primary peritonitis undergo surgery to insure that no specific cause of peritonitis is being overlooked. All patients with cirrhosis or nephrosis in whom primary peritonitis is suspected should have a paracentesis with Gram's stain and culture of any aspirate. If the Gram's stain has organisms, the patient should be treated with antibiotics and not undergo abdominal exploration. The patients with urinary tract infection or pneumonia and no x-ray evidence of abdominal disease should be treated for 12 to 24 hours with antibiotics and observed for improvement of peritoneal findings. The bacteriology of primary peritonitis has changed from that of a predominantly gram-positive infection to one with a predominance of gram-negative organisms, so antibiotics that are used should be effective against *E. coli* and *Pseudomonas* species in addition to covering for gram-positive organisms.

Up to 50% of infants with primary peritonitis still die of generalized sepsis. In a series by McDougal et al.[10] 15% of the older children died as compared to only one death in 157 other patients with peritonitis from specific causes. Complications are also frequent in those explored for primary peritonitis. Drainage of the peritoneum in these patients is not recommended.

Necrotizing Enterocolitis

Necrotizing enterocolitis (NEC) is the most frequent serious gastro-intestinal problem in newborns. The cause is not known, but premature infants who have had perinatal stress (as evidenced by low Apgar scores and difficulty in resuscitation) comprise 90% of the patients. However, NEC occurs in full-term babies and in infants as old as 3 months. No single set of factors, including the stress of prematurity, insertion of umbilical artery or vein catheters, early feeding of high osmolar formulas, or the protective effect of breast milk have been consistent findings in several reviews.[11-13] The epidemic character of NEC in various nurseries is well recognized. The spectrum of NEC can be such that the entire small bowel and colon can be affected either so mildly that ileus or mild diarrhea with hematochezia are the only symptoms followed by complete recovery, or the bowel is so severely involved that the entire gut becomes necrotic and death occurs. The classic picture is that of a premature who develops abdominal distention, passes blood and intestinal mucosa in his stools, shows signs of sepsis, becomes apneic and bradycardic, and demonstrates pneumotosis intestinalis (Figure 4) or portal vein gas on abdominal x-ray. As the enterocolitis penetrates to the serosa, peritonitis develops. However, despite necrosis of the bowel, free peritoneal gas develops in less than one third of the patients.

Kosloske[14] reported that of the 17 patients requiring surgery in a series of 25 patients who had NEC, 16 had bacteria in their blood and/or peritoneum. In only 2 patients were no organisms recovered from the peritoneum. Eight patients had *Klebsiella* species as the predominant aerobic organism and 8 patients had *Clostridium* species as a predominant anaerobic organism; however, the type of bacterium grown did not correlate with survival in these patients. It is interesting that the 8 patients not requiring surgery for NEC did not have bacterial peritonitis or bacteremia. Since the organisms recovered from newborns with NEC vary from nursery to nursery,[15,16] treating these patients should include gentamicin, ampicillin with clindamycin, or chloramphenicol as a possible third antibiotic and surgical intervention when required.

Treatment of NEC requires respiratory support, fluid and blood components (fresh frozen plasma, packed cells and platelets), and sys-

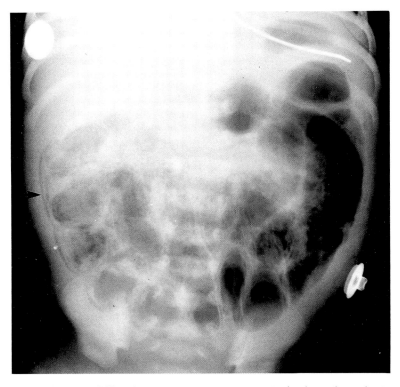

Figure 4: Abdominal film showing pneumotosis intestinalis throughout the intestine, with the characteristic "string of beads" pattern (arrow).

temic antibiotics (gentamicin, ampicillin) and nasogastric suction. Intraluminal antibiotics should not be given as the variation in absorption is very likely to give toxic blood levels while not increasing survival or decreasing morbidity. Only 40% of patients will require surgery. Free gas in the peritoneal cavity is the only absolute indication for surgery. Even then, extensive bowel necrosis often precludes definitive limited excision, and bowel diversion and limited resections are performed. Peritoneal aspiration is helpful in that brown fluid with bacteria indicates that exploration and drainage should be performed while yellow clear fluid reinforces continued nonsurgical therapy.[17] The surgeon's role is to stop contamination of the peritoneum by continued fecal soilage, divert the fecal stream with single or multiple ostomies, and get the patient over the septic phase. Three weeks of bowel rest and total parenteral nutrition followed by slow advancement of formula concentration is necessary to allow regeneration of the intestinal mucosa and limit relapses. When the patient is showing good weight gain any ostomies can be closed. At this time, careful check of the gut must be made to rule out strictures that occur in up to 20% of patients secondary to scarring of the bowel. Mortality in surgical and nonsurgical patients is the same (about 50%) and is related most closely with the size of the newborn and associated severe congenital anomalies.

Gastrointestinal Perforation

Gastrointestinal peforation without necrotizing enterocolitis occurs most often in the small bowel, colon, and stomach, in that order. These newborns are often stressed at birth and have low Apgar scores, and require umbilical artery or vein catheter insertion followed by exchange transfusions. Overdistention of the stomach and passage of nasogastric tubes have been suggested as causes of gastric perforation. The patient with a colon perforation must have Hirschsprung's disease excluded, and most sigmoid and rectosigmoid perforations are associated with enemas and thermometer insertion. Small bowel perforations are most often associated with atresias at various levels. Peptic ulcer disease causing perforation is a known, but rare entity.

The newborn with a gastrointestinal perforation is usually noted to have pronounced abdominal distention at 3 to 5 days of age and an abdominal x-ray shows free air in the peritoneum (Figures 5A and 5B); a cross table lateral is an excellent technique to see free air in a sick newborn without disturbing him too much. In contrast to necrotizing enterocolitis, the bowel is usually only involved at the site of perforation. Almost all gastric perforations occur along the greater curvature and closure of these should always have a protective Stamm-type gastrostomy. The surgeon must use his judgment in deciding whether colostomy is needed for sigmoid and rectal perforations. Although the peritoneum can be massively contaminated with formula or stool, peritoneal irrigations and debridement, closure of the perforation or diversion of the fecal stream results in survival in 50% of patients.[18] Of course, expert neonatal intensive care with skilled nurses, respirators, and long-term total parenteral nutrition are essential for this high survival rate.

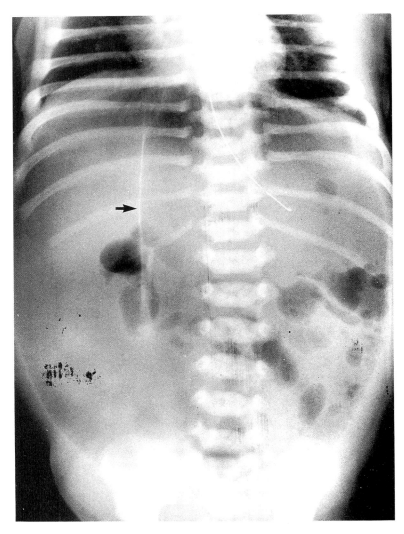

Figure 5A: Supine abdominal view showing free air and the falciform ligament (arrow).

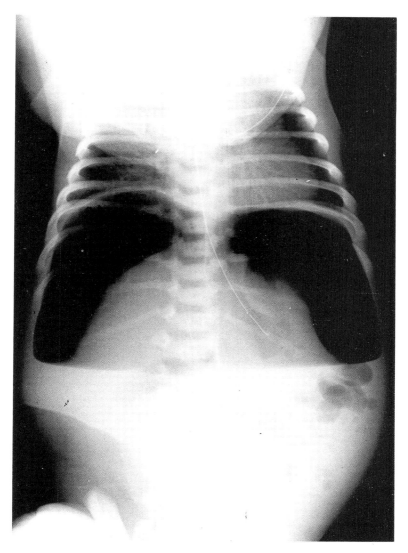

Figure 5B: Upright view of the same patient shown in Figure 5A dramatically highlighting the large amount of peritoneal air.

Peritonitis Associated With Ventriculoperitoneal Shunts

An interesting cause of peritonitis in the infant and child is contamination of the peritoneum from an infected cerebral ventriculoperitoneal shunt inserted for hydrocephalus. These children present with fever, generalized or localized signs of peritoneal irritation, and white blood count ranging from 11–17,000 per cubic millimeter. They do not normally have neurological findings.[19,20]

The problem is differentiating primary intra-abdominal sepsis from secondary peritonitis from the shunt itself. Therefore, the patient's shunt reservoir is aspirated and if gram-positive organisms (usually *Staphylococcus epidermidis* or *Staphylococcus aureus*) are found, then the shunt itself is the cause of the infection, and therapy consists of exteriorization of the shunt, antibiotics for 14 days, followed by replacement of the shunt. If gram-negative organisms are found in the shunt fluid, then an abdominal source such as ruptured appendix is sought. Occasionally, the surgeon will have to drain encysted, contaminated shunt fluid in the abdomen before a new ventriculoperitoneal[21] shunt can be inserted.

Pneumoperitoneum in Ventilated Newborns

Newborns who have high ventilator pressure settings may have air dissect into the the peritoneum causing a classic pneumoperitoneum.[22] If the infant has any suggestion of abdominal sepsis, a perforation of the gastrointestinal tract may be suspected in such cases. Several factors can help differentiate simple dissection of air from the mediastinum into the peritoneum from intra-abdominal sepsis. There is often posterior mediastinal air along the tract of the dissection into the peritoneum; if a paracentesis is performed, air flow synchronous with the ventilator cycle suggests a respiratory origin of the gas; if the oxygen content of the abdominal gas is the same as the FiO_2, this suggests a respiratory origin. If paracentesis yields no cloudy-greenish fluid this suggests a nonintestinal source for air. By applying these clinical tests, rupture of a viscus should be excluded. However, if doubts still persist, instillation of water soluble contrast material into the gastrointestinal tract with serial x-rays in the neonatal intensive care unit should rule out gastrointestinal perforation.

Bile Peritonitis

Bile peritonitis is an extremely rare event in childhood and is usually due to perforation of the bile ducts.[23,24] It may occur as two different clinical forms: (1) acute bile peritonitis that occurs in early infancy with abdominal pain, tenderness, vomiting, and occasional icterus, or (2) chronic bile peritonitis that usually presents with early icterus followed by painless abdominal distention, biliary ascites, or bile sac formation. The sac in chronic bile peritonitis may perforate into the general peritoneal cavity resulting in severe symptoms. The etiology of perforation of the bile ducts is not clear, but distal obstruction or congenital weakness of the common duct have been suggested as possible causes.[11]

The abdominal x-rays show diffuse haziness and floating small bowel suggestive of free peritoneal fluid (Figure 6). Intravenous cholangiography and I^{131} Rose bengal studies may be helpful in documenting the perforation. Paracentesis shows fluid that looks like bile, is occasionally turbid, and usually has a bilirubin content over 400 mg per 100 cc.

Laparotomy is essential in all cases of bile peritonitis as all infants not operated upon usually die. The identification of the site of perforation at operation is often not possible, however, an operative cholangiogram may reveal distal obstruction in some cases. Drainage of the peritoneal cavity is frequently all that is required without repair or identification of the distal obstruction. In one series, operative biliary drainage alone was performed in 45 infants with a survival rate of 80%.[24]

Perforated Appendicitis in Infants and Preschool Children

In the United States, appendicitis is the most common condition that requires abdominal surgery in children. It is important to establish the approximate time of onset with some accuracy since appendicitis progresses more rapidly in children than adults, resulting in early gangrene and perforation. In this preschool group, difficulty in obtain an accurate history, less typical clinical features, increased frequency of abdominal pain from various causes, and parental delay contribute to the rupture rate of 50% to 85%.[25,26] Rupture of the appendix in children is more frequently followed by diffuse peritonitis and distant intra-abdominal

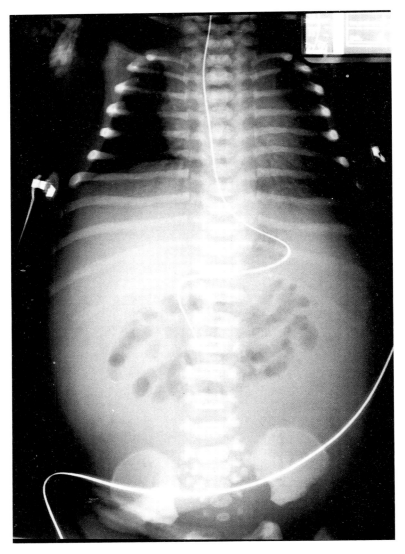

Figure 6: Plain view of the abdomen showing the bulging flanks and the central location of small bowel gas that are characteristic of peritoneal fluid as seen in bile peritonitis.

abscesses than in adults because the incompletely developed greater omentum is less efficient in walling off the inflammatory process and the small immature pelvis means the appendix is more intra-abdominal.

In preschool children, Graham et al.[25] reported the most common symptoms on initial examination were abdominal pain in 100%, fever in 81%, nausea and vomiting or both in 80%, anorexia in 60%, and diarrhea in 10%. Children 4 to 6 years of age had a mean duration of symptoms of 58 hours compared to 102 hours if less than 4 years old. Abdominal tenderness is most often diffuse in nature, but when localized, is often present in the periumbilical or right lower quadrant regions of the abdomen. The common classic description of abdominal tenderness is found more frequently in children over 4 years old. When the appendix ruptures, the pain becomes more diffuse.

Elevated temperature was present in most of the children. The child with ruptured appendicitis lies still with legs drawn up and breathes shallowly with an open mouth. Vomiting is more frequent with perforated appendicitis, and this is correlated with the frequently absent or diminished bowel sounds in children with perforated appendicitis. The white blood cell count will almost always be markedly elevated in these younger patients. X-rays of the abdomen are quite helpful in young children: 50% of children with abdominal pain and a fecalith on abdominal X-ray may have perforated appendicitis; paralytic ileus or air fluid levels in the right lower quadrant indicate peritoneal inflammation.

These sick infants must be prepared for surgery with rehydration, correction of electrolyte imbalance, preoperative antibiotics, and reduction of fever. After rehydration, prompt operation for perforated appendicitis and broad-spectrum antibiotic coverage, including clindamycin, is widely accepted by most pediatric surgeons.

Bacteriological data from Stone[27] and Marchildon and Dudgeon[28] emphasize the importance of anaerobic organisms, particularly bacteroides species in perforated appendicitis. Antibiotics have been shown to decrease the rate of intra-abdominal abscess,[29] but did not change the incidence of the infection in the study by Stone et al.[26] Randomized studies by Greenall et al.[30] and Haller et al.[31] have shown no benefit from the use of drains in perforated appendicitis with generalized peritonitis without abscess. Despite these reports, some surgeons favor routine drainage of the copious irrigation of the peritoneal cavity and delayed primary closure of the subcutaneous tissue and skin. Preoperative and postoperative use of clindamycin, gentamicin, and ampicillin has been very effective in controlling intra-abdominal sepsis in these infants.[32]

Perforated Peptic Ulcers in Infants

Peptic ulcer disease occurs infrequently in infancy.[33-36] Stress ulceration with duodenal or gastric perforation is seen in premature and sick infants. An acute ulcer is occasionally seen as an isolated presentation in the newborn without traumatic birth, delivery, or other stress. The etiology of ulceration of the stomach and duodenum in newborns is not known, but gastrlc acidity is thought to play a role. Miller[34] has reported that free and total acid increases in the first 2 days of life, falls to a lower level after several days, then gradually rises after 10 days to level off between 10 and 23 weeks. During the later half of the first year, free hydrochloric acid in the stomach decreases. The review of the literature by Bell et al.[35] in which the mean age of duodenal perforation was 10 weeks, corresponds well to these physiologic data.

Unlike adult patients in whom simultaneous perforation and hemorrhage rarely occur, hemorrhage is often seen in these newborns and infants prior to perforation. In contrast to stress ulceration in adults, stress ulceration in infants appears to have a higher frequency of (1) single ulcer, (2) perforation, (3) duodenal (rather than gastric) location, and (4) persistent vomiting as a sign of impending perforation.[33]

Bell et al.[35] reported a mortality rate of 40% in a recent series of newborns and infants with stress ulceration. Bleeding in the stressed infant may be a warning sign of perforation, but fortunately, upper gastrointestinal bleeding in the newborn is most often self-limited, does not require surgical intervention, and is usually not able to be diagnosed as being caused by an ulcer, esophagitis, or gastritis. These infants usually respond to antacids, and blood transfusions with complete recovery. If an infant bleeds massively, a peptic ulcer may be diagnosed on upper gastrointestinal series in 80%. Even those infants with severe bleeding should respond to medical management, and in Johnson's[33] series only two patients required surgery for the control of bleeding or to close a perforation.

References

1. Rickham PP: Meconium and bacterial peritonitis. In: Rickham PP, Johnston JH. *Neonatal Surgery*. New York: Appleton-Century-Crofts; 1969:348-365.
2. Bell MJ, Ternberg JL, Bower RJ: The microbial flora and anti microbial therapy of neonatal peritonitis. *J Pediatr Surg* 15(4):569-573, 1980.
3. Lorimer WS Jr, Ellis DG: Meconium peritonitis. *Surgery* 60:470, 1966.

4. Dolan TF Jr, Touloukian RJ: Familial meconium ileus not associated with cystic fibrosis. *J Pediatr Surg* 9:821-824, 1974.
5. Bishop HC, Koop CE: Management of meconium ileus: resection, Roux-en-Y anastomosis and ileostomy irrigation with pancreatic enzymes. *Ann Surg* 145:410-414, 1957.
6. Mabogunjb O, Wang CI, Mahour H: Improved survival of neonates with meconium ileus. *Arch Surg* 117:34-40, 1982.
7. Nixon HH, Tawes RW: Etiology and treatment of small intestinal atresia: analysis of a series of 127 jejunoileal atresias and comparison with 62 duodenal atresias. *Surgery* 69:41, 1971.
8. Grosfeld JL, Ballantine TVW, Shoemaker R: Operative management of intestinal atresia and stenosis based on pathologic findings. *J Pediatr Surg* 14:368-375, 1979.
9. Duggan MB, Khwaja MS: Neonatal primary peritonitis in Nigeria. *Arch Dis Child* 50:130-132, 1975.
10. McDougal WS, Izant RJ, Zollinger RM Jr: Primary peritonitis in infancy and childhood. *Ann Surg* 181(3):310-313, 1975.
11. Schullinger JN, Mollitt DL, Vinocur DC, et al: Neonatal necrotizing enterocolitis. *Am J Dis Child* 135:612-614, 1981.
12. Kliegman RM, Fanaroff AA: Neonatal necrotizing enterocolitis: a nine-year experience. *Am J Dis Child* 135:603-607, 1981.
13. Kliegman RM, Fanaroff AA: Neonatal necrotizing enterocolitis: a nine-year experience. *Am J Dis Child* 135:608-611, 1981.
14. Kosloske AM, Ulrich JA: A bacteriologic basis for the clinical presentation of necrotizing enterocolitis. *J Pediatr Surg* 14:558-563, 1980.
15. Book LS, Overall JC, Herps TJJ, et al: Clustering of necrotizing enterocolitis: interruption by infection control measures. *N Engl J Med* 297:984-986, 1977.
16. Guinan M, Schaberg D, Bruhn SW, et al: Epidemic occurrence of neonatal necrotizing enterocolitis. *Am J Dis Child* 133:594-597, 1979.
17. Kosloske AM: Paracentesis and lavage for diagnosis of intestinal gangrene in neonatal necrotizing enterocolitis. *J Pediatr Surg* 13:315-320, 1978.
18. Emanuel B, Zlotnik P, Raffensperger J: Perforation of the gastrointestinal tract in infancy and childhood. *Surg Gynecol Obstet* 146:926-928, 1978.
19. Hubschmann OR, Counter RW: Acute abdomen in children with infected ventriculoperitoneal shunts. *Arch Surg* 115:305-307, 1980.
20. Tchirkow G, Verhagen AD: Bacterial peritonitis in patients with ventriculoperitoneal shunts. *J Pediatr Surg* 14:182-184, 1979.
21. Ekong CE, Clein LJ: Formation of abdominal cyst secondary to ventriculoperitoneal shunting. *Can J Surg* 22:250-252, 1979.
22. Knight PJ, Abdenogr G: Pneumoperitoneum in the ventilated neonate: respiratory or gastrointestinal origin? *J Pediatr* 98:972-974, 1981.
23. Hendren WH, Donahoe PK: Bile duct perforation in a newborn with stenosis of the ampulla of water. *J Pediatr Surg* 11:823, 1976.
24. Prenol J, Rickham PP, Hecker WC: Acute biliary peritonitis. *Prog Pediatr Surg* 1:196, 1971.
25. Graham JM, Pokorny WT, Harberg FJ: Acute appendicitis in preschool age children. *Am J Surg* 139:247-250, 1980.

26. Stone HH, Sanders SL, Martin JD: Perforated appendicitis in children. *Surgery* 69:673-679, 1971.
27. Stone HH: Bacterial flora of appendicitis in children. *J Pediatr Surg* 11:37-42, 1976.
28. Marchildon MB, Dudgeon DL: Perforated appendicitis: current experience in a children's hospital. *Ann Surg* 185:85-87, 1977.
29. Bower RJ, Bell MT, Ternberg JL: Controversial aspects of appendicitis management in children. *Arch Surg* 116:885-887, 1981.
30. Greenall JM, Evans M, Pollock AV: Should you drain a perforated appendix. *Br J Surg* 65:880-882, 1978.
31. Haller JA, Shaker IJ, Donahoo JS, et al: Peritoneal drainage vs non drainage for generalized peritonitis from ruptured appendicitis in children. A prospective study. *Ann Surg* 177:595-600, 1973.
32. Brook I: Bacterial studies of peritoneal cavity and postoperative surgical wound drainage following perforated appendix in children. *Ann Surg* 192:208-212, 1980.
33. Johnson D, L'Heureux P, Thompson T: Peptic ulcer disease in early infancy: clinical presentation and roentgenographic features. *Acta Paediatr Scand* 69:753-760, 1980.
34. Miller RA: Gastric acidity during the first year of life. *Arch Dis Child* 17:198, 1972.
35. Bell MJ, Keating JP, Ternberg JL, Bower RJ: Perforated stress ulcers in infants. *J Pediatr Surg* 16:998-1002, 1981.
36. Berg RM: Peptic ulcer in children. *Southern Med J* 54:325, 1961.

12

Special Problems in Peritonitis:
Peritonitis from the Biliary Tract and Pancreas

Donald E. Fry, MD, and Daniel T. Martin, MD

Peritonitis secondary to the pancreatico-biliary complex is commonly encountered and is highly variable in severity. It may affect the young or the elderly patient. Because the bacteriology of the biliary tract is distinct from the gastrointestinal tract, there is a greater tendency for monomicrobial rather than polymicrobial infections. Indeed peritonitis from cholecystitis may be bacteriologically sterile and actually represents nonspecific inflammation. Similarly, pancreatitis is initially not a bacterial disease but is rather a chemical peritonitis. Nevertheless, peritoneal signs on physical examination can be as dramatic as any peritonitis of bacterial origin. These distinct features of peritonitis from the pancreatico-biliary complex require separate consideration from other causes.

Peritonitis Secondary to the Biliary Tree

Natural History

Generally speaking, peritonitis from the biliary tract begins with obstruction of the cystic duct from calculous disease. This anatomical

---

From Fry DE, (ed): *Peritonitis.* Mount Kisco NY, Futura Publishing Co., Inc., © 1993.

obstruction results in spastic contractions by the smooth muscle of the gallbladder wall to expel the blockade. Mucus production is accelerated and significant accumulation may result in the clear fluid contents of the gallbladder at cholecystectomy. Mucus production may also aggravate distention of the gallbladder. Persistent contraction of the smooth muscle results in sustained tension and a nonspecific inflammatory response in the wall. While the severity of the inflammatory changes will be increased by the presence of bacteria, it is initially the inflammation itself and not microorganisms that are responsible for peritoneal signs on the physical examination.

The localized peritoneal irritation from the adjacent inflammation of the gallbladder persists until one of several events occurs. The obstructing calculous may be dislodged either back into the gallbladder or into the common duct with temporary resolution of the obstruction. Persistence of the obstruction with entrapment of primary or secondary bacterial contamination may result in suppuration and the development of empyema. Increased pressure in the gallbladder wall may result in embarrassed venous and lymphatic drainage and a subsequent reduction in arterial inflow with ischemic necrosis of a portion or all of the gallbladder. Perforation of the gallbladder through the necrotic portion, with or without an accompanying empyema, may then occur with generalized peritonitis being the result. Perforation may occur without necrosis because of increased intraluminal pressure that exceeds the tensile strength of the gallbladder wall, although this latter mechanism is surely uncommon without some component of tissue ischemia. While the initial diffuse peritonitis following perforation is a chemical one, secondary bacterial infection usually occurs.

Acute acalculous cholecystitis has a somewhat different natural history but a common end result. Like the patient with cholelithiasis, obstruction of the cystic duct is the common denominator. However, the obstruction may occur from tumor, edema, blood clot, or fibrous occlusion of the cystic duct.[1] Commonly acute acalculous cholecystitis occurs as an intercurrent problem following surgery or in-hospital care for other illness, particularly in elderly patients.[2] It may occur in younger patients in association with shock, multiple trauma, and particularly with severe burns.[3-5] Acute acalculous cholecystitis in the absence of an organic obstruction of the cystic duct is usually associated with an antecedent low flow syndrome from either hypovolemia, cardiac failure, or sepsis. Thus, this illness differs from obstructive cholecystitis in that it is primarily an ischemic injury of the gallbladder.

Because there is litle inflammation of the gallbladder wall prior to the ischemic event, it is not surprising that there are few symptoms of localized tenderness prior to necrosis. Since the inflammation from an antecedent obstruction is not present, only necrosis results in the inflammatory response that yields peritoneal signs. The time interval from the onset of tissue ischemia until perforation and diffuse peritonitis is commonly very short (eg, 12 hours).

Diagnostic Methods

The diagnosis of peritonitis secondary to biliary tract disease is principally suspected from the history and physical examination. Because the gallbladder is a derivative of the embryonic foregut, initial symptoms of visceral pain are referred to the epigastrium. As the inflammation proceeds, the parietal peritoneum overlying the dome of the gallbladder becomes involved and pain localizes to the right upper quadrant of the abdomen. Physical examination at this point demonstrates localized tenderness, guarding, and rebound. If perforation of the gallbladder has occured, signs and symptoms are diffuse and are similar to findings of peritonitis in general.

Laboratory studies are of marginal value in the diagnosis of peritonitis secondary to the biliary tree and are generally nonspecific indicators. Leukocytosis is usually present, may exceed 20,000 cells per cubic millimeter in some cases, but may be totally absent in elderly patients. Elevations of serum glutamic-oxaloacetic transaminase (SGOT), serum glutamate pyruvate transaminase (SGPT), and lactate dehydrogenase (LDH) may be present but will not serve to differentiate biliary tract disease, hepatocellular disease, or perihepatic sepsis.

Elevations of serum bilirubin may be very misleading. The bilirubin level will rise with either acute cholecystitis,[6,7] empyema of the gallbladder,[8] gangrene of the gallbladder,[9] or ascending cholangitis from obstruction of the common duct.[10,11] Importantly, fever, leukocytosis, right upper quadrant tenderness, and rapidly evolving jaundice demand biliary exploration and no further diagnostic studies.[12]

When acute cholecystitis is suspected, several methods can be used to establish the diagnosis. Ultrasonography has been reported of value in many series,[13-15] but is of most value in the hands of those with the greatest experience in its use (Figures 1 and 2). Infusion tomography is another method reported to be of value.[16] Oral cholecystography is not

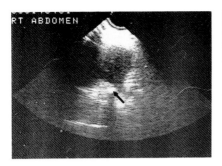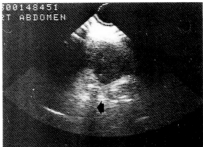

Figure 1: Demonstrates two plates from an ultrasound study of the gallbladder. The plate on the left shows the stone quite clearly. The plate on the right is a different "cut" from the same patient and does not clearly show the stone, but the echogenicity behind the stone is identified and is reasonable proof that a stone is present.

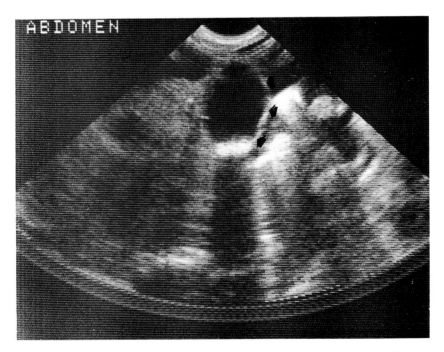

Figure 2: Demonstrates a very large stone in a patient with symptoms of acute cholecystitis. The ultrasound demonstrates a thickened wall of the gallbladder and is presumptive proof for a diagnosis of acute cholecystitis.

an option in the acute patient with biliary disease and intravenous cholangiography carries significant morbidity and variable reliability.

The advent of the 2,6 dimethylphenyl carbomoylmethyl imino-diacetic acid (HIDA) and paraisopropyl iminodiacetic acid (PIPIDA) technetium-labeled scans have introduced a new dimension in the rapid diagnosis of acute cholecystitis.[17,18] These compounds are selectively secreted by the liver into the biliary tract and with appropriate scanning techniques can quickly identify the gallbladder (Figures 3, 4, and 5). These scans also can be performed with bilirubin levels of 10 mg% or greater with reasonable accuracy. Patients with severe hepatocellular disease (eg, cirrhosis, severe hepatitis) may not excrete adequate amounts of these compounds into the biliary tract, limiting the usefulness of the method.

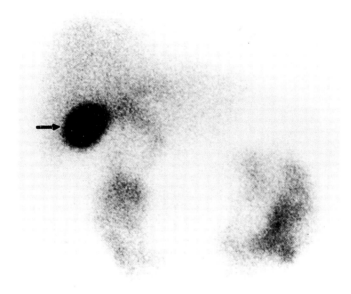

Figure 3: Demonstrates a normal HIDA scan. The gallbladder is indicated by the arrow. Contrast is noted within the duodenum.

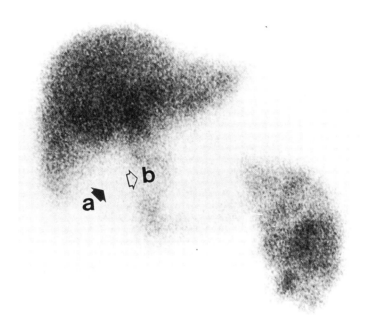

Figure 4: Demonstrates an abnormal HIDA scan. The gallbladder (a) is absent. Secondly the diameter of the common duct appears abnormally large (b) and was documented at operation to have common duct stones.

Occasionally, the diagnosis of right upper quadrant tenderness with or without hyperbilirubinemia, or the diagnosis of clinical jaundice with or without peritoneal signs may baffle the clinician. Fever and leukocytosis with generalized deterioration of the patient's condition may not permit conventional diagnostic methods. The "mini-laparotomy" has been a valuable method in such circumstances.[19] A small incision is made in the right upper quadrant under local anesthesia with general anesthesia available should circumstances warrant. The gallbladder can be identified, checked for viability, and aspirated for presence of pus.

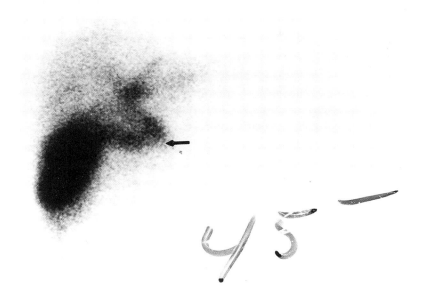

Figure 5: Demonstrates a HIDA scan in a patient without cholecystitis but with common duct obstruction. Adenocarcinoma of the pancreas was subsequently confirmed.

Cholecystocholangiography may confirm either cystic duct or common duct obstruction. On rare occasions, poor-risk patients may have either acute cholecystitis or ascending cholangitis temporized by leaving the cholecystotomy tube used for cholecystocholangiography in place for dependent drainage. Finally, a liver biopsy can also be performed if primary hepatocellular disease is a diagnostic concern. Based upon the findings of the "mini-lap", the diagnosis can usually be ascertained and a judgment to proceed, with general anesthesia and a formal exploration of the biliary tract or abdomen, may be made. As is discussed below, the revolutionary changes in laparoscopic approaches to the biliary tract have resulted in the mini-laparotomy becoming a very seldom used procedure.

Treatment

Obviously the best treatment for peritonitis secondary to the biliary tract is prevention. The diagnosis of biliary calculi should generally warrant elective cholecystectomy at the earliest possible time to avoid the onset of acute cholecystitis and its sequelae.

When the diagnosis of acute cholecystitis is established, urgent cholecystectomy is, in the judgement of the author,[8,9], the treatment of choice. Nasogastric suction is instituted, antibiotics (see below) are initiated preoperatively, and cholecystectomy is performed within 24 hours. The nonoperative management of acute cholecystitis subjects the patient to excessive pain and suffering, flirts with gangrenous or pyogenic progression of the disease, and serves only to postpone the inevitable cholecystectomy to some later date.

While some authors have advocated conservative management of acute cholecystitis if the "golden period" of 72–96 hours of symptoms has passed,[20,21] our experience and that of other authors,[22,23] suggests that excessive complications are not identified when one proceeds directly to definitive therapy at the time of the patient's presentation. Rather our experience has demonstrated an excessive frequency of catastrophic complications when conservative therapy is pursued.[8,9]

Only selected high-risk patients (eg, recent myocardial infarction) should be candidates for conservative management. Even the patient with a recent myocardial infarction and acute cholecystitis should be monitored very closely during conservative management since a high frequency of gangrene of the gallbladder may be seen in these patients. Failure of these high-risk patients to show improvement within 24 hours of conservative therapy may be cause for cholecystostomy drainage of the gallbladder under local anesthesia.

The presence of acute cholecystitis does not preclude the possibilities that calculi of the common duct may be present. Nearly 20% of patients with empyema of the gallbladder have positive common duct explorations for stones.[8] Thus routine operative cholangiography is as important in the cholecystectomy for acute cholecystitis as it is in the elective case. On the other hand, operative morbidity increases substantially when a common duct exploration accompanies the cholecystectomy for acute cholecystitis.[8] Preoperative evidence to suggest common duct pathology (eg, hyperbilirubinemia, elevated alkaline phosphatase) should not be sole indicators for choledochotomy and exploration.[6]

When empyema or gangrene of the gallbladder is present, mortality rates approximate 20%. Mortality rates are 40% to 50% when perforation of the gallbladder complicates either gangrene or empyema.[8] Operative therapy requires cholecystectomy and operative cholangiography. Indications for common duct exploration are as noted above. Extrabiliary abscess may accompany gallbladder perforation and will require drainage.

If the septic process represents suppurative cholangitis, then T tube drainage of the common duct is the treatment of choice. Generally the severely acute nature of the patients with this malady may require only drainage, with cholecystectomy and common duct exploration deferred to a future reoperation.

Cholecystostomy has had some advocates in the treatment of acute cholecystitis.[24] In particularly compromised circumstances this may be a desirable procedure. However, it is important that cholecystocholangiography documents that the common duct freely communicates with the common duct; otherwise, an alternative drainage method will be required.[25,26]

Antibiotic Therapy

In Table 1, the bacterial organisms most commonly encountered in the biliary tree are enumerated.[27-30] Generally speaking, *Escherichia coli, Klebsiella sp.,* and the enterococcus are most frequently cultured. Staphylococcus and even pseudomonas are occasionally identified. Anaerobic

Table 1

Organism	Chetlin/Elliott[27]	Fukunaga[28]	Martin*[30]
E. Coli	11%	15%	8%
Klebsiella/Enterobacter sp.	5%	9%	6%
Enterococcus sp.	4%	5%	1%
Staphylococcus sp.	2%	12%	0%
Bacteroides sp.	0%	0.4%	0%
Clostridial sp.	0.4%	4%	3%
No growth	66%	53%	82%

Indicates the frequency of isolation of major biliary tract bacteria from all patients cultured in the respective studies. (*Quantitative cultures: > 100,000 organisms used as criterion for a positive culture).

bacteria are infrequently of significance in the biliary tract, although *Clostridium species*[29] and *Bacteroides fragilis*[31] have been recognized as being of concern in the elderly. Cultures from empyema and gangrenous cholecystitis specimens follow similar microbiological patterns.[8,9]

Antibiotic therapy should principally be directed against the gram-negative rods. Drugs with such a spectrum that also are concentrated in the biliary tract have a theoretical advantage. Cefazolin has both the spectrum and biliary kinetics, and has been shown as an effective agent for prevention in patients undergoing elective biliary surgery.[32] As a single agent, cefazolin is adequate for patients with acute cholecystitis. In those patients with systemic manifestations of sepsis, the addition of an aminoglycoside may also be desirable. Some authorities have recommended ampicillin to cover the enterococcus but no evidence currently indicates that this additional drug makes any difference in results of therapy. The absence of good clinical studies in patients with established biliary infection makes any recommendation of antibiotics prone to personal preference rather than scientific data.

Laparoscopic Management of Acute Cholecystitis

In the past, cholecystectomy via laparotomy was the avenue of choice for treating acute cholecystitis. With the advent of laparoscopic cholecystectomy and subsequent developments within the field of laparoscopy, and with the evolving experience of surgeons that has liberalized the indications for laparoscopy, acute cholecystitis, and even gangrenous cholecystitis are being treated with minimal access surgery. Previously a relative contraindication, laparoscopic intervention in acute intraperitoneal pathology is now viewed as an alternative for the diagnostic and therapeutic management of these patients.

The techniques of laparoscopic cholecystectomy have been published widely,[33-35] and have been extensively practiced during routine elective cholecystectomy. More recently several authors have reported their results with this technique in the setting of acute inflammation of the gallbladder,[36-39] and have generally found that after extensive experience with laparoscopic-guided procedures, successful cholecystectomy can be achieved even in the face of acute inflammation. Espoused advantages of laparoscopic methods as opposed to traditional open laparotomy include reduced hospitalization, rapid return to normal daily activities, and less pain or need for analgesics. An added attraction from the patient's perspective is the reduction in cosmetic disfigurement.

If laparoscopic cholecystectomy is to be undertaken in patients with severe acute inflammation or gangrenous cholecystitis, respect must be given to the anatomy of the hepatobiliary triangle, particularly in the face of edema accompanying the disease process. This concern for definition of the anatomy has led to the routine use of operative cholangiography at our institution and others[40] for both elective and emergent laparoscopic or open cholecystectomy. The controversy about cystic duct cholangiography during cholecystectomy persists, but the need for radiologic delination of common duct anatomy is crucial.

In addition to the variability of common duct anatomy, there are the more prevalent variations of cystic and hepatic arterial anatomy.[41,42] Basic surgical principles must always be followed in performing the dissection around the gallbladder, identifying all arterial and ductal structures prior to division, and maintaining a willingness to convert the procedure to an open cholecystectomy should there be the slightest confusion in what structures are being dissected.

In the case of discovering common bile duct stones on operative cholangiography, the options are multiple and controversial. We prefer laparoscopic common bile duct exploration with a flexible choledochoscope and basket extraction of stones, while others[43] have championed use of postoperative endoscopic retrograde cholangiography and sphincteroplasty when that expertise is reliable and readily available in their institution.

Often when encountering acute cholecystitis, hydrops is encountered, and some have noted that decompression and aspiration of the gallbladder contents followed by endoloop control of the decompression site will facilitate retraction and exposure.[44,45] Without this maneuver it may be impossible to grasp the gallbladder. In addition to this marked distention, it is common to encounter dense adhesions around the acutely inflamed gallbladder. Adhesions are lysed with careful, blunt dissection, although sharp dissection may be required in selected circumstances. Throughout this arduous process, maintaining strict hemostasis will allow the operation to progress without unnecessary delay or risk to the patient. Electrocautery can be of assistance in this endeavor if applied cautiously and in short bursts via insulated dissecting instruments. Insertion of an additional cannula to facilitate exposure should be entertained in difficult procedures.

Although placement of drains in patients undergoing cholecystectomy is optional and varies from one surgeon to another, in the patient with acute cholecystitis, a drain placed in the gallbladder fossa is recommended. The drain can be promptly removed the following day in the absence of bilious drainage. If a common bile duct exploration has been undertaken, a drain and a T tube are utilized. Reinforcement of the cystic duct stump is advisable, so that a second pretied suture is placed over the primarily hemoclip. There may be a small amount of bilious leakage from accessory ducts, which if overlooked, further justifies the use of subhepatic drainage.

The conversion of a laparoscopic cholecystectomy to an open precedure must not be viewed as a complication, and the conversion ratio may well be higher in cases of acute cholecystitis.[46] It is imperative that any surgeon undertaking laparoscopic procedures for acute inflammation of the gallbladder should have extensive experience with both laparoscopic and open biliary procedures. In addition to expertise, proficiency can be enhanced by acquiring appropriate instrumentation and gaining familiarity with all available equipment.[47] The safety of the patient cannot be overemphasized, and if the anatomy is unclear or the tissue planes are obliterated, open cholecystectomy may remain the safest course of action.

Peritonitis Secondary to Acute Pancreatitis

Natural History

Acute pancreatitis usually arises secondary to alcoholism or calculous disease of the biliary tract. In calculous disease, lodgment of the stone at the ampulla results in obstruction to pancreatic secretion and potentially to reflux of bile salts into the pancreatic ductal system. In alcoholism, spasm of the ampulla from ethanol combined with increased stimulation of pancreatic exocrine function may set the stage for acute pancreatitis.[48] Regardless of cause, acute pancreatitis results in a severe acute inflammation within the pancreatic parenchyma. This process results in disruption of pancreatic cells and injures segments of the ductal system. Thus, varying degrees of pancreatic enzymes may be released into the surrounding tissues and the inflammatory process is further enhanced by the digestive processes of these enzymes.

The autolysis from liberated pancreatic enzymes may thrombose portions of the pancreatic vasculature and lead to necrotizing pancreatitis or this enzyme activity may actually disrupt the vasculature and initiate hemorrhagic pancreatitis. Containment of major extravasations of pancreatic secretions within the lesser sac results in pancreatic pseudocyst. The addition of bacteria to either the acutely inflamed or necrotic pancreas, with blood or pooled pancreatic secretions in the lesser sac, sets the stage for life-threatening peripancreatic sepsis.

While obstruction to the normal exocrine function of the pancreas is a somewhat unifying concept for pancreatitis of diverse causes, other factors are also important. The occurence of pancreatitis in patients with shock, sepsis, hyperlipidemia, drug therapy, open heart surgery, and other causes suggests that pancreatic ischemia and other variables may be an inciting event for some patients.[49-51]

Diagnosis

The diagnosis of peritonitis secondary to pancreatitis is principally a clinical one. Pain ordinarily begins in the epigastric and upper quadrants of the abdomen, but commonly proceeds to generalized tenderness. Nausea and vomiting are usually present. Physical examination usually demonstrates volume-depleted patients with epigastric tenderness. Unfortunately, the degree of tenderness and peritoneal signs can be fairly mild or quite severe. It is not uncommon for these patients to present with a board-like abdomen and the question of a perforated viscus becomes another source for concern.

Fever and leukocytosis are commonly present but are of varying degrees of severity. Hyperamylasemia and elevations of serum lipase are usually present but may be close to normal in those patients who have had previous severe episodes of pancreatitis. The so-called "sentinal loop" is a commonly discussed sign of pancreatitis on the abdominal roentgenogram but is probably less often seen in clinical medicine than on surgical examinations. The final determination of a given patient having pancreatitis remains a clinical distillation of all the findings at presentation and does not have a definitive diagnostic sign short of laparotomy.

The evolution of peripancreatic sepsis from an infected acute pseudocyst, or the development of true pancreatic abscess from secondary infection of the necrotic portions of parenchyma, have traditionally posed a very difficult diagnostic problem. Some have recommended the use of ultrasound for establishment of the diagnosis of a peripancreatic collection (Figure 6). The technology with computerized tomography (CT) has significantly aided the earlier diagnosis of fluid or suppurative collections, within or about the pancreas, and when correlated with other clinical parameters may facilitate prompt surgical intervention in these difficult patients[52] (Figures 7 and 8).

Treatment

The treatment of the patient with diffuse peritonitis secondary to acute pancreatitis is nonsurgical by design. When the diagnosis is reasonably certain, management consists of nasogastric suction and intravenous support of extracellular fluid volume. Anticholinergic agents have been used but probably do not facilitate recovery. Trasylol has

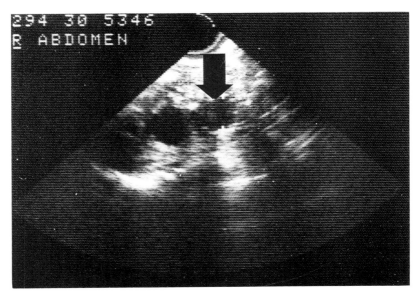

Figure 6: Demonstrates an ultrasound of the pancreas that identifies a "dumbbell" shaped pseudocyst. Such examinations with ultrasound may occasionally be of benefit.

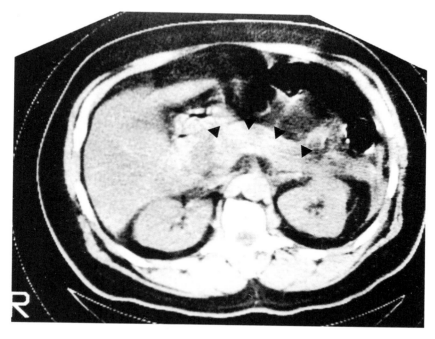

Figure 7: Demonstrates a computed tomography (CT) scan that clearly identifies a very large and edematous pancreas in a patient with severe acute pancreatitis.

commonly been used in the patient with acute pancreatitis in Europe but enthusiasm for this agent is not present in the United States.[53] Some have advocated systemic antibiotics for prevention of infected pseudocysts or pancreatic abscess.[54,55] A prospective randomized trial of ampicillin versus a placebo has failed to demonstrate any benefit in patients with alcoholic pancreatitis.[56] Sustained use of preventive antibiotics to prevent infection is only likely to change the infecting organism, but not the frequency of the complication.

In patients with mild pancreatitis, the conventional therapy identified above will prove to be satisfactory for most patients. However, Ranson[57] has identified those clinical variables that predict poor results in patients with fulminant pancreatitis (Table 2). For this latter group of patients, continuous peritoneal lavage appears to improve the results from initial resuscitation and management.[58] This methodology requires placement of a peritoneal catheter and hourly irrigation of the peritoneal

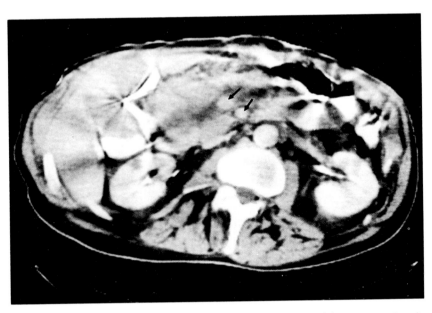

Figure 8: Demonstrates a computed tomography (CT) scan of the same patient in Figure 7 after 2 weeks. The pancreas is now beginning to fragment and is good evidence when correlated with clinical events that reoperation is indicated. The arrows indicate the superior mesenteric artery and vein.

cavity in much the same fashion that peritoneal dialysis is performed. The clinical data with this technique indicate improved results in acute management of these patients, but overall survival is apparently unchanged because of the high frequency and lethality of subsequent pancreatic sepsis.

The correct diagnosis of patients with severe peritonitis, leukocytosis, and hyperamylasemia may not always be pancreatitis. Patients with perforated peptic ulcers and elderly patients with ischemic intestine from a vascular insult may appear to have pancreatitis but truly need surgical intervention. Data by Diaco and associates[59] indicate that the overall results of acute pancreatitis are not adversely affected by laparotomy. When confidence in the primary diagnosis of pancreatitis is not satisfactory, laparotomy should be strongly entertained.

If laparotomy is chosen and the patient has only acute pancreatitis, intraoperative placement of a Tenckhoff catheter may prove desirable for postoperative peritoneal irrigation. Peritoneal lavage when per-

Table 2
Adverse Prognostic Signs in Pancreatitis at Presentation:

Age > 55 Years
WBC Count > 16,000/ Cubic MM.
Blood Glucose > 200 MG%
Serum LDH >350 IU/L
SGOT > 250 Sigma units
Within Initial 48 Hours:
Hematocrit Fall > 10%
BUN Increase > 5 MG%
Serum Calcium < 8 MG%
Arterial pO_2 < 60 mm Hg
Base Deficit > 4 mEq/L
"Third space" > 6000 ml

Indicates the grave prognostic signs of acute pancreatitis as defined by Ranson.[57]

formed with optimal aseptic technique will obviate the liabilities of the conventionally advocated drainage methods of the lesser sac. Penrose drains poorly evacuate fluid collections and may serve as a conduit for bacterial contamination of the acutely inflammed pancreas. Sump drains are more effective in the evacuation of peripancreatic fluid, but actively expose the pancreatic bed to the environmental contaminants of the intensive care unit and may facilitate bacterial lodgement about the pancreas.

When lesser sac bacterial infection intervenes in the patients with severe pancreatitis, surgical drainage must be used. Acute pseudocysts may become infected and have traditionlly required laparotomy and external drainage. Even if a mature wall is present, internal drainage of infected pseudocysts is contraindicated.[60] Infected pseudocysts may be effectively drained by percutaneous methods, guided by continuous imaging with computerized tomography as has been previously reported.[61] The liquid content of such collections makes this a potential option when clinicians with appropriate skills are available to use this technique.

However, true pancreatic abscess represents a far more difficult problem. Mortality rates for these patients vary from 20% to greater than 50%.[62-67] These infections involve the dissolution of necrotic pancreatic parenchyma. Surgical drainage and mechanical debridement of pus, fibrinous debris, and devitalized pancreas is essential. External drainage of the abscess bed with suction drains is necessary because of the continued dissolution of fragments of the infected pancreas. Because of the major blood vessels that are adjacent to the lesser sac, sump drains are preferred to closed suction devices in draining these infected areas (Figure 8).

Sequential operations are usually necessary to achieve survival in the patient with pancreatic abscess. The timing of these sequential operations is very difficult and in former years was based only on clinical criteria when the patient was deteriorating. Computerized tomography has been very effective in the identification of abscess collections in the lesser sac and has improved the timing of these reoperations prior to catastrophic deterioration of the patient (Figure 8). While CT is useful in diagnosis and may facilitate better timing of sequential operations, the multiloculated nature of these abscesses with dead pancreatic debris makes these purulent collections not amenable for percutaneous drainage.

The bacteriology of pancreatic suppuration is illustrated in Table 3. Of special interest in this bacteriology is the frequency of Staphylococci, and opportunistic gram-negative rods. These organisms occur more often in this setting than in abscesses of colonic origin and illustrate the importance of cultures in guiding systemic antibiotic

Table 3

Organism	Carner et al.[48] n = 88	Others[47,50–52] n = 53
E. Coli	45%	34%
Nonenteric gram positives (Streptococcus sp./Staphylococcus sp.)	9%	36%
Klebsiella sp./Enterobacter sp.	35%	28%
Proteus sp.	17%	17%
Enterococcus sp.	19%	17%
Monomicrobial abscess	47%	47%
Polymicrobial abscess	53%	53%

Indicates pathogens isolated from pancreatic abscesses in several series of patients. Only patients with known bacteriological reports are counted. The totals add to more than 100% because of the polymicrobial isolates in certain cases.

therapy. Furthermore the frequency of Staphylococcus and Pseudomonas organisms also suggests that secondary contamination from exogenous sources plays an important role in peripancreatic sepsis, and may reflect poor management of drains placed in the lesser sac from prior operations during the acute phase of pancreatitis. Antibiotics are usually begun empirically for these patients and usually demand broad-spectrum coverage until culture data are available. The only prospects for antibiotics to significantly affect the outcome of these patients are when they are combined with aggressive surgical debridement and drainage.

References

1. Anderson A, Bergdahl L, Boquist L: Acalculous cholecystitis. *Am J Surg* 122:3-7, 1971.
2. Glenn F, Wantz GE: Acute cholecystitis following the surgical treatment of unrelated disease. *Surg Gynecol Obstet* 102:145-153, 1956.
3. Alawneh I: Acute non-calculous cholecystitis in burns. *Br J Surg* 65:243-245, 1978.
4. Howard FJ, Delaney JP: Posttraumatic cholecystitis. *JAMA* 218:1006-1007, 1971.
5. Weeder RS, Bashant GH, Muir RW: Acute noncalculous cholecystitis associated with severe injury. *Am J Surg* 119:729-732, 1970.
6. Cheung LY, Maxwell JG: Jaundice in patients with acute cholecystitis. *Am J Surg* 130:746-748, 1975.
7. Dumont AE: Significance of hyperbilirubinemia in acute cholecystitis. *Surg Gynecol Obstet* 142:855-857,1976.
8. Fry DE, Cox RA, Harbrecht PJ: Empyema of the gallbladder: a complication in the natural history of acute cholecystitis. *Am J Surg* 141:366-368, 1981.
9. Fry DE, Cox RA, Harbrecht PJ: Gangrene of the gallbladder: a complication of acute cholecystitis. *South Med J* 74:666-668, 1981.
10. Dow RW, Lindenauer SM: Acute obstructive suppurative cholangitis. *Ann Surg* 169:272-276, 1969.
11. Haupert AP, Carey LC, Evans WE, Ellison EH: Acute suppurative cholangitis. *Arch Surg* 94:460-468, 1966.
12. Welch JP, Donaldson GA: The urgency of diagnosis and surgical treatment of acute suppurative cholangitis. *Am J Surg* 131:527-532, 1976.
13. Bartrum RJ Jr, Crow HC, Foote SR: Ultrasonic and radiographic cholecystography. *N Engl J Med* 296:538-541, 1977.
14. Prian GW, Norton LW, Eule J Jr, Eiseman B: Clinical indications and accuracy of gray scale ultrasonography in the patient with suspected biliary tract disease. *Am J Surg* 134:705-711, 1977.
15. Thal ER, Weigelt J, Landay M, Conrad M: Evaluation of ultrasound in the

diagnosis of acute and chronic biliary tract disease. *Arch Surg* 113:500-503, 1978.
16. Danley RB, Love L, Pickleman JR: Rapid roentgenologic diagnosis of acute cholecystitis. *Surg Gynecol Obstet* 143:602-604, 1976.
17. Bennett MT, Sheldon MI, dos Remedios LV, Weber PW: Diagnosis of acute cholecystitis using hepatobiliary scan with technetium-99 PIPIDA. *Am J Surg* 142:338-343, 1981.
18. Weissman HS, Rosenblatt R, Sugarman LA, Freeman LM: An update in radionuclide imaging in the diagnosis of cholecystitis. *JAMA* 246:1354-1357, 1981.
19. Stein HD, Saalfrank V, Meng C-H: Minilaparotomy as an aid to diagnosing liver disease. *Surg Gynecol Obstet* 145:49-54, 1977.
20. Haff RC, Butcher HR Jr, Ballinger WF: Biliary tract operations, a review of 1000 patients. *Arch Surg* 98:428-434, 1969.
21. Wright HK, Holden WD: The risks of emergency surgery for acute cholecystitis. *Arch Surg* 81:341-347, 1960.
22. van der Linden W, Sunzel H: Early versus delayed operation for acute cholecystitis. *Am J Surg* 120:7-13, 1970.
23. Gardner B, Masur R, Fujimoto J: Factors influencing the timing of cholecystectomy in acute cholecystitis. *Am J Surg* 125:730-733, 1973.
24. Glenn F: Cholecystostomy in the high risk patient with biliary tract disease. *Ann Surg* 185:185-191, 1977.
25. Gayic N, Frey CF: The results of cholecystostomy for the treatment of acute cholecystitis. *Surg Gynecol Obstet* 140:255-257, 1975.
26. Saik RP, Greenburg AG, Peskin GW: cholecystostomy hazard in acute cholangitis. *JAMA* 235:2412-2413, 1976.
27. Chetlin SH, Elliott DW: Biliary bacteremia. *Arch Surg* 102:303-307, 1971.
28. Fukunaga FH: Gallbladder bacteriology, histology, and gallstones. *Arch Surg* 106:169-171, 1973.
29. Keighley MRB, McLeish AR, Bishap HM, et al: Identification of the presence and type of biliary microflora by immediate gram stains. *Surgery* 81:469-472, 1977.
30. Martin LF, Zinner SH, Kagan JP, et al: Bacteriology of the human gallbladder in cholelithiasis and cholecystitis. *Am Surg* 49:151-154, 1983.
31. Pitt HA, Postier RG, Cameron JL: Biliary bacteria, significance and alterations after antibiotic therapy. *Arch Surg* 117:445-449, 1982.
32. McLeish AR, Strachan CJL, Powis SJA, et al: The influence of biliary disease on the excretion of cefazolin in human bile. *Surgery* 81:426-430, 1977.
33. Reddick E, Olsen D: Laparoscopic laser cholecystectomy: a comparison with mini-lap cholecystectomy. *Surg Endosc* 3:34-39, 1989.
34. Zucker KA, Bailey RW, Gadacz TR, Imbembo AI: Laparoscopic guided cholecystectomy. *Am J Surg* 161:336-344, 1991.
35. Zucker KA: Laparoscopic guided cholecystectomy with electrocautery dissection. In: Zucker KA, Reddick EJ, Bailey RW, eds. *Surgical Laparoscooy*. St. Louis, Mo: Quality Medical Publishing; 1991:164-191.
36. Flowers JL, Bailey RW, Scovill WA, Zucker KA: The Baltimore experience with laparoscopic management of acute cholecystitis. *Am J Surg* 161:388-392, 1991.

37. Ferzli R, Kloss DA: Laparoscopic cholecystectomy in both chronic and acute cholecystitis: a report of 165 cases. *Contemporary Surg* 40:17-19, 1992.
38. Cooperman A: Laparoscopic cholecystectomy for severe acute, embedded and gangrenous cholecystitis. *J Laparoendoscopic Surg* 1:37-40, 1990.
39. Reddick EJ, Frasier W: Laparoscopic cholecystectomy: a report on 500 consecutive cases. *Surg Endosc Laparosc* 1:2-7, 1991.
40. Phillips EH, Berci G, Carroll B, et al: The importance of intraoperative cholangiography during laparoscopic cholecystectomy. *Am Surg* 56:792-795, 1990.
41. Scott-Conner CEH, Hall TJ: Variant arterial anatomy in laparoscopic cholecystectomy. *Am J Surg* 163:590-592, 1992.
42. Hugh TB, Kelly MD, Li B: Laparoscopic anatomy of the cystic artery. *Am J Surg* 163:593-595, 1992.
43. Stockmann PT, Soper NJ: Early results of laparoscopic cholecystectomy at a teaching institution. *Perspect Gen Surg* 2:1-19, 1991.
44. Goodman GR, Hunter JG: Results of laparoscopic cholecystectomy in a university hospital. *Am J Surg* 162:576-579, 1991.
45. Reddick EJ, Olsen D, Spaw A, et al: Safe performance of difficult laparoscopic cholecystectomies. *Am J Surg* 161:377-381, 1991.
46. Stoker ME, Vose J, O'Mara P, Maini BS: Laparoscopic cholecystectomy: a clinical and financial analysis of 280 operations. *Arch Surg* 127:589-595, 1992.
47. Phillips E, Dayhovsky L, Carroll B, et al: Laparoscopic cholecystectomy: instrumentation and technique. *J Laparoendoscopic Surg* 1:3-15, 1990.
48. Schapiro H, Wruble LD, Britt LG: The possible mechanism of alcohol in the production of acute pancreatitis. *Surgery* 60:1108-1111, 1966.
49. Warshaw AL, O'Hara PJ: Susceptibility of the pancreas to ischemic injury in shock. *Ann Surg* 188:197-201, 1978.
50. Cameron JL, Capuzzi DM, Zuidema GD, Margolis S: Acute pancreatitis with hyperlipemia, the incidence of lipid abnormalities in acute pancreatitis. *Ann Surg* 177:483-489, 1975.
51. Cornish AL, McClellan JT, Johnston DH: Effects of chlorthiazide on the pancreas. *N Engl J Med* 265:673, 1961.
52. Haaga JR, Alfidi RJ, Havrilla TR, et al: Definitive role of CT scanning of the pancreas. *Radiology* 124:723-730, 1977.
53. Geokas MC: Acute pancreatitis. *Ann Intern Med* 76:105-117, 1972.
54. Feller JH, Brown RA, Toussant GP, Thompson AG: Changing methods in the treatment of severe pancreatitis. *Am J Surg* 127:196, 1974.
55. Geokas MC: Pancreatitis: mortality, antibiotics. *Ann Intern Med* 76:1045, 1972.
56. Finch WT, Sawyers JL, Schenker S: A prospective study to determine the efficacy of antibiotics in acute pancreatitis. *Ann Surg* 183:667-671, 1976.
57. Ranson JHC, Rifkind KM, Roses DF, et al: Prognostic signs and the role of operative management in acute pancreatitis. *Surg Gynecol Obstet* 139:69, 1974.
58. Ranson JHC, Spencer FC: The role of peritoneal lavage in severe acute pancreatitis. *Ann Surg* 187:565-575, 1978.
59. Diaco JF, Miller LD, Copeland EM: The role of early diagnostic laparotomy in acute pancreatitis. *Surg Gynecol Obstet* 129:263-269, 1969.
60. Polk HC Jr, Zeppa R, Warren WD: Surgical significance of differentiation between acute and chronic pancreatic collections. *Ann Surg* 169:444, 1969.

61. Aeder MI, Wellman JL, Haaga JR, Hau T: Role of surgical and percutaneous drainage in the treatment of abdominal abscesses. *Arch Surg* 118:273-280, 1983.
62. Jones CE, Polk HC Jr, Fulton RL: Pancreatic abscess. *Am J Surg* 129:44-47, 1975.
63. Carner SJ, Tan EGC, Warren KW, Braasch JW: Pancreatic abscess, a critical analysis of 113 cases. *Am J Surg* 129:486-492, 1975.
64. Ranson JHC, Spencer FC: Prevention, diagnosis, and treatment of pancreatic abscess. *Surgery* 82:99-106, 1977.
65. Altemeier WA, Alexander JW: Pancreatic abscess. *Arch Surg* 87:96-105, 1963.
66. Evans FC: Pancreatic abscess. *Am J Surg* 117:537-540, 1969.
67. Donahue PE, Nyhus LM, Baker RJ: Pancreatic abscess after alcoholic pancreatitis. *Arch Surg* 115:905-908, 1980.

13

Endometritis-Salpingitis Peritonitis

John A. Carlson, Jr, MD, Thomas G. Day, Jr, MD, and Byron J. Masterson, MD

Acute pelvic infections in women due to sexually transmissable diseases have a significant impact on the health care industry in the United States. Recent reports indicate that there are 500,000 to 850,000 annual cases generating 2.5 million physician visits, 200,000 hospital admissions, and 115,000 surgical procedures annually.[1-3] Consequently, there are many patients with this acute pelvic infections treated daily in most busy offices, clinics, and emergency rooms. The proper management of these patients demands a correct diagnosis and treatment based upon a current knowledge of this type of infection. In this chapter, the microbiology of acute endometritis-salpingitis peritonitis is updated, the clinical presentations reviewed, diagnostic techniques reintroduced, and a management program outlined.

An acute pelvic infection in the female patient resulting from sexually transmissable disease has become known as endometritis-salpingitis peritonitis, also called pelvic inflammatory disease.[4] Endometritis-salpingitis peritonitis often begins as an infection involving the endocervical glands that then ascends through the reproductive organs producing a peritonitis as the purulent exudate spills from the fallopian tubes and contaminates the pelvis.[1,4,5] Occasionally, acute endometritis-salpingitis peritonitis may be associated with organisms capable of transmural penetration of the reproductive tract so that a regional cellulitis may develop involving the lateral supporting structures of the uterus, known as a parametria. Since the internal iliac vessels are located on the lateral aspect of the parametria a prolonged,

From Fry DE, (ed): *Peritonitis.* Mount Kisco NY, Futura Publishing Co., Inc., © 1993.

serious, or neglected infection may be associated with a septic pelvic thrombophlebitis.[5] The vaginal microbial flora is a source of many of the organisms secondarily involved in pelvic infections, including acute endometritis-salpingitis peritonitis.[1,3-13] The bacterial composition of the vagina remains reasonably constant in healthy women, although quantitative differences have been noted relative to the hormonal milieu, the presence of an intrauterine device or postoperatively.[10,14-16] In the healthy vagina, anaerobic bacteria are more common than aerobic organisms.[7,10] The most common anaerobes include *Peptoccus saccharolyticus* and *Peptostreptococcus anaerobious*. The *Bacteroides* species identified most commonly are *B. melaninogenicus, B. bibius, B. dissiens,* and *B. fragilis*. Gram-negative facultative aerobes represent a highly significant subgroup of organisms commonly cultured from the vagina. *Escherichia coli* is the predominant coliform, *Proteus* species and *Klebsiella* species have also been identified. Other organisms frequently cultured from the healthy vagina include *Staphylococcus epidermidus, Staphylococcus aureus,* enterococcus, group B β-hemolytic *Streptococcus, Lactobacillus, Diptheroids,* nongonococcal *Niesseria* species, *Clostridia sp.,* and *Candida albicans.*[6,7,14-16]

Despite the bacterial colonization of the vagina and the potential anatomical communication between the vagina and the upper reproductive organs, most women do not develop infections of the endometrium, uterine tubes, or ovaries. This is presumably due to the anatomical and physiologic characteristics of the endocervix and the cervical mucus that are believed to protect against ascending infections.[1,5] The viscosity and lymphocyte concentration of the cervical mucus are postulated protective factors, as well as the local immunoglobins secreted into the endocervical mucus.[17] This physiologic barrier, however, is temporarily weakened during the menstrual period, at which time an especially virulent organism (for exampie, *Neisseria gonorrhea*), may migrate cephalad to establish an infection in the uterine cavity. The patient with an intrauterine device is at risk for ascending infections at any time during the menstrual cycle, since the physiologic barrier is violated by the presence of a foreign body that projects from the endometrial cavity into the vagina.[1,13,18]

Microbiology of Acute Endometritis-Salpingitis Peritonitis

Nonhospital acquired acute pelvic infections have been recently termed endometritis-salpingitis peritonitis. Endometritis-salpingitis peritonitis was previously considered a monoetiologic condition signifying a gonococcal infection. Recent improvements in microbiological techniques and the expanding role of culdocentesis have redefined this clinical infection as a polymicrobial process in many patients with the participation of several anaerobic and aerobic organisms in each infectious episode.[1,3-13] Currently, *Neisseria gonorrhea* is identified in about one half of endocervical cultures obtained from patients with acute endometritis-salpingitis peritonitis.[1,3,13,19] Although the failure to culture this fastidious organism from the endocervix was once thought to reflect improper collection or transport techniques, it is likely that the low rate of recovery of *Neisseria gonorrhea* in current studies reflects the true absence of the gonococcus and the significance of other organisms in the etiology of acute endometritis-salpingitis peritonitis. In particular, *Chlamydia trachomatis* has been isolated in 20% to 30% of endocervical cultures in patients with acute endometritis-salpingitis peritonitis (as opposed to 3% to 13% of controlled populations).[1,3,12,13,20,21] The virulence of *C. trachomatis* has been documented. This organism has been the sole pathogen recovered from cultures of the endocervix, cul-de-sac, and peritoneai cavity in some patients with acute endometritis-salpingitis peritonitis.[20,22,23] *Mycoplasma hominis* has also been incriminated as a possible primary infecting agent.[3,12,13,20,24]

As the principal pathogen establishes the primary infection in the endocervix, there is a sufficient disruption of the local anatomical and physiologic barriers to permit other less virulent organisms that inhabit the vagina to migrate into the upper reproductive organs and promote a synergistic infection. Consequently, many anaerobic and aerobic bacteria gain access to the peritoneal cavity. As the infection progresses in the upper reproductive organs and pelvic cavity, inflammatory debris accumulates and the redox potential shifts to produce an unfavorable environment for many of the aerobic bacteria, including possibly the initial infecting organism. Consequently, the bacterial composition of the infection is continuously undergoing change.[1,4,5]

The bacteriology of acute endometritis-salpingitis peritonitis can be studied by cul-de-sac cultures obtained either by transvaginal needle aspiration or laparoscopy.[1,3,9,12,22,23,25] In 84 patients with acute endometritis-salpingitis peritonitis treated at the University of Louisville, 64 underwent culdocentesis prior to antibiotic therapy (Table 1). In 27 of 64 patients (42%), bacteria were isolated from the cul-de-sac. Forty-eight organisms were identified in these 27 patients, or 1.78 organisms per positive culture. *Neisseria gonorrhea* was recovered in 10 of 27 positive cultures and was the sole isolate in 5. There were an additional 24 aerobic

Table 1
Culdocentesis in Patients with Acute Endometritis-Salpingitis Peritonitis

Total Number Patients		84
Patients Having Culdocentesis		64 (76%)
No. culdocentesis specimens positive	27 (42%)	
Neisseria gonorrhea only	5	
Neisseria gonorrhea plus other organisms	5	
Organisms other than *N.* gonorrhea	17	

Table 2
Culdocentesis Bacteriology of Patients with Acute Endometritis-Salpingitis Peritonitis

Aerobic		Anaerobic	
Neisseria gonorrhoeae	10	Bacteroides	9
Escherichia coli	8	Bacteroides fragilis	3
Enterococci	4	Bacteroides melaninogenicus	1
Streptococcus viridans	2	Bacteroides oralis	1
Haemophylus influenzae	1	Bacteroides asacchyrolyticus	2
Lactobacillus species	1	Bacteroides ovatus	1
Proteus acchyrolyticus	1	Bacteroides urelyticus	1
Nonhemolytic streptococcus	1	Clostridium clostridiforms	1
Staphylococcus epidermidis	2	Bifidocacterium eriksonii	1
Diphtheroides	2	Peptococcus	
TOTAL	32	asacchyrolyticus	1
		niger	1
		Peptostreptococcus	
		anerobius	1
		species	1
		Propriana bacterium jensenii	1
		TOTAL	16

and 14 anaerobic organisms recovered (Table 2). These findings are compatible with other studies.[3-13,26]

Clinical Presentations and Diagnosis

Patients with acute endometritis-salpingitis peritonitis have bilateral lower abdominal and pelvic pain that is aggravated by activity.

Symptoms usually begin 5–10 days after the most recent menstrual period and gradually worsen over 24–72 hours.[5,27] Dysuria, tenesmus, anorexia, and constipation are more common than nausea or vomiting. There may be a heavier than usual vaginal discharge. One of four patients may give a history of previous gonorrhea or pelvic infection.[1] Chronic infertility may be acknowledged.[27] It is most important to identify the patient with an intrauterine device, the patient who has had recent uterine instrumentation, or pregnancy evacuation, or the patient with a missed menstrual period who may have evidence to suggest the infection of an early intrauterine pregnancy.

On physical examination, the patient should be febrile, although, in some studies, as many as 50% of patients have had temperatures less than 38°C upon initial presentation.[1,5,27,29] Tachycardia is common, but unless the patient has a septicemia or ruptured pelvic abscess, tachypnea and hypotension are usually absent.[29] On abdominal examination there is tenderness to palpation in both lower quadrants with or without rebound tenderness.[3,27,29] An ileus is recognized as abdominal distention, tympany, and hypoactive or absent bowel sounds.

The pelvic examination is essential in establishing the diagnosis of acute endometritis-salpingitis peritonitis. A purulent exudate from the uterine cervix is almost pathognomic and a Gram's stain of the exudate may demonstrate intracellular gram-negative diplococci suggesting acute gonococcal endometritis-salpingitis peritonitis.[1,5,27,29] The uterus and adnexae are tender when palpated. The rectal-vaginal examination is essential in defining parametrial and adnexal tenderness or identifying a pelvic abscess. Palpating a mass in the pelvis, however, does not unequivocally establish the diagnosis of a pelvic abscess since a mass may reflect other pelvic pathology or a phlegmon produced by the sigmoid colon, omentum, and small bowel. Unilateral pelvic tenderness, especially in the absence of a purulent cervical exudate, is more consistent with a noninfectious gynecologic process or a nongynecologic infection. The exception to this rule is the patient with an intrauterine device in whom unilateral pelvic infections have been well documented.[1,30,31]

Once the purulent exudate has spilled from the fallopian tube into the pelvis, the exudate can spread up the pericolonic gutters and collect in the hepatorenal and subdiaphragmatic spaces. Consequently, there can be prominent upper abdominal pain and tenderness. This presentation of acute endometritis-salpingitis peritonitis has been termed the Fitz-Hugh-Curtis syndrome.[5,32-34] The prevalence of this entity cannot be accurately stated, but is believed to be fairly common since many patients undergoing unrelated abdominal surgery years after an episode of acute endometritis-salpingitis peritonitis will have adhesions between the liver capsule and the parietal peritoneum. These 'violin string' adhesions are believed to represent the repair from previous infection and indicate that patients with this syndrome can be cured with antibiotics.[27,34]

When examining the patient with presumed acute endometritis-salpingitis peritonitis, the contraceptive and menstrual history should be obtained in some detail. Although many patients with acute endometritis-salpingitis peritonitis will have irregular uterine bleeding, a history of missed or delayed menses may reveal the patient presenting with a septic abortion instead of acute endometritis-salpingitis peritonitis. Since many septic abortions result from illegal operations, the patient may not acknowledge the fact.[35] On physical examination, however, a septic abortion can be suspected if the cervical os is dilated and if tissue or clots are seen passing from the uterus. It is vitally important to recognize the patient with a septic abortion since the organisms involved are inherently more invasive than those encountered in acute endometritis-salpingitis peritonitis. *Group A, hemolytic streptococcus, Staphylococcus aureus*, and *clostridia species* (especially tetani and perfringens) have been frequently cultured from these acute infections.[36,37] Retained intrauterine products offer a luxuriant culture media for these organisms. The trauma of instrumentation has sheared blood vessels within the uterus, providing direct access to the circulatory system that has been stimulated by the pregnancy-related hormones. Proper management of septic abortion includes broad-spectrum antibiotics and evacuation of the uterus immediately.[36]

The female patient with acute bilateral pelvic and lower abdominal pain is suspected to have acute endometritis-salpingitis peritonitis, but other conditions need to be considered. Appendicitis and diverticulitis need to be excluded as well as cholecystitis, pancreatitis, and duodenal ulcer in the patient with the Fitz-Hugh-Curtis syndrome.[5,27,32,38] Some noninfectious gynecologic conditions may also masquerade as acute endometritis-salpingitis peritonitis, including ovarian tortion, rupture of an ovarian cyst or neoplasm, ectopic pregnancy, or endometriosis. Guidelines that may prove helpful in excluding these alternative diagnoses are revealed in the history and physical examination. Particularly suggestive of acute endometritis-salpingitis peritonitis is a gradual onset of symptoms, a history of chills and fever, bilaterality of symptoms, and the secondary onset of gastrointestinal symptoms. On physical examination, the patient should be febrile (greater than 38'C), have predominant lower abdominal signs, and should demonstrate an exudate from the cervix, and uterine and bilateral adnexal tenderness. The clinical laboratory should support the diagnosis with a leukocytosis including an increase in polymorphonuclear cells and either an elevated sedimentation rate or C-reactive protein.[27,38,39]

Prior to initiating therapy in a patient with acute endometritis-salpingitis peritonitis, appropriate cultures should be obtained. At the onset of the vaginal examination, a culture should be taken from the endocervical canal for *Neisseria gonorrhea*. Cultures for *N. gonorrhea* should be inoculated onto Thayer-Martin plates immediately, or, if this is not possible, then a thioglycolate media may be used to transport the specimen to the microbiology laboratory. If *C. trachomatis* is suspected, then McCoy cell culture should be used. (A more detailed description of culturing techniques may be found in the recent literature.[8,9,20]) After the bimanual and rectal-vaginal pelvic examination, a 23-gauge, 3-inch needle is passed into the cul-de-sac transvaginally, following the appropriate cleansing of the vagina with an antibiotic solution.[8,9,12] The culdocentesis should avoid direct puncture of a pelvic mass. If exudate is obtained, it should be immediately transferred from the closed needle syringe unit to the appropriate aerobic and anaerobic cultures. If exudate is not obtained, then the peritoneal cavity may be irrigated with 5-cc sterile saline that can be reaspirated. This microbiological information may assist in clinical management should the patient fail to respond to the initial antimicrobial agents. The oropharynx and anal canal might also be cultured for *Neisseria gonorrhea* in the appropriate patients.[5] Although blood cultures are obtained in most patients with acute endometritis-salpingitis peritonitis, it is uncommon for these cultures to be positive.[37]

When acute endometritis-salpingitis peritonitis is suspected, but not confirmed by culdocentesis, laparoscopy may be a valuable diagnostic tool, although it should not be used in patients with significant intestinal distention.[1,25,27,38] The first report on the use of laparoscopy in endometritis-salpingitis peritonitis included 814 patients.[40] When judged against the laparoscopic criteria of visualizing erythema, edema, or purulent exudate spilling from the fallopian tube, the clinical accuracy of establishing the diagnosis of endometritis-salpingitis peritonitis was only 65%. Twenty-three percent of those patients laparoscoped with the presumptive diagnosis of acute endometritis-salpingitis peritonitis had no abnormal anatomical findings and 12% had other clinical diagnosis, including appendicitis, ovarian cyst, and ectopic pregnancy. Although the error rate observed in the study would suggest that a laparoscopic evaluation was important in all patients suspected to have acute endometritis-salpingitis peritonitis, the diagnostic criteria were not stringent in that some patients were laparoscoped without fever or leukocytosis. Other investigators have demonstrated a clinical accuracy of almost 90% when more rigid criteria were observed.[41] Furthermore, the risk of general anesthesia and laparoscopy in patients with peritonitis must be strongly considered, especiaiiy when the pelvic structures cannot always be visualized in acute endometritis-salpingitis peritonitis due to pelvic adhesions. Therefore, it seems prudent to reserve laparoscopy for those patients in whom a definitive diagnosis cannot be made due to inconsistent physical examination, lack of laboratory confirmation, or negative culdocentesis.

Endometritis-salpingitis peritonitis is a spectrum of clinical infection.[4,5,13] The initial infection in a patient who presents promptly for treatment may be limited to the mucosa and submucosa of the involved tissue and secondary invading organisms may not have had sufficient time to enter into the infectious process. Consequently, even though inflammatory exudate spills freely into the cul-de-sac, the patient responds promptly to an antibiotic regimen. An infection of longer duration that has become polymicrobial may be more resistant in that different antimicrobial sensitivities may necessitate broad-spectrum antibiotic coverages.[3,4,8,42] If the fallopian tube has been previously damaged and the fimbriated distal tube agglutinated, then pus accumulates within the fallopian tube, distending the lumen, and creating a pyosalpinx. Pronounced distention of a hollow viscus interferes with the microcirculation in the wall of the tube and transmural migration of bacteria may occur. Rupture of a pyosalpinx, however, is uncommon. Patients with previous infections may have patent fallopian tubes, but also may have significant adhesions between the fallopian tube, ovary, and other pelvic structures so that when they acquire an acute reinfection, the purulent exudate that spills from the fallopian tube will loculate to form a tubo-ovarian abscess.[29,43] The infection can gain access to the ovarian parenchyma through a site of recent ovulation and establish an intraovarian abscess. The rupture of a tubo-ovarian abscess can be catastrophic and demands early surgical exploration and extirpation of the pelvic organs.[29,43]

Surgery is seldom necessary in patients with acute endometritis-salpingitis peritonitis. However, hospitalization with the administration of intravenous fluid, analgesics, and parenteral antibiotics is often the preferred treatment.[5,19,42,43] Antibiotic selection is critical to patient care. Formerly, many investigators recommended a combination of antibiotics for the treatment of this disease. Penicillin was the agent for treating the gonococcus and anaerobic gram-positive cocci. Aminoglycosides provided coverage for the gram-negative coliforms, and chloramphenicol or clindamycin treated the penicillin-resistant, gram-negative anaerobe *Bacteroides fragilis*.[3-7,44-47] Due to the potential toxicity of these agents on the kidneys, bone marrow, gastrointestinal tract, and eighth cranial nerve, clinical investigators have been examining the role of single agent antibiotics capable of providing sufficient antibacterial activity with less toxicity.[48-50] To date, there is no consensus as to the preferred antibiotic regimen for acute endometritis-salpingitis peritonitis. Creditable response rates have been obtained with single agent doxycycline,[51] cefoxitin,[52,53] cefotaxime,[54] and amoxicillin.[3] In an ongoing prospective clinical trial at the University of Louisville, single agent cefamandole appears as efficacious as penicillin-gentamicin.[26] Newer antibiotics such as ticarcillin, moxalactam, and piperacillin need more clinical investigation, but claim to have good coverage against both the Enterobacteriaceae and the gram-negative anaerobes.[55-57] Metronidazole may be of particular benefit since it is highly active against all anaerobes, including *B. fragilis*.[58, 59]

The patient with acute endometritis-salpingitis peritonitis requires a thorough diagnostic evaluation, a thoughtful selection of antibiotics, and a diligent evaluation for therapeutic response. During the initial 48–72 hours after the onset of antibiotic therapy, the patient should subjectively experience a dramatic improvement, defervesce, and objectively demonstrate less peritoneal and pelvic tenderness. Any mass structure present on the initial pelvic examination should resolve in accordance with the clinical improvement. Accordingly, the laboratory evaluation should demonstrate a resolving leukocytosis and, if followed, a declining C-reactive protein. Parenteral antibiotics should be maintained in the patient who is demonstrating a clinical and laboratory response until she has been afebrile (less than 99.6°F) for 48–72 hours. Once these criteria have been satisfied, all antibiotics can be discontinued. The prolonged use of oral antibiotics has not been proven to be clinically efficacious once the infection has been eliminated by higher dose systemic antibiotics.

Surgical intervention becomes necessary in those patients who fail to improve clinically on appropriate antibiotic therapy. The decision to operate must be based upon serial evaluations of the patient by the same examiner. Indications for laparotomy include continued febrility, progressive peritonitis, enlarging or nonresolving pelvic mass, or rupture of a tubo-ovarian abscess.[3,5,60] The surgical intervention should not be postponed to satisfy mandatory time specifications in patients who are not improving clinically. Aggressive surgical intervention will reduce patient morbidity and exposure to ineffective antibiotics, as well as protect the patient from the rupture of a pelvic abscess.[29,43,60]

Surgical intervention in the patient with nonresponding acute endometritis salpingitis peritonitis should be performed through a vertical incision that can be extended to the upper abdomen to allow for a complete evaluation of the peritoneal cavity, including the hepatorenal and subdiaphragmatic spaces. At the time of exploration, purulent exudate is often identified in the upper abdomen as well as the pelvis. The omentum is frequently adherent to the pelvic structures and it is not uncommon to find the sigmoid colon and small bowel similarly involved. Once identified, the fallopian tubes are often edematous, convoluted, and densely adherent to the ovaries producing bilateral tubo-ovarian abscesses. Since both adnexae are involved, a total abdominal hysterectomy and bilateral salpingo-oophorectomy is the usually performed operation for the management of nonresponding pelvic infections. The operation is best performed by first isolating and ligating the infundibulopelvic vessels and mobilizing the pelvic mass from its lateral attachments prior to attempting the specific identification of central structures through dissection. Following the extirpation of the pelvic organs, copious irrigation of the pelvis and abdomen with 8–10 L of physiologic saline is imperative. The addition of antibiotic solutions or betadine into the peritoneal lavage has no documented efficacy and may produce undesirable toxicities.[61,62] The peritoneal cavity should be debrided of significant incrustations of exudate. Saratoga sump drains may be placed in the pelvis or subdiaphragmatic spaces to evacuate an abscess or areas at high risk for fluid accumulation. The ventral abdominal wall should be closed with a nonabsorbable monofilament suture utilizing a Smead-Jones internal retention technique.[63] If gross contamination of the abdominal incision has occurred, a secondary closure of the subcutaneous tissue and skin may be necessary. Postoperatively, parenteral antibiotics should be maintained to treat the bacterial cellulitis that persists until the patient has been afebrile for 48–72 hours. Intestinal tract decompression becomes necessary in many patients. If a lengthy recovery is contemplated, nutritional support should be considered.

When a disease process is predominantly unilateral, as may occur in endometritis-salpingitis peritonitis associated with an intrauterine device, and the patient desires future pregnancies, then a unilateral adnexectomy may be performed.[1,30,31] Conservational surgery in acute endometritis-salpingitis peritonitis, however, requires that the surgeon and patient recognize the very real potential for surgical re-exploration during the same hospitalization for persistent infection unresponsive to postoperative antibiotic use or subsequent surgery for the late sequela of acute endometritis-salpingitis peritonitis, which are chronic pelvic pain, infertility, and ectopic pregnancy.[28,29,43,64]

Occasionally, a patient with acute endometritis-salpingitis peritonitis will develop a large cul-de-sac abscess amenable to drainage by a colpotomy. Such an abscess should be midline, fluctuant, and dissect the rectal-vaginal septum. Attempting to drain a cul-de-sac abscess before it has dissected the rectal-vaginal septum sufficiently may predispose to intraperitoneal rupture. The abscess is drained by performing a posterior colpotomy, which is a transverse incision made in the vaginal wall. The abscess is entered sharply, cultured, loculations are joined, and a drain is placed to allow continued postoperative drainage.[63,65,66]

When acute endometritis-salpingitis peritonitis is diagnosed during a laparotomy initially performed for another diagnosis (appendicitis, perforated duodenal ulcer, ectopic pregnancy, etc.), the surgeon should culture the pelvic exudate and the fallopian tube lumen, suction any free exudate, copiously irrigate and conclude the operative procedure, unless there is a ruptured tubo-ovarian abscess, or if a future pregnancy is not desired by the patient. Since most patients with acute endometritis-salpingitis peritonitis are successfully treated with antibiotics, there is no indication to categorically remove the reproductive organs without a trial of appropriate antibiotics in the patient desiring fertility. Although a second operative procedure may be necessary in some patients, most patients will not require re-exploration. For ethical reasons, there is, of course, no randomized clinical study to support this thesis, but the personal clinical experiences of the authors recommend this approach.

Conclusion

Acute pelvic infection in the female patient due to sexually transmissable diseases can be associated with generalized peritonitis. This peritonitis is fundamentally different from that which results from the contamination of the peritoneal cavity by intestinal contents, bile, or urine.[67-71] The obvious difference is that the peritoneal contamination in acute endometritis-salpingitis peritonitis does not result from a perforation, fistula, or traumatic injury to the intestinal tract, but results from bacterial invasion along normally patent organs. Consequently, if the infecting organisms can be eliminated with bacteriacidal drugs, then recontamination of the peritoneal cavity is unlikeiy unless the patient becomes reinfected with another purulent organism. Second, acute endometritis-salpingitis peritonitis usually occurs in otherwise healthy women under the age of 34, which is a significantly different population from the general surgery patients with intra-abdominal infection who are frequently older, have associated diseases, and are more likely to have reduced immune defenses.[28,67,70,71] Third, although both gynecologic and nongynecologic intra-abdominal infections are polymicrobial, involving both aerobic and anaerobic bacteria, there are significant qualitative and quantitative differences between the microorganisms isolated. In acute endometritis-salpingitis peritonitis, *Neisseria gonorrhea*, *Chlamydia trachomitis*, and enterococcus are frequently encountered aerobes. The more common anaerobic species are *Peptococcus*, *Peptostreptococcus*, and *Bacteroides*, although B. *fragilis* is uncommon.[1,3-13] In nongynecologic intra-abdominal infections, the predominant anaerobes include *Bacteroides fragilis* and *Clostridial* species. The more common aerobic species are *Escherichia coli*, *Klebsiella*, *Proteus*, and *Pseudomonas*. The virulence of these organisms is reflected by the fact that bactermia is more common in nongynecologic intra-abdominal infections.[37,67-71] Finally, mortality rates in nongynecologic intra-abdominal infections range from 24% to 53%, despite vigorous antibiotic and surgical treatment, and survivors of these infections often require extended hospitalizations.[67-71] The mortality rate in acute endometritis-salpingitis peritonitis, however, is 0% to 1%, even though most patients are treated nonsurgically and are frequently hospitalized for less than 1 week.[28]

The incidence of acute endometritis-salpingitis peritonitis has been steadily increasing since the 1960s and so this clinical entity will continue to present in the offices, clinics, and emergency rooms in epidemic proportions. The material offered in this chapter reviews the clinical presentation of this infection, and presents a basis for the thoughtful management of patients with acute peritonitis, secondary to sexually transmitted diseases.

References

1. Eschenbach DA: Epidemiology and diagnosis of acute pelvic inflammatory disease. *Obstet & Gynecol* 55(suppl):142S, 1980.
2. Curren JW: Economic consequences of pelvic inflammatory disease in the United States. *Am J Obstet Gynecol* 138:848, 1980.
3. Thompson SE, Hager WD, Wong K: The microbiology and therapy of acute pelvic inflammatory disease in hospitalized patients. *Am J Obstet Gynecol* 136:179, 1980.
4. Monif GRG: Significance of polymicrobial bacterial superinfection in the therapy of gonococcal endometritis-salpingitis-peritonitis. *Obstet & Gynecol* 55(suppl):154S, 1980.
5. Schwarz RH: Acute pelvic inflammatory disease, In: Monif GRG, ed. *Infectious Diseases in Obstetrics and Gynecology*. Harper & Row; 1974:381-395.
6. Chow AW, Marshall JR, Guze LB: Anaerobic infections of the female genital tract: prospects and perspectives. *Obstet & Gynecol Survey* 30:477, 1975.
7. Sweet RL: Anaerobic infections of the female genital tract. *Am J Obstet Gynecol* 122:891, 1975.
8. Monif GRG, Welkos SL, Baer H, et al: Cul-de-sac isolates from patients with endometritis-salpingitis-peritonitis and gonococcal endocervicitis. *Am J Obstet Gynecol* 126:158, 1976.
9. Chow, AW, Malkasian KL, Marshall JR, et al: The bacteriology of acute pelvic inflammatory disease. *Am J Obstet Gynecol* 122:876, 1976.
10. Louria DB, Sen P: Anaerobic infections of the pelvis. *Obstet & Gynecol* 55(suppl):114S, 1980.
11. Larsen B, Galask RP: Vaginal microbial flora: practical and theoretic relevance. *Obstet & Gynecol* 55(suppl):100S, 1980.
12. Eschenbach DA, Buchanan TM, Pollock HM, et al: Polymicrobial etiology of acute pelvic inflammatory disease. *N Engl J Med* 293:166, 1975.
13. Holmes KK, Eschenbach DA, Knass JS: Salpingitis: overview of etiology and epidemiology. *Am J Obstet Gynecol* 138:893, 1980.
14. Osborne NG, Wright RC, Grubin L: Genital bacteriology: a comparative study of premenopausal women with postmenopausal women. *Am J Obstet Gynecol* 135:195, 1979.
15. Goldacre MJ, Watt B, Loudon N: Vaginal microbial flora in normal young women. *Br Med J* 1:1450, 1979.
16. Grossman JH, Adams RL: Vaginal flora in women undergoing hysterectomy with antibiotic prophylaxis. *Obstet & Gynecol* 53:23, 1979.
17. Moghissi S: Composition and function of cervical secretion. *Handbook of Physiology—Endocrinology 2*. 1973:25-48.
18. Kaufman DW, Shapiro S, Rosenberg L: Intrauterine contraceptive device use and pelvic inflammatory disease. *Am J Obstet Gynecol* 136:159, 1980.
19. Rees E: The treatment of pelvic inflammatory disease. *Am J Obstet Gynecol* 138:1042, 1980.
20. Mardh P: An overview of infectious agents of salpingitis, their biology, and recent advances in methods of detection. *Am J Obstet Gynecol* 138:933, 1980.

258 · PERITONITIS

21. Osser S, Persson K: Epidemiologic and serodiagnostic aspects of Chlamydial salpingitis. *Obstet Gynecol* 59:206, 1982.
22. Henry-Suchet J, Catalan F, Loffredo V, et al: Microbiology of specimens obtained by laparoscopy from controls and from patients with pelvic inflammatory disease or infertility with tubal obstruction: *Chlamydia trachomatis* and *Ureaplasma urealyticum. Am J Obstet Gynecol* 138:1022, 1980.
23. Mardh P, Ripa T, Svensson V, et al: *Chlamydia trachomatis* infection in patients with acute salpingitis. *N Engl J Med* 296:1377, 1977.
24. Mardh P, Lind I, Svensson L, et al: Antibodies to *Chlamydia trachomatis, Mycoplasma laminis* and *Neisseria gonorrhaeae* in sera from patients with acute salpingitis. *Br J Vener Dis* 57:125, 1981.
25. Sweet RL, Draper DL, Schacter J, et al: Microbiology ond pathogenesis of acute salpingitis as determined by laparoscopy: what is the appropriate site to sample? *Am J Obstet Gynecol* 138:985, 1980.
26. Day TG: Personal communication.
27. Jacobson L: Differential diagnosis of acute pelvic inflammatory disease. *Am J Obstet Gynecol* 138:1006, 1980.
28. Westrom L: Incidence, prevalence and trends of acute pelvic inflammatory disease and its consequences in industrialized countries. *Am J Obstet Gynecol* 138:880, 1980.
29. Daly JW, Monif GRG: Tubo-ovarian and ovarian abscesses. In: Monif SRG, ed. *Infectious Diseases in Obstetrics and Gynecology.* Harper & Row; 1974:396-403.
30. Burkman RT: Intrauterine device use and the risk of pelvic inflammatory disease. *Am J Obstet Gynecol* 138:861, 1980.
31. Golde Sh, Israel R, Ledger WJ: Unilateral tubo-ovarian abscess: a district entity. *Am J Obstet Gynecol* 127:807, 1977.
32. Van Knorring J, Nieminen J: Gonococcal perihepatitis in a surgical ward. *Ann Clin Res* 11:66, 1979.
33. Onsrud M: Perihepatitis in pelvic inflammatory disease—association with intrauterine contraception. *Acta Obstet Gynecol Scand* 59:69, 1980.
34. Kornfeld SJ, Worthington MG: Culture-proved Fitz-Hugh-Curtis Syndrome. *Am J Obstet Gynecol* 139:106-107, 1981.
35. Gold J, Cates W, Nelson M, et al: A cluster of septic complications associated with illegal induced abortions. *Obstet & Gynecol* 56:311, 1980.
36. Ledger WJ: Septic abortion and septic pelvic thrombophlebitis in infectious diseases. In: Monif G, ed. *Obstetrics and Gynecology.* Harper and Row; 1974:275.
37. Ledger WJ, Norman M, Gee C, et al: Bacteremia on an Obstetric-Gynecologic Service. *Am J Obstet Gynecol* 121:205, 1975.
38. Ledger WJ: Laparoscopy in the diagnosis and management of patients with suspected salpingo-oophoritis. *Am J Obstet Gynecol* 138:1012, 1980.
39. Angerman NS, Evans MI, Moravec WD, et al: C-reactive protein in the evaluation of antibiotic therapy for pelvic infection. *J Reprod Med* 25(2):63, 1980.
40. Jacobsen L, Westrorn L: Objectionalized diagnosis of acute pelvic inflammatory disease. *Am J Obstet Gynecol* 105:1088, 1969.
41. Sweet RL, Mills J, Hadley KW, et al: Use of laparoscopy to determine the microbiologic etiology of acute salpingitis. *Am J Obstet Gynecol* 134:68, 1979.

42. Monif GRG, Welkos SL, Baer H: Clinical response of patients with gonococcal endocervicitis and endometritis-salpingitis-peritonitis to Doxycycline. *Am J Obstet Gynecol* 129:614, 1977.
43. Ginsburg DS, Stern JL, Hamod KA, et al: Tubo-ovarian abscess: a retrospective review. *Am J Obstet Gynecol* 138:1055, 1980.
44. Kirby BD, George WL, Sutta VL, et al: Gram-negative anaerobic Bacilli: their role in infection and patterns of susceptibility to antimicrobial agents. I. Little-known *Bacteroides* species. *Rev Infect Dis* 6:914, 1980.
45. Martin WJ, Gardner M, Washington JA: In vitro antimicrobial susceptibility of anaerobic bacteria isolated from clinical specimens. *Antimicrob ChemoTher* 1:148, 1972.
46. Ledger WJ, Gee CL, Lewis WP, et al: Comparison of Clindamycin and Chloramphenicol in treatment of serious infections of the female genital tract. *J Infect Dis* 135(suppl):S30, 1977.
47. Hermans P: General principles of antimicrobial therapy. *Mayo Clin Proc* 52:603, 1977.
48. Brewer NS: The amnioglycosides. Streptomycins, kanamycin, gentamicin, tobramycin, amikacin, neomycin. *Mayo Clin Proc* 52:675, 1977.
49. Wilkowske CJ: The penicillins. *Mayo Clin Proc* 52:616, 1977.
50. Wilson WR: Tetracyclines, chloramphenicol, erythromycin, and clindamycin. *Mayo Clin Proc* 52:635, 1977.
51. Chow AW, Malkasian KL, Marshall JR, et al: Acute pelvic inflammatory disease and clinical response to parenteral doxycycline. *Antimicrob Agents Chemo Ther* 7:133, 1975.
52. Sweet RL, Robbie M, Hadley K: Cefoxitin in treatment of obstetric and gynecologic infections. *Rev Infect Dis* 1:202, 1977.
53. Ledger WJ, Smith D: Cefoxitin in obstetric and gynecologic infections. *Rev Infect Dis* 1:199, 1979.
54. Monson TP, Miller TT, Nolan CM: Cefotaxine treatment of pelvic inflammatory disease. *Antimicrob Chemo Ther* 20:847,1981.
55. Snepar R, Poporad G, Romano J, et al: In vitro activity, efficacy and pharmacology of moxalactan, a new β-lactam. *Antimicrob Agents Chemo Ther* 20:642, 1981.
56. Yu VL: Enterococcal superinfection and colonization after therapy with moxalactan, a new broad-spectrum antibiotic. *Ann Intern Med* 94:784, 1981.
57. Winston DJ, Murphy W, Young LS, et al: Piperacillin therapy for serious bacterial infections. *Am J Med* 69:255-261, 1980.
58. Tally FP, Goldin B, Sullivan NE: Nitromidazoles: in vitro activity and efficacy in anaerobic infections. *Scand J Infect Dis Suppl* 26:46, 1981.
59. George WL, Kirby BD, Sutter VL, et al: Intravenous metronidazole for treatment of infections involving anaerobic bacteria. *Antimicrob Agents Chemo Ther* 21:441, 1982.
60. Ledger WJ: The surgical care of severe infections in obstetrics and gynecologic patients. *Surg Gynecol & Obstet* 136:753, 1973.
61. Lores ME, Ortiz JR, Rossello PJ: Peritoneal lavage with povidone-iodine solution in experimentally induced peritonitis. *Surg Gynecol & Obstet* 153:33, 1981.
62. Ericsson CD, Duke JH, Pickering LK: Clinical pharmacology of intravenous

and intraperitoneal aminoglycoside antibiotics in the prevention of wound infections. *Ann Surg* 188:66, 1978.

63. Masterson BJ: *Manual of Gynecologic Surgery*. Springer-Verlag, New York, 1979:34.
64. Rivlin ME, Hunt JA: Ruptured tubo-ovarian abscesses. *Obstet & Gynecol* 50:518, 1977.
65. Westrom L: Effect of acute pelvic inflammatory disease on fertility. *Am J Obstet Gynecol* 121:707, 1975.
66. Mattingly RF: Pelvic inflammatory disease and its sequelae. In: *Telinde's Operative Gynecology*. 5th Edition. Philadelphia, PA: J.B. Lippincott Company; 1977:259-289.
67. Stephen M, Loewenthal J: Generalized infective peritonitis. *Surg Gynecol & Obstet* 147:231, 1978.
68. Swenson RM, Lorber B, Michaelson TC, et al: The bacteriology of intra-abdominal infections. *Arch Surg* 109:398, 1974.
69. Pitcher WD, Musher DM: Critical importance of early diagnosis and treatment of intra-abdominal infection. *Arch Surg* 117:328, 1982.
70. Polk HC: Generalized peritonitis: a continuing challenge. *Surgery* 86:777, 1979.
71. Polk HC, Fry DE: Radical peritoneal debridement for established peritonitis. *Ann Surg* 192:350, 1980.

14

Nosocomial Infection in the Peritonitis Patient

Donald E. Fry, MD

Patients with peritonitis are at increased risk for developing infectious complications at other anatomical sites during the management of the peritonitis event itself. These patients have numerous catheters and tubes that transgress normal barriers of the body, and represent portals of bacterial entry. Infection itself at a remote site will increase the probability of the patient developing a second infection. For example, patients with remote infections have an increased risk of surgical wound infection following elective procedures.[1] Peritonitis and intra-abdominal abscess similarly appear to be associated with increased frequency and severity of postoperative pulmonary infection.[2,3] Finally, peritonitis patients are being treated with systemic antibiotics that result in changes in the character of bacterial colonization globally throughout the body. Accordingly, nosocomial infection in peritonitis patients under treatment tends to be with highly resistant, hospital-acquired bacteria.

Following a surgical procedure for peritonitis, it is assumed that postoperative fever and signs of infection are related to the intraperitoneal compartment. While evolving abscess is indeed a concern, other sites of infection may well be present. Recognition and appropriate management of these alternative sites may prevent needless reoperations for presumed intra-abdominal complications.

Wound Infection

Infection of the surgical wound is a fairly common complication in the peritonitis patient. The surgical wound represents the access route

From Fry DE, (ed): *Peritonitis.* Mount Kisco NY, Futura Publishing Co., Inc., © 1993.

for the treatment of the patient's peritonitis. It will be contaminated with the same bacteria that infect the patient's peritoneal cavity. The probability of infection of the surgical wound will correlate with the density of bacteria encountered during the operation. Thus, perforations of acute peptic ulcers will have low rates of wound infection, while colonic perforations can be expected to have very high wound complication rates.

Pathogenesis

Surgical wound infections generally begin within the subcutaneous tissues of the abdominal wound. The subcutaneous interface of the surgical wound is essentially avascular fat. Bacterial contaminants from the peritonitis within the abdominal cavity assault the wound edges throughout the course of the operative procedure. As bacteria make contact with the subcutaneous wound surface, they become embedded in the fibrin matrix, which is the consequence of activated fibrinogen that is present within the wound. This "carpet" of bacteria-fibrin matrix will result in bacterial proliferation and infection after closure of the wound, if the bacterial contamination exceeds a threshold density. That density is generally viewed as 10^5 bacteria per gram of subcutaneous tissue.[4]

The threshold number of bacteria necessary to cause infection can be reduced by the presence of adjuvant factors in the wound. Free hemoglobin and wound hematoma will significantly reduce the number of bacteria necessary to cause a wound infection.[5,6] Dead tissue from devascularized pieces of tissue and fat, or necrotic tissue from liberal use of the electrocautery will promote infection.[1] Foreign bodies, particularly braided suture material, will change the probability of infection from a given inoculum of bacterial contamination.[7]

With wound closure, those bacteria within the wound interface will elicit a phagocytic response. Local chemotactic signals from complement activation, activation of the coagulation cascade, and inflammatory proteins from mast cells result in margination of neutrophils around the perimeter of the contaminated wound area. The gradient of chemotactic signals from the area provides direction for the chemotactic diapedesis of neutrophils toward the contamination. Small numbers of bacteria are readily ingested by the process of phagocytosis and are internally digested by the neutrophil.[8-10] Larger concentrations of bacteria will overload the capacity of the neutrophils with resultant death of those cells that have ingested excessive numbers of microorganisms.

The magnitude of bacteria, foreign bodies, and dead tissue as a summed biological insult dictates the magnitude of the phagocytic cell response. Following the initial response of the neutrophil, macrophage infiltration of the area occurs within 24–48 hours of the injury. The macrophage serves as a "barometer" of the severity of the contamination. In mild circumstances, such as would be seen in a clean surgical wound, the number of bacteria or other stimuli for an inflammatory response are minimal and activation of the macrophage essentially does not occur. With severe contamination mast cell inflammatory proteins, complement cleavage products, and bacterial cell products stimulate the macrophage through membrane receptors to a heightened level of activation. This results in the release of cytokines that promote the febrile and acute phase response via interleukin-1 and other cytokines. The local release of tumor necrosis factor (TNF) results in the paracrine stimulation/activation of neutrophils, and the autocrine self-stimulation of macrophages in the environment. This TNF stimulation provokes frenzied phagocytic activity by the neutrophils that results in extracellular release of reactive oxygen intermediates. The phagocytosis of large numbers of bacteria results in death of many neutrophils. The result of dead neutrophils, extracellular digestion of tissues, fibrin, inflammatory proteins, and bacteria is well known to the clinician as pus. The discharge of pus becomes the definitive finding of wound infection.

Prevention

In the patient with peritonitis, prevention of wound infection is a vitally important consideration. At the very least, wound infections retard recovery and prolong hospitalization. Fascial necrosis may occur from necrotizing infection that results in additional need for operative debridement, and places the patient at-risk for dehiscence and/or evisceration. Gastrointestinal fistulae then become an added risk that can be a major cause of death in the peritonitis patient.

The surgical wound is assaulted with large numbers of bacteria in the patient who is undergoing laparotomy for peritonitis. Barrier protection of the wound edges with laparotomy pads makes sense, although is will not be a complete barrier to bacterial penetration. Effective hemostasis with discrete use of the electrocautery will minimize the risk of wound hematomas, but will also minimize the amount of dead tissue in the wound. Avoidance of braided suture material for hemostasis and for fascial closure is desirable.

In the peritontis patient, the most effective preventive measure is delayed primary closure.[11] The fascia is closed and the skin/subcutaneous tissue remains open. The open surgical wound is then managed with coarse gauze, wet-to-dry saline dressings that are changed every 6–8 hours. At 4–5 days postoperatively, the wound is evaluated for delayed closure. If a clean wound with "buds" of granulation tissue is present, then the wound can be closed with tape and benzoin at the patient's bedside. If the wound has evidence of pus and shaggy exudate, then secondary closure will be necessary. The open wound is commonly a source of emotional distress and concern to the patient and the family, but remains a preferred method for the management of severely contaminated surgical wounds in peritonitis patients. The scar of secondary closure is usually not a severe cosmetic problem, and certainly is not nearly the problem that attends resection of the abdominal wall for necrotizing fasciitis.

Topical antiseptics have been used to facilitate the reduction of viable bacteria within the open surgical wound. None have been shown to be superior to saline wet-to-dry dressings, but several have been shown to have injurious effects upon viable tissue or negative effects upon phagocytic cells of the host defense.[12]

Preventive systemic antibiotics have been demonstrated to be of value in the prevention of wound infection following clean and clean-contaminated surgical procedures.[13-17] In contaminated cases, the data are somewhat less clear, but generally favor the use of preventive systemic antibiotics in acute appendicitis[18] or following intestinal perforation from penetrating abdominal trauma.[19] Preventive antibiotics are of unproven value in the prevention of infectious wound morbidity when the wound is managed by delayed primary closure. Nevertheless, antibiotics need to be initiated prior to operation in the peritonitis patient regardless of wound considerations, but the drugs probably only benefit wound morbidity for those selected number of cases where primary closure is undertaken.

Diagnosis

The diagnosis of postoperative wound infection is strictly a clinical one. The wound is examined for the classic signs of inflammation. Cellulitis will commonly be present as the infection is beginning to evolve. The wound edges will be warm to the touch as the vasodilation of the microcirculation about the wound provides increased blood flow to the area. The wound will usually have palpable evidence of induration that is clearly painful to the patient in a fashion much greater than would be seen with the usual postoperative incisional discomfort. In obese patients, all findings can be quite subtle and systemic fever may be the only objective sign that a wound infection is evolving. The discharge of pus from the wound clearly indicates that a wound infection has occurred.

Culturing surgical wound infections has been a somewhat controversial subject in recent years. Traditional teaching has dictated that cultures should be done in every case. In more recent years, the value of these cultures has been questioned since systemic antibiotic therapy has infrequently been necessary for most infections. In the peritonitis patient, cultures are advisable given the fact that a wound infection is frequently a harbinger of a deeper seated infection within the patient's abdominal compartment. The wound culture information will commonly provide useful information in antibiotic selection for the abdominal abscess patient.

Treatment

The treatment of a wound infection is to open the wound and drain the pus. All skin sutures should be removed to eliminate any adjuvant effects. The wound edges are separated and all pus and fibrin are mechanically removed. This can usually be done at the bedside and only the most severe infections require a return to the operating room for surgical debridement. Antibiotics are reserved for only the most severe infections. When considerable cellulitis is present about the wound or when advancing wound necrosis from infection is present, then systemic antibiotics are used.

Superficial exudate and pus are commonly encountered in the open surgical wound because the contamination from the original abdominal procedure was so severe. Daily local debridement of the wound is frequently necessary for these complex wounds. Again, antibiotic therapy is not necessary if no progressive necrosis or cellulitis develop.

When fascial necrosis occurs, the surgeon is faced with a serious life-threatening complication. A return to the operating room for aggressive debridement of the fascia and other necrotic tissue is necessary. A major mistake that can be made in the management of fascial necrosis is to "cheat" on the debridement in the interest of achieving fascial and wound closure. The debridement needs to reach viable, bleeding tissue with removal of all necrosis. Closure may be achieved with the use of synthetic mesh material and reconstruction can then be undertaken at a subsequent time after the acute crisis of intra-abdominal infection and abdominal wall necrosis have been controlled.

Pulmonary Infection

Postoperative pulmonary infection is a common complication in the patient with peritonitis. Pulmonary infection has even been identified as a more common cause of death in peritonitis patients than the peritoneal process itself.[20] These infections have three separate patterns of occurrence and need to be discussed individually.

Nonventilator-Associated Pneumonitis

Pathogenesis

Nonventilator-associated pneumonitis is the consequence of the patient having an inadequate tidal volume of ventilation in the postoperative period. Peritonitis patients have a painful abdomen from the primary inflammation and from the surgical incision. The patients have undergone a general anesthetic. They are receiving narcotics for pain control in the postoperative period. The net consequence of these variables is reduced minute volume of ventilation and atelectasis.

Atelectasis is the collapse of small airways and alveoli. The bacteria that colonize the small airways are entrapped within the collapsed segment, and bacterial proliferation is the result. The alveolar macrophage responds in a fashion similar to the tissue macrophage described above. The result is inflammation. Without reexpansion of the collapsed segment of lung, invasive infection is the result with progression of the bacterial infection and an attendant inflammatory response through other previously unaffected areas of the lung tissue. Progressive loss of functional pulmonary units results in the inability of the patient to oxygenate red cells. Ventilator support and even death now attends the progressive process.

Prevention

Prevention of nonventilator-associated pneumonia requires the prevention of atelectasis. The prevention of atelectasis requires coughing, deep breathing, and early ambulation of the postoperative surgical patient. In peritonitis patients, achieving these goals can be very difficult. Nevertheless, it is essential that tidal volume be maintained. In selected difficult cases, nasotracheal suctioning will be useful not because anything is really being suctioned, but rather because the tracheal stimulation produces a paroxysm of coughing.

During the last 20 years there have been multiple devices and techniques that have been advocated for the prevention of postoperative atelectasis and pneumonia. Intermittant positive pressure breathing was popular at one point for this purpose. More recently, incentive spirometry has been used extensively. These gimmicks have more of a commercial flair rather than being methods that have been shown to reduce postoperative pneumonia. Coughing, deep-breathing, and early ambulation remain the best methods for prevention.

Preventive systemic antibiotics for prevention of pneumonia have no place in the management of the postoperative patient. The entire concept of preventive antibiotics is predicated on the premise that the period of bacterial contamination and risk for a given patient is brief. Preventive antibiotics given over several days will result in changes in the patient's colonization of the airways so that if infection occurs, it will be with resistant bacteria. Furthermore, preventive antibiotics do not change the basic pathophysiologic conditions (ie, atelectasis) that are responsible for the evolution of pneumonia. This practice cannot be advocated.

Diagnosis

The diagnosis of atelectasis is a clinical one. It is essential that the clinician recognize and respond to the development of atelectasis, otherwise clinical pneumonia will be the consequence. Atelectasis most commonly presents as early postoperative fever. This is customarily an event of the first postoperative evening. The patients may or may not have an associated leukocytosis. Small areas of inflammation are occasionally recognized as linear areas of "plate-like" atelectasis on the chest roentgenogram, which actually represent focal areas of pneumonia. For the most part, the diagnosis of atelectasis must be made by criteria of early postoperative fever in a patient who clinically has an inadequate tidal volume. Re-expansion of the atelectatic segments of lung are essential if invasive pneumonia is to be avoided. Antibiotic treatment of atelectasis is inappropriate and will not avoid the evolving pneumonia.

The diagnosis of invasive pneumonia is made by the correlation of several clinical variables. Fever and leukocytosis are usually present. Chest roentgenograms will usually demonstrate significant infiltration. Purulent sputum will usually be present for culture documentation of the pathogen. Once a clinical diagnosis of pneumonia is established, then the treatment strategy becomes very different from that of the management of atelectasis.

Treatment

Established pneumonia in the postoperative peritonitis patient requires aggresive efforts to evacuate the purulent material from the

Table 1	
Organism	# Isolates
Pseudomonas sp.	41
Klebsiella sp.	29
Staphylococcus sp.	25
E. coli	24
Proteus sp.	18
Enterobacter sp.	16
Streptococcus pneumoniae	13
Serratia sp.	10
Group A Streptococci	5
Hemophilus influenzae	4
Other gram-negative organisms	9

Identifies the pulmonary pathogens that were cultured in 136 cases of postoperative pneumonia. Because some patients had more than one isolate, the total exceeds the total number of patients.

patient's pulmonary tree, and the initiation of antibiotic therapy. Purulence in the lung is like pus in any other setting and requires drainage. Expectorants, pulmonary suctioning, and even bronchoscopy for purposes of evacuating purulent material may be necessary. Postural drainage is likewise a useful method in those patients who can be physically moved into a head-down position for chest physiotherapy.

The pathogens likely to be encountered in postoperative pneumonia are identified in Table 1.[21] Antibiotic therapy needs to be addressed to the identified pathogen. Empirical treatment may be necessary until such time as the sputum cultures are returned. Since peritonitis patients will have been hospitalized for many days prior to the development of pneumonia and will have already been on antibiotic therapy during their hospitalization for the management of the peritonitis, the selection of antibiotics for postoperative pneumonitis can be difficult. Patients who develop pneumonia in the face of antibiotic therapy for peritonis, will likely have resistant organisms that are responsible for their pneumonia. Prolonged hospitalization and lengths of stay in the surgical intensive care unit will also increase the probability that *Pseudomonas sp., Serratia sp.,* or resistant Enterobacteriaceae will be the likely pathogens. Aminoglycosides, quinolones, aztreonam, or ceftazidime are commonly used antibiotics for the treatment of pneumonia under these circumstances.

When patients still require antibiotic therapy to manage the peritonitis, then expanded spectrum β-lactam antibiotics with coverage of both aerobic and anaerobic pathogens may be desirable in an effort to cover both the needs of the peritonitis and the pneumonia in a single selection. Expanded spectrum penicillins, cephalosporins, and carbapenems are potential choices to provide coverage for both the peritoneal and the pulmonary pathogens. Combination therapy to cover all treatment objectives may be necessary. The duration of antibiotic therapy for postoperative pneumonia will need to be judged based upon the patient's clinical response.

Ventilator-Associated Pneumonia

Pathogenesis

Patients have numerous reasons to require ventilator support. Intrinsic lung disease, acute pulmonary infection, pulmonary contusion from trauma, and large volume resuscitation after hemorrhage are all associated with the need to support systemic oxygenation.

The patient with acute peritonitis may have several variables that require ventilator support. The peritonitis process is similar to a large peritoneal "burn" and large volume administration of crystalloid solution is commonly necessary. The patient's age and predisposing lung disease are also issues. The septic response from the peritonitis itself may result in pulmonary shunting that provokes systemic hypoxemia.

The placement of a patient onto ventilator support breeches the first line of host defenses of the lung; specifically, the glottis. The endotracheal tube provides a direct access from the external environment of the intensive care unit into the patient's airway. Colonization of the ventilator tubing and air conduits permits the aerosolization of bacteria for direct delivery into the lung.

Since the lung is commonly edematous secondary to the generalized edema that attends the volume-expanded peritonitis patient, not only do bacteria have easy access, but tissue level host defense is compromised. Edematous tissues become a fertile ground for bacterial lodgment and proliferataion. Edema renders the normal mucociliary action of the lung less efficient. Alveolar macrophages may well function less effectively in this environment. Indeed, pulmonary bacterial clearance within the lung tissue is inefficient.

Prevention

The prevention of ventilator-associated pneumonia requires optimization of aseptic technique in the management of the ventilator and the patient's endotracheal appliance. Appropriate gloves are to be worn when suctioning the endotracheal appliance. This will prevent contamination of the airway from the hand flora of the intensive care unit personnel. Hand washing between patient contacts prevents cross contamination within the intensive care unit environment. Changing the ventilator tubing every 24 hours prevents colonization of the equipment of ventilation. The colonization of the airway of the ventilator patient commonly comes from the environment of the intensive care unit. All efforts need to be focused upon the prevention of the personnel or ventilator equipment from being the means of introduction of potential pathogens.

As has been identified in other postoperative situations, systemic antibiotics are not effective in the prevention of ventilator-associated pneumonia. However, antibiotic aerosols have been advocated for the prevention of ventilator-associated pneumonia.[22] Studies have demonstrated that in the short run, reduced rates of pneumonia can be identified. Unfortunately, but not unexpectedly, aerosolization of antibiotics into the environment of the intensive care unit sets the stage for resistance to emerge to those antibiotics that are employed in the aerosolization procedure. In the long term, infection rates are not reduced because of the emergence of resistance.

The most effective preventive measure is rapid weaning of the patient from ventilator support. Once the conduit for direct bacterial access to the lung is eliminated, then the period of risk for ventilator-associated pneumonia is past. Weaning parameters using intermittent mandatory ventilation should be implemented at the earliest possible time in these patients to effect elimination of ventilatory support.

Diagnosis

The diagnosis of ventilator-associated pneumonia can be quite elusive. The peritonitis patient who is having ventilation support after a major operation for peritonitis has numerous potential sources for postoperative fever and leukocytosis. Cultures of the tracheal aspirate of the patient who has been on the ventilator for longer than 48 hours will almost always be positive, but the differentiation of colonization from invasive infection is not answered by the tracheal culture. By the time that the patients demonstrate advancing infiltrates on chest roentgenography, the physician will be quite delayed in the initiation of antibiotic therapy.

Numerous different methods have been used to facilitate diagnosis and differentiate colonization versus invasive pneumonia. Quantitative cultures have been advocated with the idea that tracheal quantities of bacteria that exceed a given threshold ($> 10^6$) are representative of bacterial infection.[23] However, this method has been challenged.[24] Examination of the sputum by Gram's stain to identify elastin fibers has been demonstrated to be quite accurate, but may be a late finding of pneumonia in that elastin fibers obviously reflect late findings of lung necrosis.[25] Bronchoalveolar lavage or protected-brush sampling of the smaller airways of the lung via the bronchoscope have been advocated,[26,27] but remain of unproven value in separating the issue of colonization versus invasive infection in the ventilator-dependent patient. Certainly, bronchoalveolar lavage can be a complicating study itself in that the chest roentgenogram commonly looks worse following the diagnostic effort than previously. The identification of bacteria within polymorphonuclear cells on the Gram's stain is probably as reliable as any other diagnostic method, but has the advantage of being simple to perform and provides very quick results following acquisition of the sputum specimen.

Treatment

Treatment of the ventilator-associated pneumonia in the peritonitis patient is a formidable problem. The isolated pathogens in this situation are invariably the resistant gram-negative organisms of the intensive care unit. Antibiotic therapy needs to be addressed to those bacteria. In the severely ill and immunosuppressed patient, cultures will demonstrate *Staphylococcus epidermidis* and *Candida albicans*. Resistance patterns for the commonly isolated nosocomial bacteria within a given intensive care unit should be known by the physician to guide antibiotic therapy. Combination therapy is commonly used even when only one pathogen is cultured in an effort to optimize antimicrobial synergism. Mortality rates may exceed 50% in the severe ventilator-associated pneumonia, and treatment requires early diagnosis and aggresive antibiotic therapy.

Aspiration-Associated Pneumonia

Pathophysiology

Aspiration-associated pneumonia may be the consequence of gross or occult aspiration of contents of the upper aerodigestive tract. Gross aspiration is well appreciated by surgeons as a cause of morbidity in postoperative patients. Gross aspiration usually occurs in the patient who has an altered sensorium either from the associated disease (eg, peritonitis), from organic causes (eg, the elderly), or from medications (eg, analgesia) used in management of the patient. Gross aspiration of gastric contents in the postoperative peritonitis patient will usually reflect the normal gastric fluids and will not have particulate food matter. Gross aspiration results in a chemical injury of the lung that if severe enough, will require ventilatory support. The patient then assumes all the risks associated with ventilator-associated pneumonitis by virtue of having an injured lung with direct access to the environment of the intensive care unit.

Occult aspiration of saliva and other pooled fluids within the patient's mouth and oropharynx have been a source of concern for postoperative pneumonia. Saliva and other fluids of the upper aerodigestive tract customarily have a limited concentration of fairly innocuous microorganisms. However, in the peritonitis patient who has been on systemic antibiotic therapy, colonization of the mouth and hypopharynx with resistant hospital-acquired bacteria has been a potential reservoir for infectious pathogens for the lung. Considerable concern has recently focus upon the consequences of alkalinization of the upper aerodigestive tract through the use of antacids and H-2 histamine antagonists.[28] The data to support the adverse consequences of alkalization are tenuous, although this area needs additional study.

Prevention

The prevention of gross aspiration events can be quite difficult. It is important to recognize the patient who is at-risk. Nasogastric decompression of the stomach of those postoperative patients with an altered sensorium can reduce the risks of aspiration. Prudent use of narcotics and analgesics, particularly in the elderly patient, will hopefully avoid confusion episodes and altered mental status.

Some have advocated the use of alternative agents to antacids and H-2 histamine antagonists to avoid the potential deleterious effects of alkalinization. Sucralfate has been recommended for this purpose.[29] It remains unclear whether sucralfate is as effective as other regimens in the prevention of stress-associated gastritis, and whether pneumonia rates will really be reduced.

Aspiration that has occurred has been seen as an indication for the use of preventive antibiotics to prevent the evolution of pneumonia. Efforts to study the use of preventive antibiotics have generally shown the practice to be a failure in preventing pneumonia, but to increase the probability that resistant pathogens will likely infect the patient if pneumonia does develop. Thus, preventive antibiotics are not recommended to prevent pneumonia in the wake of an aspiration event

Diagnosis

In many circumstances, the diagnosis of an aspiration event is readily apparent. Vomiting occurs and the patient has an abrupt deterioration of pulmonary function which rapidly leads to entubation. Particulate matter or bilious stained fluids are then aspirated from the airway.

In postoperative patients, this diagnosis may be considerably more subtle. The rapid evolution of new reticular infiltrates in the lung, usually bilaterally, is strong evidence to support aspiration as an event. Bronchoscopy may actually be required to examine for evidence of lung injury. Bronchoscopy has the potential advantage of also being therapeutic in that lavage of the airways to remove particulate matter may also be possible.

Treatment

The treatment of established aspiration pneumonia is very difficult. The physician is faced with the combined effects of a chemical injury of the lung with a superimposed invasive infection. In peritonitis patients, they will have already likely been the recipients of several days of antibiotic therapy at the time of the aspiration and pneumonia. Resistant bacteria are likely to be encountered. Aggressive antibiotic therapy is necessary. Daily cultures performed from the lung following an aspiration event will provide a profile of likely bacteria to cause infection and can be very useful in antibiotic selection. Because these patients may be undergoing antibiotic management of the peritonitis process as well, double or even triple antiobiotic combinations may be required to address all problems. Mortality rates for full-blown aspiration pneumonia in peritonitis patients will exceed 50%.

Urinary Tract Infection

Pathogenesis

Urinary tract infection is a fairly common complication that will be encountered in the peritonitis patient. Essentially all peritonitis patients will require the placement of the Foley catheter to monitor urine output during the early phases of management. The breech of the urinary tract by the Foley catheter becomes the avenue for bacterial access to the otherwise sterile environment of the urinary bladder.

Infection of the bladder occurs via retrograde migration and proliferation of bacteria in the pericatheter space within the urethra. The nonspecific inflammation that is created by the foreign body within the urethra eliminates the beneficial effects of bacteriostatic urethral mucins and IgA antibody. The Foley catheter abrades the urethral mucosa, and may lead to compression necrosis and injury of the transitional epithelium about the bladder trigone from the inflated catheter balloon. Loss of the normal epithelial integrity provides sites for bacterial attachment, proliferation, and invasive infection.

Prevention

Prevention of urinary tract infection complicating the management of the peritonitis patient is achievable. Aseptic placement of the catheter initially reduces the introduction of bacteria into the bladder and the urethra. The catheter needs to be anchored and immobilized to prevent to-and-fro "piston-like" movements of the catheter within the urethra. Such movements of the catheter literally draw bacteria into the urinary bladder by this sump action. Maintenance of the closed drainage system of the catheter system is important to prevent contamination of the internal lumen of the catheter. Finally, removing the catheter as soon as its purpose has been served is of paramount importance. Maintenance of the urine volume during and following catheterization actively eliminates would-be pathogens from the bladder and urethral spaces.

Systemic antibiotics for prevention of urinary tract infection have not been useful and should not be employed. Considerable interest has focused upon the use of urinary tract irrigation for the prevention of urinary tract infection in the catheterized patient. While the use of the three-way irrigation Foley catheter may be of value in the treatment of certain difficult urinary tract infections, irrigants have not been shown to prevent infection, but do adversely affect the types of pathogens that will be subsequently seen when infection does occur.[30]

Diagnosis

The accepted "gold standard" for the diagnosis of urinary tract infection has been the quantitative urinary tract culture. The culture may be done because of fever, leukocytosis of unknown origin, or because patients are having symptoms of postcatheterization dysuria. The post-catheterization dysuria is commonly a consequence of catheter trauma and does not necessarily mean infection. When the culture demonstrates greater than 10^5 bacteria per milliliter of urine, then a presumptive diagnosis of urinary tract infection is established.[31]

It should be emphasized that the sanctity of the 10^5 bacteria per milliliter as the threshold for infection has been established in community-acquired urinary tract infection, and not in patients with in-dwelling Foley catheters. In a previous study of postcatheterization infections in surgical patients, many patients had their apparent infection resolve despite inadequate or even no treatment.[32] It raises the serious question of whether removal of the catheter and adequate subsequent flow of urine volume is often sufficient to clear the bacteruria. Clearly, some patients do have clinically significant infection that requires specific treatment.

Treatment

Antibiotic therapy is necessary for the patient with postcatheterization urinary tract infection. While *E. coli* is the most common urinary tract pathogen among patients with community-acquired infections, more resistant bacteria will be identified in the peritonitis patient with this complication (Table 2).[32] The patients will have developed this infectious complication under the influence of the antibiotic therapy that was used for the treatment of the peritonitis. Sensitivity data are necessary to direct therapy. The author prefers alternatives to aminoglycosides in the treatment of these infections. Quinolones have become popular since intravenous administration is not necessary if the patient has reached a point of convalescence from the peritonitis to permit oral administration.

Intravascular Device Infections

The utilization of intravascular devices in the management of critically-ill surgical patients has dramatically increased during the last two decades. Central venous catheters, Swan-Ganz catheters, and arterial lines have become commonplace. When these additional intravascular lines are added to the routine use of conventional peripheral intravenous catheters, a given patient may have four or more intravascular catheters,

Table 2

Organism	# Isolates
E. coli	56
Klebsiella sp.	38
Pseudomonas sp.	37
Proteus sp.	30
Enterobacter sp.	22
Enterococcus sp.	22
Serratia sp.	16
Citrobacter sp.	10
Streptococcus sp.	9
Staphylococcus epidermidis	8
Providencia sp.	5
Candida sp.	3

Identifies the cultured isolates from 212 postoperative urinary tract infections in 153 surgical patients. The total number of isolates exceeds the total number of infections because of polymicrobial infections in a significant number of patients.

each of which can become a portal for bacterial entry into the patient's vascular system.

Pathogenesis

The common feature of all intravascular devices is that they transgress the patient's skin and provide a direct access route from the external environment into the vascular compartment. Colonization of the foreign body device can then occur either from cutaneous resident microflora of the patient's skin, or from bacterial contamination during the process of catheter placement or management subsequent to placement. The pericatheter space about the barrel of the catheter then becomes the critical avenue for bacterial migration and proliferation. Migration of these microorganisms along the barrel of the catheter ultimately results in bacterial access to the intravascular component of the catheter. At this point the bacteria find an environment that is very conducive to proliferation. The foreign body itself, fibrin on the catheter, and clot on the vascular wall at the site of the vascular puncture each become major adjuvant effects which will result in dissemination of the microorganisms with clinical bacteremia being the result.

Prevention

Prevention of catheter-associated bacteremia requires that several measures be consistently applied. Aseptic technique in the placement of the catheter is essential. Careful cleansing of the skin is important, although the topical antiseptic that is used on the skin at the time of placement remains a source of debate in terms of which effectively reduces infection rates.[33] Central venous catheters and Swan-Ganz catheters require careful management by having the dressing changed and the skin about the site of catheter entry cleansed and redressed at least every 48 hours. The use of long-term catheters (eg, Groshong catheters) that are tunneled under the skin and have a "collar" to facilitate tissue in-growth should be considered for those patients requiring long-term central venous catheterization for nutritional support and other indications.

Finally, it should be emphasized that peripheral intravenous lines remain the most common site of catheter-associated bacteremia. These catheters are subject to constant movement and the dressings over these catheters are constantly assaulted with moisture and other insults. The best way to prevent peripheral catheter bacteremias is to simply change the catheter site every 48–72 hours.

Diagnosis

The diagnosis of catheter-associated bacteremia requires that the clinician maintains a high index of suspicion for this complication in the peritonitis patient. Catheter-associated bacteremia is an event that occurs more than 72 hours into the patient's management for peritonitis. A common scenario has a patient who is making satisfactory progress following laparotomy and antibiotic therapy who develops a spiking temperature on the fourth postoperative day or later. When blood cultures grow *Staphylococcus aureus*, then the clinician must conclude that the diagnosis is catheter-associated bacteremia until proven otherwise.

The diagnosis of catheter-associated bacteremia is documented by the semi-quantitative culture of the catheter.[34] The catheter is removed, and the catheter tip is amputated and sent to the microbiology laboratory for culture. The catheter is then "rolled" across blood agar. After 24 hours of incubation, the identification of greater than 15 colony forming units confirms the diagnosis. In most cases, the colony count on the culture will be very large and leaves no doubt about the diagnosis. Obviously, the cultured organism from the catheter tip and the blood culture should be with the same organism.

Treatment

The treatment of an intravascular device infection is first and foremost the removal of the offending catheter.[35] This will prove sufficient for the management of many patients alone without any additional treatment. Approximately 20% to 25% of patients with peripheral intravenous catheter infections will require excision of the infected vein or local incision and drainage of a subcutaneous abscess at the site of the catheter. Suppurative thrombophlebitis will most commonly be seen when the pathogen is *Staphylococcus aureus*.

Antibiotic therapy needs to be chosen for the offending pathogen, but requires different durations of treatment (Table 3).[35] When a gram-negative rod is encountered, it is the author's opinion that antibiotic coverage needs to only cover the 2 or 3 days following catheter removal. Antifungal therapy should be extended for a longer period of time. The most problematic issue is staphylococcal bacteria. The *Staphylococcus aureus* pathogen can cause metastatic sites of infection, with bacterial

Table 3	
Organisms	*# Identified*
Staphylococcus aureus	41
Staphylococcus epidermidis	22
Klebsiella sp.	12
Serratia marcescens	11
Candida sp.	11
Enterobacter sp.	6

Identifies the cultured pathogens from 100 intravascular device infections. In three cases, there were multiple isolates.

endocarditis being the site of greatest concern. For this reason, intravenous antibiotic therapy should be continued for a full 7 days. When antibiotic failures are apparent, the clinician must look for other sites of infection to account for the patient's continued problems. *Staphylococcal bacteremia* after catheter removal should alert the physician to examine the patient for either septic thrombophlebitis at an intravenous site or acute bacterial endocarditis.

Candida Sepsis

A major intercurrent nosocomial infection that is seen in patients with peritonitis is Candidemia. The *Candida sp.* are uncommon colonists of the normal human skin or gastrointestinal tract. However, the influence of broad spectrum antibiotics, such as are used in the peritonitis patient will result in colonization of the skin and of the gastrointestinal tract with these fungal organisms. This sets the stage for Candidemia as a complication that arises either from central venous catheters or from the gastrointestinal reservoir as a primary organism of microbial translocation.

Pathogenesis

Colonization of the skin and the gastrointestinal tract is principally bacterial in nature. Colonization of the skin is principally gram-positive, except for those areas about the perineum. Gastrointestinal colonization is essentially sterile within the stomach lumen itself, but becomes more densely colonized with gram-negative bacteria at the more distal parts of the small bowel. At the most distal part of the small bowel and through the length of the human colon, anaerobic species are not only identified, but become the prevailing colonists in the left colon.

Systemic antibiotic therapy changes the normal colonization. In the peritonitis patient, the comprehensive aerobic and anaerobic coverage changes the colonization by eliminating those microbes that are sensitive to the antibiotics that are being used. Fungal species can become frequent skin and gut colonists and become sources of potential pathogens. The *Candida* species will be contaminants of central venous catheters and become sources of fungemia by the mechanisms that have been previously described.

Candida species are the prototype organisms that can translocate out of the intestinal lumen and result in systemic candidemia.[35] The gastro-intestinal barrier that contains colonization within the gut lumen becomes defective secondary to biological stress, malnutrition, and many other biological stimuli all of which are present in the peritonitis patient.[36-39] Anaerobic bacteria are felt to be major components of the gut barrier, in part because they are competitive inhibitors of the overgrowth of adverse species of bacteria.[40] Most antibiotic regimens for the treatment of peritonitis will have appropriate anaerobic coverage, but will also adversely affect the barrier function of the gut. Candida overgrowth occurs and candidemia is the consequence as fungal organisms invade the portal circulation and the mesenteric lymph nodes.

Prevention

Several preventive measures have been emphasized to prevent candidemia in the peritonitis patient. A more restrictive attitude about the duration of antibiotic therapy is certainly warranted. While comprehensive antibiotic therapy is important in the management of peritonitis, the duration of antibiotic therapy can be excessive. Earlier cessation of systemic antibiotics may be desirable.

Antifungal chemotherapy for suppressing fungal overgrowth within the gut lumen has been advocated. Oral mycostatin, or more recently, fluconazole has been used. Whether these regimens truly reduce the frequency of candidemia is not clear. A major problem in using oral preventive chemotherapy has been the problem of case selection. Certainly, all peritonitis patients do not need preventive chemotherapy. Well-stratified studies of patients who are truly at-risk may demonstrate effectiveness for this strategy.

A recent area of interest in the prevention of microbial translocation in general and Candidemia in specific has been nutritional manipulation. Enteral nutrition, when possible, is felt to support gastrointestinal barrier function by providing intraluminal nutrients and by fostering normal colonization.[41] Peritonitis patients will commonly not be able to tolerate enteral support. Recent interest in the use of glutamine nutritional support for the enterocyte is another promising area of support for the gut barrier that may reduce the risk of microbial translocation.[42] The entire area of nutritional support of the gut will be an area of considerable change in the future, as efforts to support barrier function of the gastrointestinal tract are increased.

Diagnosis

The diagnosis of Candidemia generally requires documentation of the organism on blood culture. While conventional blood cultures are generally used for this purpose, there is some clinical and experimental data that would suggest that arterial cultures are more efficient in the isolation of these organisms.[43] Additional studies are necessary to validate this interesting idea.

A dilemma that is constantly seen in peritonitis and other seriously ill patients is the positive urine culture for Candida. Does this constitute a pathogen in urine or not? Almost all candidemia patients will have the organism in the urine, but not all positive urine cultures reflect Candidemia. In seriously ill patients with positive urine cultures for *Candida sp.*, a vigilant effort to culture the blood for fungal organisms may be advisable. If only a Candida urinary tract infection appears to be the problem, then topical drug therapy with amphotericin irrigation may be the preferred treatment.

Candida peritonitis appears to be an unusual, but identified site of infection with this fungal organism.[44] Since transmural migration of microorganisms from the gut appears to be a real clinical phenomenon, the patient with severe peritonitis and long-term antibiotic therapy may well develop Candida peritonitis as an intercurrent infection. This diagnosis is made by heavy growth of *Candida sp.* on peritoneal culture. Systemic amphotericin treatment is then necessary for this relatively small number of patients.

Treatment

The treatment of Candidemia is principally that of amphotericin antifungal therapy, despite the specific Candida isolate that is encountered (Table 4).[45] It is essential that all in-dwelling central lines be removed to eliminate this possible cause, but systemic chemotherapy is necessary. Recent trends in management have been to accelerate nutritional strategies, reduce systemic antibiotic therapy as much as possible, and employ amphotericin doses at 0.5 mg/kg per day. While reducing systemic antibiotic therapy makes good sense, these patients will commonly have other bacterial pathogens in the blood culture and require antibiotic therapy to be continued (Table 5).

Table 4

Candida Species Isolated	# Cultures
Candida albicans	73
Candida parapsilosis	28
Candida tropicalis	14
Candida rugosa	2

Identifies the common *Candida sp.* that were recovered from the blood cultures of 83 patients with 117 episodes of Candidemia.

Table 5

Bacterial Isolate	# Isolates
Staphylococcus sp.	25
Enterococcus sp.	25
Klebsiella sp.	22
Serratia sp.	20
Pseudomonas sp.	11
Bacteroides sp.	9
Enterobacter sp.	7
Proteus sp.	6
E. coli	6
Others	15

Identifies the bacterial isolates that were identified in the blood cultures at the same time that the Candida species were cultured.

Summary

Nosocomial infection remains a major source of fever and leukocytosis in the peritonitis patient. The surgical wound, the lung, the urinary tract, and intravascular devices will account for over 90% of infectious complications in this group of patients. All nosocomial infections are potentially preventable and certainly their frequency can be reduced.

Prompt diagnosis and treatment can optimize the outcome of these very difficult complications in the peritonitis patient.

References

1. Cruse PJE, Foord R: A five-year prospective study of 23,649 surgical wounds. *Arch Surg* 107:206-211, 1973.
2. Richardson JD, Fry DE, Van Arsdall LR, Flint LM: Pulmonary bacterial clearance in peritonitis. *J Surg Res* 26:499-503, 1979.
3. Richardson JD, DeCamp MM, Garrison RN, Fry DE: Pulmonary infection complicating intraabdominal sepsis: clinical and experimental observations. *Ann Surg* 195:732-738, 1982.
4. Robson MC, Krizek TJ, Heggers JP: Biology of surgical infections. In *Current Problems in Surgery*. Chicago, IL: Year Book Medical Publishers; 1973:1-8.
5. Polk HC Jr, Miles AA: Enhancement of bacterial infection by ferric iron: kinetics, mechanisms, and surgical significance. *Surgery* 70:71-77, 1971.
6. Pruett TL, Rotstein OD, Fiegel VD, et al: Mechanisms of the adjuvant effect of hemoglobin in experimental infections: VIII. A leukotoxin is produced by Escherichia coli metabolism of hemoglobin. *Surgery* 96:375-383, 1984.
7. Elek SD, Conen PE: The virulence of Staphylococcus pyogenes for man: a study of the problem of the wound. *Br J Exp Pathol* 38:573-580, 1975.
8. Stossel TP: Phagocytosis. *N Engl J Med* 290:717, 1974.
9. Stossel TP: Phagocytosis. *N Engl J Med* 290:774, 1974.
10. Stossel TP: Phagocytosis. *N Engl J Med* 290:833, 1974.
11. Bernard HR, Cole WR: Wound infection following potentially contaminated operations: effect of delayed primary closure of the skin and subcutaneous tissue. *JAMA* 184:290-294, 1963.
12. Lineaweaver W, Howard R, Soucy D, et al: Topical antimicrobial toxicity. *Arch Surg* 120:267-272, 1985.
13. Polk HC Jr, Lopez-Mayor JF: Postoperative wound infection: a prospective study of determinant factors and prevention. *Surgery* 66:97-103, 1969.
14. Stone HH, Hooper CA, Kolb LD, et al: Antibiotic prophylaxis in gastric, biliary and colonic surgery. *Ann Surg* 184:443-449, 1976.
15. Stone HH, Haney BB, Kolb LD, et al: Prophylactic and preventive therapy: timing, duration and economics. *Ann Surg* 189:691-697, 1979.
16. Kaiser AB, Clayson KR, Mulherin JL Jr, et al: Antibiotic prophylaxis in vascular surgery. *Ann Surg* 188:283-289, 1978.
17. Platt R, Zaleznik DF, Hopkins CC, et al: Perioperative antibiotic prophylaxis for herniography and breast surgery. *N Engl J Med* 322:153-157, 1990.
18. Foster PD, O'Toole RD: Primary appendectomy: the effect of prophylactic cephaloridine on postoperative wound infection. *JAMA* 239:1411-1414, 1978.
19. Fullen WD, Hunt J, Altemeier WA: Prophylactic antibiotics in penetrating wounds of the abdomen. *J Trauma* 12:282-287, 1972.
20. Hunt JL: Generalized peritonitis: to irrigate or not to irrigate the peritoneal cavity? *Arch Surg* 117:209-214, 1982.

21. Martin LF, Asher EF, Casey JM, Fry DE: Postoperative pneumonia: determinants of mortality. *Arch Surg* 119:379-383, 1984.
22. Feeley TW, du Moulin GC, Hedley-White J, et al: Aerosol polymyxin and pneumonia in seriously ill patients. *N Engl J Med* 293:471-475, 1975.
23. Polk HC Jr: Quantitative tracheal cultures in surgical patients requiring mechanical ventilatory assistance. *Surgery* 78:485-489, 1975.
24. Johanson WG, Pierce AK, Sanford J, et al: Nosocomial repiratory infection with gram-negative bacilli: the significance of colonization of the respiratory tract. *Ann Intern Med* 77:701-706, 1972.
25. Salata RA, Lederman MM, Shlaes DM, et al: Diagnosis of nosocomial pneumonia in intubated intensive care unit patients. *Am Rev Respir Dis* 135:426-432, 1987.
26. Stover DE, Zaman MB, Hajdu SI, et al: Bronchoalveolar lavage in the diagnosis of diffuse pulmonary infiltrates in the immunosuppressed host. *Ann Intern Med* 101:1-7, 1984.
27. Wimberly N, Faling LJ, Bartlett JG: A fiberoptic bronchoscopic technique to obtain uncontaminated lower airway secretions for bacterial cultures. *Am Rev Respir Dis* 119:337-342, 1979.
28. Driks MR, Craven DE, Celli BR, et al: Nosocomial pneumonia in intubated patients given sucralfate as compared with antacids or histamine type 2 blockers: role of gastric colonization. *N Engl J Med* 317:1376-1381, 1987.
29. Tryba M: The risk of acute stress bleeding and nosocomial pneumonia in ventilated ICU patients: sucralfate vs. antacids. *Am J Med* 83:117-123, 1987.
30. Warren JW, Platt R, Thomas RJ, et al: Antibiotic irrigation and catheter-associated urinary tract infections. *N Engl J Med* 299:570-573, 1978.
31. Kass EH: Bacteriuria and the diagnosis of infections of the urinary tract. *Arch Intern Med* 100:709-714, 1957.
32. Asher EF, Oliver BG, Fry DE: Urinary tract infections in the surgical patient. *Am Surg* 54:466-469, 1988.
33. Maki DG, Band JD: A comparative study of polyantibiotic and iodophor ointments in prevention of vascular catheter-related infection. *Am J Med* 70:739-744, 1981.
34. Maki DG, Weise CE, Sarafin HW: A semiquantitative culture method for identifying catheter-related infection. *N Engl J Med* 296:1305-1309, 1977.
35. Fry DE: The positive blood culture. In: Wilmore DW, Brennan MF, Harken AH, et al: eds. *Care of the Surgical Patient*. New York, NY: Scientic American, Inc.; 1989:1-9.
36. Baker JW, Deitch EA, Li M, et al: Hemorrhagic shock induces bacterial translocation from the gut. *J Trauma* 28:896-906, 1988.
37. Deitch EA, Berg RB, Specian R: Endotoxin promotes the translocation of bacteria from the gut. *Arch Surg* 122:185-190, 1987.
38. Deitch EA, Winterton J, Berg RB: Thermal injury bacterial translocation from the gastrointestinal tract in mice with impaired T-cell-mediated immunity. *Arch Surg* 121:97-101, 1985.
39. Li M, Specian RD, Deitch EA: Effects of protein malnutrition and endotoxin on the intestinal mucosal barrier to the translocation of indigenous flora in mice. *JPEN* 13:572-578, 1989.

40. van der Waaij D: Colonization resistance of the digestive tract: clinical consequences and implications. *J Antimicrob Chemother* 10:263-270, 1982.
41. Moore FA, Moore EE, Jones TN, et al: TEN versus TPN following major abdominal trauma-reduced septic morbidity. *J Trauma* 29:916-923, 1989.
42. Wilmore DW, Smith RJ, O'Dwyer ST, et al: The gut: a central organ after surgical stress. *Surgery* 104:917-923, 1988.
43. Stone HH, Kolb LD, Currie CA, et al: Candida sepsis: pathogenesis and principles of treatment. *Ann Surg* 179:697-711, 1974.
44. Solomkin JS, Flohr AB, Quie PG, Simmons RL: The role of Candida in intraperitoneal infections. *Surgery* 88:524-529, 1980.
45. Dyess DL, Garrison RN, Fry DE: Candida sepsis: implications of polymicrobial blood-borne infection. *Arch Surg* 120:345-348, 1985.

15

Peritonitis and Multiple Organ Failure

Donald E. Fry, MD

Multiple organ failure describes the most common pattern of death among patients who have a fatal outcome from peritonitis. This syndrome has included combinations and permutations of pulmonary failure, hepatic failure, renal failure, and stress-associated gastric mucosal ulceration. Studies of patients who have developed multiple organ failure have consistently reported increased mortality rates as the number of involved organ systems increased.[1-4]

Numerous clinical variables have been associated with multiple organ failure. Hemorrhagic shock, massive resuscitation, systemic hypoxemia, long-bone fractures (ie, fat embolism), central nervous system injury, and many others have been suggested. However, the presence of apparent bacterial infection and attendant "sepsis" have been most frequently and most convincingly associated with multiple organ failure. In no other clinical setting is the relationship between the septic response and multiple organ failure more apparent than the patient with severe peritonitis.

While "sepsis" and uncontrolled infection were incriminated as putative driving forces in multiple organ failure,[2,5] some overzealous conclusions made this correlation entirely too simple. "Sepsis" as the syndrome of fever, leukocytosis, glucose intolerance, gastrointestinal ileus, and positive blood cultures appeared to be very convincing evidence to associate multiple organ failure with severe invasive infection. However, more recent recognition that bacteremia can be present without infection (eg, microbial gastrointestinal translocation) and that ster-

From Fry DE, (ed): *Peritonitis.* Mount Kisco NY, Futura Publishing Co., Inc., © 1993.

ile injury without bacteria at all can provoke the "sepsis" syndrome, has led to the understanding that the septic response is a nonspecific response of the host to the systemic dissemination of mediator and effector signals, that ordinarily have beneficial local effects. Hence, the septic response is associated with multiple organ failure and not simply severe infection. In the peritonitis patient, the septic response can be provoked by the peritonitis process itself, abdominal abscess that provides both bacteria and devitalized debris, intercurrent sites of infection (eg, pneumonitis), and by translocated microorganisms or cell products of microorganisms from the gastrointestinal tract. This multiplicity of potential stimuli can make the management of the peritonitis patient with a septic response and incipient multiple organ failure most difficult.

The significance of multiple organ failure in the patient with intra-abdominal infection is illustrated in the data presented in Tables 1 and 2. A group of 143 patients with severe intra-abdominal infection resulting in abscess was studied to identify clinical risk variables that were associated with a fatal outcome.[2] These data identified the emergence of multiple organ failure as the most important single variable. In Table 1, the frequency of organ failure by organ system is identified. When pulmonary failure, hepatic failure, renal failure, or stress-associated gastric mucosal bleeding is identified, the mortality rates are quite high.

What is more important than the specific organ system that fails is the additive effects of multiple system failure. In Table 2, the data and death rates are rearranged to examine the effects of the number of involved organ systems rather than the specific organ system per se. It would appear that a linear relationship exists between the number of organ systems that are involved rather than which specific system

Table 1

Organ System	No. Patients	Deaths
Pulmonary	46	34 (74%)
Hepatic	66	33 (50%)
Renal	38	31 (82%)
Stress gastrointestinal bleeding	17	11 (65%)

Identifies the mortality rates that were observed in the study of 143 peritonitis patients who proceeded to develop an intra-abdominal abscess during their hospital course. Mortality rates by organ system are quite high.

Table 2

No. Failed Organ Systems	No. Patients	Deaths
One	31	7 (23%)
Two	15	8 (53%)
Three	29	23 (79%)
Four	4	4 (100%)

Identifies the progressively increasing mortality rate of peritonitis patients who develop an intra-abdominal abscess as a function of the number of failed organ systems.

actually fails. In these data, as has been identified in other series of organ failure patients whom we have studied, renal failure has generally been the prediction of a fatal outcome.

Hemodynamic and metabolic features of the septic response clearly identify that the peripheral utilization of oxygen is problematic.[6] Patients experience an elevated cardiac output, a reduced peripheral vascular resistance, and narrowing of arteriovenous oxygen differences. This exaggerated stress response is identified with increased concentrations of lactate species in the peripheral blood even though metabolic acidosis may not be evident because of respiratory and other compensatory mechanisms. When peripheral blood lactate accumulation occurs, then failure of critical organ function is at hand. These temporal associations of apparently reduced oxygen consumption, apparently adequate oxygen delivery, lactate accumulation, and multiple organ failure have led to the hypothesis that failed cellular utilization of oxygen may be a central mechanism of multiple organ failure.

Cellular Hypoxia Versus Primary Cellular Injury

Numerous mechanisms have been advocated to explain the defective oxygen utilization of the septic response in peritonitis and other critically-ill surgical patients. Abnormal oxyhemoglobin dissociation,[7] altered red blood cell deformability,[8] arteriovenous shunts,[9] damage to cellular oxidative phosphorylation,[10,11] regional redistribution of blood flow,[12] and microaggretaion[13] of cellular elements of the blood have all been proposed.

During the 1970s, injury of the mitochondrion by the septic process was, and in many quarters remains, the most enthusiastically embraced theory to explain defective oxygen metabolism. Experimental studies by Schumer et al.[10] and Mela et al.[11] demonstrated uncoupling and inhibition of hepatic mitochondrial isolates following endotoxemia in rats. Siegel and associates[6] demonstrated equimolar increases in lactate and pyruvate concentrations in the peripheral blood of "septic" patients that they associated with defective activity of pyruvate dehydrogenase complex. They argued that were defective oxygen delivery an issue, lactate species would increase in molar concentrations in an exaggerated fashion compared to pyruvate, as the hypoxic cell would attempt to generate NAD^+ from $NADH^+$ in order to sustain cytoplasmic glycolysis. Thus, the primary cellular injury hypothesis emanated from endotoxic rat experiments and from inferences drawn from human *peripheral* blood samples.

Our initial experiments with acute bacterial peritonitis,[14,15] intraperitoneally-administered endotoxemia,[16] and gram-negative bacteremia[17] failed to support the concept of defective mitochondrial function. Indeed, our experiments with peritonitis and *Escherichia coli* bacteremia demonstrated increased coupling efficiency of hepatic mitochondrial isolates. This identification of "super" mitochondria had been previously reported by Mela et al.[18] among hepatic mitochondria from rats subjected to hypoxemic atmospheric conditions. The observation of a hypoxic mitochondrial response when arterial blood pressure was normal and arterial oxygenation was normal suggested that oxygen delivery rather than oxidative phosphorylation was the operative mechanism.

These observations led to experiments where hepatic tissue oxygenation was directly measured. Rats with peritontis and bacteremia had surface hepatic pO_2 measured directly with a platinum electrode.[14,17] These studies confirmed the observations of the mitochondrial experiments in that dramatic reductions of tissue pO_2 were identified during the septic course. As in the mitochondrial experiments, the rats maintained normal arterial blood pressure and normal arterial pO_2.

The hypoxic response led to experiments in peritonitis, bacteremia, and endotoxemia where efforts were made to directly measure hepatic blood flow. The initial experiment used clearance measurement of indocyanine green (ICG).[15,16,19] Indocyanine green is cleared in accordance with Michalis-Menten kinetics, with low concentrations of dye being cleared in a flow-dependent fashion. These experiments demonstrated marked prolongation of ICG clearance in peritonitis, bacteremia, and endotoxemia that were consistent with the fundamental hypothesis that hepatic nutrient blood flow was dissociated from systemic hemodynamics. Hypoperfusion was occurring even though systemic measurements of blood pressure were apparently normal.

Indocyanine green clearance as a means of measuring hepatic blood flow proved inadequate. Back-diffusion of the dye into the circulation with repeated measurements in the same animal led to concern about the accuracy of the measurements. In addition, flow was not really measured with the bolus administration technique but was rather implied by the changes that were occurring with the biological elimination half-life of the dye. This led to a search for a better method of measuring systemic hemodynamics and better methods for measuring hepatic blood flow.

Galactose clearance proved to be a better method for the measurement of nutrient hepatic blood flow. This clearance technique was readily validated, and was clearly demonstrated to obey Michalis-Menten kinetics.[20,21] Maintenance of blood concentrations beneath 200 μmol/L were within first-order clearance kinetics. In most experiments, blood concentrations were beneath 100 μmol/L where the first-order clearance curves of both control and septic rats were superimposed.[20] With our development of thermodilution cardiac output measurements in the rat, we were able to truly pursue the relationship of hepatic perfusion and systemic hemodynamics.

Using the cecal-ligation and perforation model of peritonitis, rats were demonstrated to have normal to elevated cardiac outputs with the septic peritonitis state.[22] The effective hepatic blood flow demonstrated a steady reduction over time. Tissue energy charge only changed after the flow defect was identified, suggesting that it was secondary to cellular ischemia. Hepatic tissue lactate concentrations increased dramatically while tissue pyruvate concentrations were minimally increased. The observations of tissue lactate were particularly interesting since systemic lactate:pyruvate ratios increased in unity as has been identified in septic humans. Since skeletal muscle energy charge was unchanged, we concluded that the hyperperfusion and the unaffected microcirculation of the muscle was serving as a potential "sink" for lactate consumption. The large mass of hyperperfused and normally oxygenated muscle was dictating the systemic relationship of lactate:pyruvate, while the liver and splanchnic circulation were the major source of production. Histologic examination of the liver from bacteremic rats demonstrates the evolution of microaggregates that provided visual evidence that microcirculatory arrest was a feature of the experimental septic picture.[19] Similar experiments that examined the blood flow of the kidney in peritonitis confirmed that this target organ of multiple organ failure was similarly sustaining a microcirculatory injury in the septic state.[23]

The Microcirculatory Hypothesis of Multiple Organ Failure

The experiments described above provided evidence that microcirculatory arrest in a focal distribution, within those organs known to be the target of multiple organ failure, appeared to be a potential explanation for the defective oxidative metabolism of the septic state. This led to a search for potential mechanisms that might explain these observations. Since leukocytes were consistently identified within the focal lesion of the septic liver, potential activators of leukocytes appeared to be a reasonable direction to pursue.

Activation of the complement cascade has been identified by several authors as being associated with both clinical and experimental models of severe infection.[24,25] We examined total hemolytic complement activity in rats with peritonitis and found that significant activation of complement indeed was present in these experiments.[26,27] The degree of complement activation correlated in a statistically significant fashion with the degree of nutrient blood flow reduction in both liver and kidney. Because complement cleavage products serve as chemotactic and up-regulatory signals for neutrophils and macrophages, activation of complement via the properdin pathway appeared to have real credibility as a potential "trigger" of the septic response.

This led to experiments where the septic response was re-created in rats without bacteria or endotoxin, but simply by activation of the alternative pathway of complement.[28] Rats received a dilute infusion of zymosan, a yeast extract known to activate complement through the alternative pathway. Rats demonstrated a hyperdynamic circulation and reduced peripheral vascular resistance. Of particular significance, the effective hepatic blood flow declined in these rats at the same time that cardiac output increased.

Enthusiasm for the complement "trigger" of the septic response became less plausible when experiments were completed with cobra venom factor.[29] Cobra venom factor is a potent activator of the complement cascade. However, it did not demonstrate any abnormality of liver perfusion. This led to a search for other potential mediator signals that might amplify complement activation by cobra venom factor. Indeed, platelet activating factor appears to be that amplification factor that makes activation of complement by cobra venom appear similar to that seen with zymosan or endotoxin. It is likely that other chemical signals may have this same amplification effect. Thus, it would appear that biological stimuli of significant enough magnitude to activate the complement cascade may well provoke a septic response without the presence of bacteria or endotoxin.

With the emergence of cytokines as chemical autocrine, paracrine, and endocrine signals that were released by activated macrophage cells, considerable interest focused upon tumor necrosis factor (TNF) as a potential mediator of the septic response. Human recombinant TNF when given to rats produced a septic response similar to that seen in animals subject to peritonitis.[30] An interesting difference was the absence of the activation of the complement cascade in the septic response that was elicited by TNF. These data supported the supposition that complement activation was an event that may well provoke cytokine release, but that TNF did not activate complement. Macrophage stimulation that is independent of complement activation can be a stimulus to the septic response.

A common feature of both complement activation and TNF is the activation of neutrophils. Activation of neutrophils in a systemic and indiscriminate fashion appears to result in the critical sequestration of neutrophils within the microcirculation of the organ systems known to fail in the multiple organ failure syndrome. Histologic evidence validates the microcirculatory sequestration by binding of neutrophils to the endothelial cell. Thus, the systemic activation of neutrophils by complement cleavage products, TNF, and perhaps direct neutrophil activation by endotoxin[31] (which is bound to lipopolysaccharide binding protein via the CD 14 receptor on the neutrophil), results in the neutrophil being the efferent agent in the injury of the microcirculation in the septic response.

The systemically activated neutrophil mediates neutrophil and microcirculatory injury by the release of toxic reactive oxygen intermediates.[32,33] Membrane peroxidation of lipids results in the microcirulatory activation of the coagulation cascade and platelets that lead to the microaggregate that embarrasses microcirculation and results in a focal ischemic injury of the affected tissue. The microcirculatory activation of platelets results in the local release of thromboxane A_2. Thromboxane A_2 then becomes a microcirculatory vasoconstrictor. The tandem effects of a biomechanical plug and the vasconstrictive effects of thromboxane A_2 results in microcirculatory arrest.

Tissue necrosis then becomes a stimulus to further activate the tissue level inflammatory response. In essence, the end product (ischemia) now becomes the stimulus to reactivate the inflammatory cascade. Ischemia causes inflammation, which causes more ischemia. A self-energized cycle is thus created that represents a biological point of no return (Figure 1). This hypothesis emphasizes that a point is reached in patient management where successful elimination of the initial provacateur of the septic response may not down-regulate the self-energized, tissue level inflammatory response. The septic response is self-destructive inflammation.

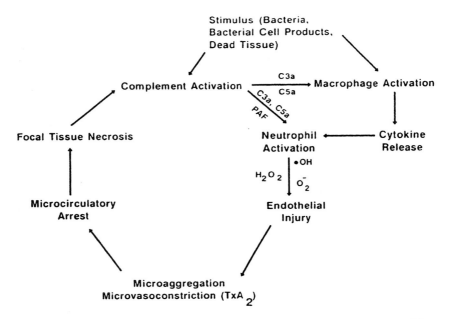

Figure 1: This schematic representation identifies the self-energizing aspect of the microcirulatory hypothesis of multiple organ failure. The inflammatory stimulus results in neutrophil activation, which results in endothelial cell damage. The ischemic injury of the microcirculatory arrest creates focal necrosis, which results in a stimulus that recycles the entire process.

Biologic Rationale for Multiple Organ Failure

A critical assessment of the microcirculatory hypothesis of multiple organ failure includes the question of why should our own inflammatory response be the means for destruction and death of the host tissues. A rationale for this response can be identified by examination of the basic function of the inflammatory response when tissue injury occurs.

When a soft tissue injury occurs, the inflammatory process is activated. Disruption of collagen, extravasation of red cells, and activation of coagulation proteins result in two seminal events to provoke the inflammatory response. Mast cells are activated that release inflammatory protein mediators that have several effects. These inflammatory proteins increase the capillary and microcirculatory permeability in the immediate area of the injury, which results in the extravasation of plasma into the injured area.[34] Hence the edema of inflammation is initiated. The same local variables that activate the degranulation of mast cells also activate the complement cascade. Cleavage products from complement activation further stimulate mast cell degranulation, but also serve as potent chemotactic and opsonic signals.[35] The summed effects of the numerous chemotactic signals from the site of the injury and contamination result in a biochemical signal to draw neutrophils to the area of the injury.

The diffusion of inflammatory proteins and endotoxins from the area of injury results in the stimulation of endothelial cells of the microcirculaton about the area of injury. Acetylcholine stimulation of these endothelial cells as part of the neuroendocrine response to injury may similarly occur. The stimulation of the endothelial cell results in the release of nitric oxide as the chemical mediator which relaxes vascular smooth muscle and vasodilates the area of injury.[36,37] This results in the redness and warmth of the wounded area as the inflammatory process matures. This vasodilation facilitates the delivery of more plasma and phagocytic cells to the area of injury.

Diffusion of chemotactic signals into the adjacent microcirculation provokes the margination of neutrophils to endothelial cells. The chemotactic gradient then serves as a biological "beacon" that provides a directional signal to direct neutrophil diapedesis toward the area of injury and contamination. Neutrophil contact with foreign particles (particularly bacteria), activates the process of phagocytosis that results in the creation of phagosomes that become internalized compartments with ingested tissue debris or would-be pathogenic microorganisms. The process is then completed by intracellular killing of microorganisms and intracellular digestion of foreign particles.

The infiltration of the injured tissue with neutrophils is a prompt response that occurs within 24 hours of injury. A second phagocytic cell response is that of the macrophage that occurs 24–48 hours following injury. The same chemotactic signals provide the directional stimulus for the macrophage cell. While the neutrophil is the principal cell for actual phagocytic "cleansing" of the injured area, the macrophage becomes the barometer of severity of the contamination. When concentrations of foreign particles and chemotactic signals exceed a certain critical threshold, the macrophage is then stimulated to release critical , paracrine, and endocrine signals that then escalate the aggregate host response to the soft tissue insult.

The release of TNF is one of the most notable cytokine signals that is produced by the activated macrophage. This is principally an autocrine and paracrine biological signal. The autocrine effects result in heightened activation of the macrophage cell itself and activation of other macrophage cells in the immediate area. Most importantly, the paracrine effects result in a "frenzied" level of neutrophil activation. Phagocytic activity of the neutrophil is provoked, with extracellular elaboration of toxic oxygen intermediates being the result. This extracellular release of toxic oxygen intermediates promotes extracellular digestion and killing. In this fully activated state, the neutrophil becomes the principal producer of pus in the area, while the macrophage becomes the conductor of the process.

Additional endocrine signals are released by the macrophage to mobilize a systemic level response to contain the local tissue injury. Interleukin-1 and other cytokines become mediators of the acute phase response that include fever, neutrophilia, up-regulation of acute phase reactants from the liver, and down-regulation of albumen synthesis. This endocrine signal by the macrophage becomes a message to mobilize a second order of response by the host to the injury event.

The summed effects of these numerous responses are the containment of the contaminants at the primary site of injury. If the severity of contamination and tissue response is sufficiently severe, the marginated neutrophil may receive chemical signals of sufficient magnitude to provoke full activation while the neutrophil remains within the microcirculation. This results in the release of toxic oxygen intermediates that damage endothelial cells that in turn provoke an intravascular inflam-

systemic septic response. Scavengers of these toxic oxygen intermediates have been studied for many years, although trials in septic humans have not emerged. Experimental evidence appears to favor the use of superoxide dismutase, with or without catalase, as being effective.[48] However, neutralization of neutrophil oxygen free radical production is not necessarily a desirable treatment objective in that intracellular killing of phagocytosed pathogens would be compromised.

A major area of speculation in the treatment of the septic response has been the inhibition of prostaglandin metabolism. The prostaglandin metabolites have a broad array of functions both as intracellular signals and as intercellular autocrine and paracrine signals. Experimental studies with prostaglandin synthetase inhibition have demonstrated favorable effects in severe models of infection.[49,50] The neuroendocrine and metabolic effects of bolus endotoxin in human subjects have been blocked by pretreatment with ibuprofen.[51] Studies of thromboxane synthetase inhibition have suggested that specific inhibition of thomboxane A_2, may eliminate adverse vasoconstrictive effects of prostaglandin metabolism, but preserves the favorable vasodilatory benefits of postacyclin (PgI).[52,53] Yet other studies have advocated the administration of PgE as treatment for the adult respiratory distress syndrome.[54] The vast array of prostaglandin effects makes a generalized inhibition very unlikely to be beneficial to septic man. Clearly, additional research in this complex area is necessary before a reasonable treatment regimen can be advocated.

As can be seen from the foregoing discussion, the number of potential treatments of the septic response, septic shock, and multiple organ failure are large but of unproven efficacy. Many will be emphasizing very expensive recombinant and molecular biology techniques. Therapy has been promising in the laboratory but is largely untested in people. Recollections of the fanfare and expectations that attended corticosteroid therapy for septic shock should provide a sobering influence about the need for human trials to document efficacy before such treatments reach any level of clinical application. A common thread in the above new treatments is the inhibition or alteration of the normal biological response. A constant awareness must be preserved that inhibition of an adverse systemic response may have very negative consequences at the local tissue level of the inflammatory response. The next decade will be interesting as the riddle of the septic response and its treatment unfolds.

Summary

The hypothesis is presented that the septic response, septic shock, and the multiple organ failure syndrome are portions of the continuum of the same biological process; specifically, systemic activation of the inflammatory cascade. This systemic inflammatory response results in a microcirculatory injury that results in tissue destruction and local ischemia as the pathophysiologic injury of multiple organ failure. Newer treatments are necessary to improve the current management of the multiple organ failure patient. Newer treatments will need to address specific biochemical aspects of this disease. The design of newer therapies must maintain a constant cognizance that manipulation of the inflammatory response to reduce or eliminate deleterious systemic effects, may created adverse local consequences.

References

1. Fry DE, Pearlstein L, Fulton RL, Polk HC Jr: Multiple system organ failure: the role of uncontrolled infection. *Arch Surg* 115:136-140, 1980.
2. Fry DE, Garrison RN, Heitch RC, et al: Determinants of death in patients with intraabdominal abscess. *Surgery* 89:517-523, 1980.
3. Fry DE, Garrison RN, Polk HC Jr: Clinical implications in bacteroides bacteremia. *Surg Gynecol Obstet* 149:189-192, 1979.
4. Fry DE, Garrison RN, Williams HC: Patterns of morbidity and mortality in splenectomy for trauma. *Am Surg* 46:28-32, 1980.
5. Eiseman B, Beart R, Norton L: Multiple organ failure. *Surg Gynecol Obstet* 144:323-326, 1977.
6. Siegel JH, Cerra FB,Coleman B, et al: Physiologic and metabolic correlations in human sepsis. *Surgery* 86:163-193, 1979.
7. Miller LD, Oski FA, Diaco JF, et al: The affinity of hemoglobin for oxygen: its control and in vivo significance. *Surgery* 68:187-195, 1970.
8. Hurd T, Dasmahapatra K, Rush B, et al: Red blood cell deformability in human and experimental sepsis. *Arch Surg* 123:217-220, 1988.
9. Siegel JH, Greenspan M, Del Guercio LR: Abnormal vascular tone, defective oxygen transport and myocardial failure in human septic shock. *Ann Surg* 165:504-513, 1967.
10. Schumer W, Das Gupta TK, Moss GS, et al: Effect of endotoxemia on liver cell mitochondria in man. *Ann Surg* 171:875-879, 1970.
11. Mela L, Bacalzo LV, Miller LD: Defective oxidative metabolism of rat liver mitochondria in hemorrhage and endotoxin shock. *Am J Physiol* 220:571-576, 1971.
12. Rutherford RB, Balis JV, Trow RS, et al: Comparison of hemodynamic and regional blood flow changes at equivalent stages of endotoxin and hemorrhagic shock. *J Trauma* 16:886-897, 1976.

13. Saba TM, Blumenstock FA, Scovill WA, et al: Cryoprecipitate reversal of opsonic alpha-2 surface binding glycoprotein deficiency in septic surgical and trauma patients. *Science* 201:622-623, 1978.
14. Fry DE, Silver BB, Rink RD, et al: Hepatic cellular hypoxia in murine peritonitis. *Surgery* 85:652-661, 1979.
15. Garrison RN, Ratcliffe DJ, Fry DE: Hepatocellular function and nutrient blood flow in experimental peritonitis. *Surgery* 92:713-719, 1982.
16. Asher EF, Garrison RN, Ratcliffe DJ, Fry DE: Endotoxin, cellular function and nutrient blood flow. *Arch Surg* 118:441-445, 1983.
17. Fry DE, Kaelin CR, Giammara BL, Rink RD: Alterations of oxygen metabolism in experimental bacteremia. *Adv Shock Res* 6:45-54, 1981.
18. Mela L, Olofsson K, Miller LD, et al: Effect of lysosomes and hypoxia on mitochondria in shock. *Surg Forum* 22:19-21, 1971.
19. Asher EF, Rowe RL, Garrison RN, Fry DE: Experimental bacteremia and nutrient hepatic blood flow. *Circ Shock* 20:43-49, 1986.
20. Schirmer WJ, Townsend MC, Schirmer JM, et al: Galactose elimination kinetics in sepsis: correlations of hepatic blood flow with function. *Arch Surg* 122:349-354, 1987.
21. Schirmer WJ, Townsend MC, Schirmer JM, et al: Galactose clearance as an estimate of effective hepatic blood flow: validation and limitations. *J Surg Res* 41:543-556, 1987.
22. Townsend MC, Hampton WW, Haybron DM, et al: Effective organ blood flow and bioenergy status in murine peritonitis. *Surgery* 100:205-213, 1986.
23. Haybron DM, Townsend MC, Hampton WW, et al: Alterations in renal perfusion and renal energy charge in murine peritonitis. *Arch Surg* 122:328-331, 1987.
24. Fearon DT, Ruddy S, Schur PH, et al: Activation of the properdin pathway of complement in patients with gram-negative bacteremia. *N Engl J Med* 292:937-940, 1975.
25. Jacob HS, Craddock PR, Hammerschmidt DE, et al: Complement-induced granulocyte aggregation: an unsuspected mechanism of disease. *N Engl J Med* 302:259-263, 1980.
26. Schirmer WJ, Schirmer JM, Naff GB, Fry DE: Complement activation in peritonitis: association with hepatic and renal perfusion abnormalities. *Am Surg* 53:683-687, 1987.
27. Schirmer WJ, Schirmer JM, Naff GB, Fry DE: Visceral perfusion abnormalities following complement activation: clues to the mediators of organ ischemia in trauma and sepsis. *Am Surg* 54:687-692, 1988.
28. Schirmer WJ, Schirmer JM, Naff GB, Fry DE: Systemic complement activation produces hemodynamic changes characteristic of sepsis. *Arch Surg* 123:316-321, 1988.
29. Schirmer WJ, Schirmer JM, Fry DE: Hepatic perfusion abnormalities produced by synergism between platelet activating factor (PAF) and complement. *Circ Shock* 27:366, 1989.
30. Schirmer WJ, Schirmer JM, Fry DE: Recombinant human tumor necrosis factor produces hemodynamic changes characteristic of sepsis and endotoxemia. *Arch Surg* 124:445-448, 1989.
31. Vosbeck K, Tobias P, Mueller H, et al: Priming of polymorphonuclear

granulocytes by lipopolysaccharides and its binding complexes with lipopolysaccharide binding protein and high density lipoprotein. *J Leukocyte Biol* 47:97-104, 1990.

32. Schirmer WJ, Schirmer JM, Naff GB, Fry DE: Contribution of toxic oxygen intermediates to complement-induced reductions in effective hepatic blood flow. *J Trauma* 28:1295-1300, 1988.

33. Schirmer WJ, Schirmer JM, Naff GB, Fry DE: Effects of allopurinol and lodoxamide on complement induced hepatic ischemia. *J Surg Res* 45:28-36, 1988.

34. Yurt RW: Mast cells and inflammatory peptides. In Fry DE, ed. *Multiple System Organ Failure.* Chicago, IL: Mosby Year Book Publishing; 1992:205-211.

35. Clevenger FW, Fry DE: Complement. In Fry DE, ed. *Multiple System Organ Failure.* Chicago, IL: Mosby Year Book Publishing; 1992:167-177.

36. Ignarro LJ: Biosynthesis and metabolism of endothelium-derived nitric oxide. *Ann Rev Pharmacol Toxicol* 30:535-560, 1990.

37. Moncada S, Palmer RMJ, Higgs AE: The discovery of nitric oxide as the endogenous nitrovasodilator. *Hypertension* 12:365-372, 1989.

38. Goris RJA, te Boekhorst TPA, Nuytinck JKS, et al: Multiple-organ failure: generalized autodestructive inflammation? *Arch Surg* 120:1109-1115, 1985.

39. Ziegler EJ, Fisher CJ, Sprung CL, et al: Treatment of gram negative bacteremia and septic shock with HA-IA human monoclonal antibody against endotoxin. *N Engl J Med* 324:429-436, 1991.

40. Greenman RL, Schein RM, Martin MA, et al: A controlled clinical trial of E5 murine monoclonal IgM antibody to endotoxin in the treatment of gram-negative sepsis. The XOMA sepsis study group. *JAMA* 266:1097-1102, 1991.

41. Tracey KJ, Fong Y, Hess DG, et al: Anticachectin/TNF monoclonal antibodies prevent septic shock during lethal bacteremia. *Nature* 330:662-664, 1987.

42. Spinas GA, Bloesch D, Kaufmann MT, et al: Induction of plasma inhibitors of interleukin-1 and TNF-alpha activity by endotoxin administration to normal humans. *Am J Physiol* 259:R993-997, 1990.

43. Wakabayashi G, Gelfand JA, Burke JF, et al: A specific receptor antagonist for interleukin 1 prevents *Escherichia coli*-induced shock in rabbits. *FASEB J* 5:338-343, 1991.

44. Ohlsson K, Bjork P, Bergenfeldt M, et al; Interleukin-1 receptor antagonist reduces mortality from endotoxin shock. *Nature* 348:550-551, 1990.

45. Weisman HF, Bartow T, Leppo MK, et al: Soluble human complement receptor Type I: in vivo inhibitor of complement suppressing post-ischemic myocardial inflammation and necrosis. *Science* 249:146, 1990.

46. Cheadle WG, Polk HC Jr: Immune modulation. In Fry DE, ed. *Multiple System Organ Failure.* Chicago, IL: Mosby Year Book Publishing; 1992:313-323.

47. Carlos TM, Harlan JM: Membrane proteins involved in phagocytic adherence to endothelium. *Immunol Rev* 114:5-28, 1990.

48. McKechnie K, Furman BL, Parratt JR: Modification by oxygen free radical scavengers of the metabolic and cardiovascular effects of endotoxin infusion in conscious rats. *Circ Shock* 19:429-439, 1986.

49. Fink MP, MacVittie TJ, Casey LC: Inhibition of prostaglandin synthesis

restores normal hemodynamics in canine hyperdynamic sepsis. *Ann Surg* 200:619-626, 1984.

50. Feuerstein G, Dimicco JA, Ramu A, et al: Effect of indomethacin on the blood pressure and plasma catecholamine response to endotoxemia. *J Pharm Pharacol* 33:576-579, 1981.
51. Michie HR, Manogue KR, Spriggs DR, et al: Detection of circulating tumor necrosis factor after endotoxin administration. *N Engl J Med* 318:1481-1486, 1985.
52. Wise WC, Cook JA, Halushka PV, et al: Protective effects of thromboxane synthetase inhibitors in rats in endotoxic shock. *Circ Res* 46:854-859. 1980.
53. Schirmer WJ, Schirmer JM, Townsend MC, et al: Imidazole and indomethacin enhance hepatic perfusion in sepsis. *Circ Shock* 21:253-259, 1987.
54. Holcroft JW, Vassar MJ, Weber CJ: Prostaglandin E1 and survival in patients with the adult respiratory distress syndrome: a prospective trial. *Ann Surg* 203:371-376, 1986.

Index